Study Guide for

Bailey & Scott's Diagnostic Microbiology

Twelfth Edition

Betty A. Forbes
Daniel F. Sahm
Alice S. Weissfeld
Irene A. Brown

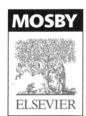

ELSEVIER

MOSBY
ELSEVIER

11830 Westline Industrial Drive
St. Louis, Missouri 63146

Study Guide for BAILEY & SCOTT'S DIAGNOSTIC
MICROBIOLOGY, Twelfth Edition

ISBN 13: 978-0-323-04780-7
ISBN 10: 0-323-04780-7

Notice

Neither the Publisher nor the Authors assume any responsibility for any loss or injury and/or damage to
persons or property arising out of or related to any use of the material contained in this book. It is the
responsibility of the treating practitioner, relying on independent expertise and knowledge of the patient,
to determine the best treatment and method of application for the patient.

The Publisher

ISBN 13: 978-0-323-04780-7
ISBN 10: 0-323-04780-7

Publishing Director: Andrew Allen
Executive Editor: Loren Wilson
Developmental Editor: Lynda Huenefeld
Publishing Services Manager: Patricia Tannian
Senior Project Manager: Anne Altepeter
Senior Designer: Julia Dummitt

Printed in the United States of America

Last digit is the print number: 9 8 7 6 5 4 3 2 1

Introduction

This study guide is designed to help you master the information and skills presented in your textbook, *Bailey & Scott's Diagnostic Microbiology*. The various exercises will challenge your knowledge, help further reinforce key concepts, and allow you to gauge your understanding of the subject matter you have studied in the respective chapters of your textbook. The following list explains the components of this study guide:

- *Chapter Objectives:* Chapter objectives presented at the beginning of each chapter in this guide help you to understand exactly what concepts you should have a firm grasp of upon completion of the chapter.
- *Summary of Key Points:* The summary of key points presented in each chapter provides a brief, yet detailed synopsis of the main concepts presented within each chapter.
- *Key Terms and Abbreviations:* These matching exercises provide you with essential practice in matching common terms relating to each chapter with their abbreviations. Ease of recognition is essential in diagnostic microbiology. If you are uncertain about some of your responses, you can then refer back to your textbook for further study.
- *True or False:* Test your knowledge of the validity of the statements. If you think a statement is true, write a "T" in the blank that precedes the statement; if you believe a statement is false, write in an "F". Completing these exercises helps you immediately to recognize content of which you are unsure. You can then review and strengthen your understanding of the material by reading again that particular section in your textbook.

ADDITIONAL RESOURCES

You can also refer to the textbook's companion website at http://evolve.elsevier.com/Forbes for chapter-specific weblinks that include general information on various topics, in addition to links to appropriate journals, associations, organizations, and agencies.

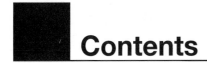

Contents

1 Microbial Taxonomy

OBJECTIVES

Upon completion of this chapter, the reader should be able to:
1. Explain the nomenclature system used for all living things.
2. Explain how relatedness of organisms is determined.

SUMMARY OF KEY POINTS

Taxonomy is the systematic classification and grouping of organisms. This grouping system has been applied to all living things. The phylogeny (evolutionary history) and the genotypic and phenotypic similarities are used in the classification scheme. There is a hierarchy to the organization. The broadest groups are kingdoms and the smallest subsets are species.
- Kingdom
- Division
- Class
- Order
- Family
- Genus
- Species
- Subspecies (biotype, serotype, phagotype)

All organisms are given two names, *genus* and *species*. This nomenclature system derives the names from Latin and Greek. The genus name is always capitalized while the species name never is. Organisms are placed in these groups based on genotypic (genetic) and phenotypic (observable) characteristics. With the advent of molecular technology, microbial organisms are being looked at from a new perspective. DNA sequence analysis is used to determine relatedness. Consequently, there has been much rearranging and renaming. To transition these classification changes and name changes more smoothly, microbiologists frequently report both names (e.g., *Burkholderia [Pseudomonas] cepacia*).

TRUE OR FALSE

1. _____ The genus name is never abbreviated.
2. _____ Classification is the organization of similar organisms into taxonomic groups.
3. _____ The genus name is always italicized.
4. _____ The family name is more specific than the genus name.
5. _____ Modern identification methods use the guanine and cytosine content and base sequence to determine relatedness.

ANSWERS

True or False
1. F
2. T
3. T
4. F
5. T

2 Bacterial Genetics, Metabolism, and Structure

OBJECTIVES

Upon completion of this chapter, the reader should be able to:
1. Explain the processes of DNA replication, transcription, and translation.
2. Explain the concept of the genetic code.
3. Describe how bacteria mutate and display such genetic diversity.
4. Explain oxidation-reduction reactions in terms of respiration and fermentation.
5. Describe the differences between prokaryotes and eukaryotes.
6. Describe the structure of the cell wall and its differences in gram-negative and gram-positive bacteria.

SUMMARY OF KEY POINTS

A basic understanding of bacterial biology is necessary for the microbiologist. Genetics, metabolism, and structure underlie the testing done in microbiology and form the foundation for susceptibility testing.

BACTERIAL GENETICS

The molecular basis of heredity is nucleic acids. The two major classes are deoxyribonucleic acid (DNA) and ribonucleic acid (RNA). DNA contains three main components: sugar, phosphate groups, and bases. The bases are the key to the genetic code. The nitrogen bases are the purines, adenine (A) and guanine (G), and the pyrimidines, cytosine (C) and thymine (T). In RNA, thymine is replaced by uracil (U). A sugar, phosphate, and base together form a unit called a *nucleotide*. The nucleotides are joined to form strands similar to the structure of a ladder, These strands coil into a helix configuration. The backbone of these strands are the bases. The order of the bases is called the *base sequence* (e.g., AAG). The base sequence provides the genetic code.

A strand of DNA makes up a chromosome. Chromosomes carry genetic information that is passed from one cell to the next as the cell divides. On the chromosome are discrete packets of information that carry the code for production of proteins. This packet or section of DNA is a gene.

In bacteria, there is one chromosome composed of double-stranded DNA that is closed or circular. The macromolecule is naked, that is, not enclosed within a membrane. Eukaryotes have linear chromosomes within a nucleus, but bacteria have one naked circular chromosome. There are also smaller circular pieces of DNA in the cytoplasm that are called plasmids. These plasmids are important because they often contain genes that encode for antibiotic resistance. There are also small pieces of DNA that can move between plasmids and the chromosome. These are transposable elements. Plasmids and transposable elements move within the bacterial cell and can be transferred to other cells. There is documentation that the gene for vancomycin resistance has been transferred from *Enterococcus* to *Staphylococcus aureus*.

Bacterial cell division produces two daughter cells. The genome must replicate in this process. Basically, the double strand of DNA in the chromosome unwinds and loses the helical shape. The strands unzip, beginning at a point of origin. The two strands become exposed to act as templates for the building of new strands. Enzymes, such as DNA polymerase, work to add nucleotide bases to the exposed (parent) strands. Two new DNA strands are built and this replication process terminates. One chromosome goes into each daughter cell.

The information encoded on the chromosome must be expressed. The bacterial cell must produce the proteins necessary for cellular structure and function. Proteins are made on the ribosomes. There are three types of RNA: ribosomal RNA (rRNA), messenger RNA (mRNA), and transfer RNA (tRNA). Genetic information must go from the chromosome to the ribosome. This is accomplished by mRNA. *Transcription* is the process of converting or transcribing the information in DNA into mRNA. On the ribosome, the information (base sequence) in mRNA is used to build a protein. *Translation* is the actual synthesis of protein from mRNA. When this occurs, there has been gene expression.

Transcription begins when the enzyme RNA polymerase binds to a particular site called a *promoter* that is located at the beginning of a gene. RNA polymerase moves along the DNA strand. As it encounters a DNA nucleotide, it adds the corresponding RNA nucleotide. The bases pair up A to T and C to G, except in RNA where thymine is replaced by uracil. A DNA sequence of ATTG would produce the mRNA sequence of UAAC. When the RNA polymerase reaches the end of the gene and a transcriptional stop code, it disengages from DNA and releases the newly transcribed mRNA.

On the ribosome, the mRNA information is translated into an amino acid sequence. Amino acids are encoded by 3 base pairs called a codon. The process begins when a rRNA molecule at the ribosome recognizes a start sequence on the mRNA. The ribosome moves along the mRNA three nucleotides (codon) at a time. Each three bases code for an amino acid. A tRNA molecule carrying an amino acid bonds to the mRNA. As additional codons are read and tRNA molecules bring additional amino acids, a polypeptide chain forms. At a translational stop

4

signal, the ribosome disengages from mRNA and releases the polypeptide.

Genetic expression must be under tight control. There are several ways to regulate gene expression. Genes that are always expressed are called constitutive. These genes code for the products essential for growth and metabolism. Genes that are expressed only under certain conditions are called *inducible*. Inducible genes produce an enzyme only if its corresponding substrate is present; this conserves the cell's resources. Genes that encode for biosynthesis (anabolic process) are repressed; they are not transcribed in the presence of the particular product.

There is great diversity in the microbial world. Change happens quickly. Genetic change in bacteria can occur by mutation, through genetic recombination, and gene exchange. Mutation is a change in the original nucleotide sequence. A change as small as one base can change the corresponding message that gets translated into an amino acid. This change can be negligible or devastating. If there is no observable change in the organism, its phenotype has not changed. In genetic recombination, one bacterial cell exchanges a segment of DNA with another cell. This happens frequently within bacteria and may go unnoticed. There are several mechanisms for gene exchange: transformation, transduction, and conjugation. Conjugation (cell-to-cell contact) allows cells to transfer plasmids. Antimicrobial resistance can spread because of plasmid-mediated transfer of resistance genes.

BACTERIAL METABOLISM

An understanding of cellular processes is necessary to understand how we use those processes to identify organisms in the microbiology laboratory. An organism that is fastidious cannot be grown on culture media without the addition of a particular nutrient. This indicates the organism cannot manufacture that nutrient and must derive it from its environment. Bacterial metabolism involves four processes: fueling, biosynthesis, polymerization, and assembly. The last three processes rely on anabolic metabolism. This is the building process of putting compounds together to make large polymers. Amino acids are the building blocks of proteins, which are macromolecules. These proteins may then be used to build structures, such as flagella. These processes are dependent on the fueling process.

The fueling process involves acquiring nutrients from the environment, producing precursor metabolites, and producing energy. The production of precursor metabolites and energy production are catabolic processes. Large molecules are broken down into intermediate compounds with the production of energy in the form of ATP. Getting nutrients from the environment into the cell may involve active transport across the cell membrane. Another transport process is known as *group translocation*, which is used by many purines and fatty acids.

The production of precursor metabolites, such as pyruvate, acetyl CoA, and pentose 5-phosphate, occurs by three central pathways. These are the Embden-Myerhof-Parnas (EMP) pathway, the tricarboxylic acid (TCA) cycle, and the pentose phosphate shunt. Please refer to Figure 2-12 in the text

Energy is stored in chemical bonds. When an electron is transferred from one molecule to another, it carries energy with it. Energy is transferred in oxidation-reduction reactions. The source molecule (substrate) is oxidized when it donates electrons to an acceptor molecule. The molecule that gains the electron is said to be reduced. Cells use the carrier molecules NAD^+ and $NADP^+$ to carry out oxidation-reduction reactions. NAD^+ oxidizes energy-rich molecules by acquiring their hydrogen atoms. It then reduces other molecules by giving them the hydrogen atom. The energy released in these reactions is transferred to high-energy phosphate bonds, such as those in adenosine triphosphate (ATP). This stored energy in ATP is released under controlled conditions in cellular reactions.

ATP can be produced by substrate-level phosphorylation and oxidative phosphorylation (electron transport). In oxidative phosphorylation, an electron transport system moves electrons to a terminal electron acceptor. If that terminal electron acceptor is oxygen, the process is aerobic respiration. If the final electron acceptor is not oxygen, anaerobic respiration or fermentation has occurred. Strict aerobes cannot grow in the absence of oxygen; they carry out aerobic respiration. Strict anaerobes cannot utilize oxygen and carry out anaerobic respiration. Facultative anaerobes can switch pathways depending on the availability of oxygen.

STRUCTURE AND FUNCTION OF THE BACTERIAL CELL

The two basic cell types are prokaryotic (bacteria) and eukaryotic (fungi and parasites). Eukaryotic cells, by definition, have a nucleus (*caryon* in Greek) that is membrane-bound and contains chromosomes. These cells have membrane-enclosed organelles, such as the mitochondria, lysosomes, and Golgi body. Enzymes for respiration are packaged in the mitochondria. Prokaryotic cells do not contain organelles. Enzymes are not packaged separately. The cytoplasm does not contain internal compartments or cytoskeleton. There is a nucleoid, which is a tightly coiled chromosome with RNA and protein. The only organelles that prokaryotes have are ribosomes. Prokaryotes have a cell wall composed of peptidoglycan, but eukaryotes do not.

Bacterial morphology varies greatly. Bacteria are small, 0.25 to 1 μm, but vary in size and cell wall structure. The cell wall is rigid and maintains the shape of the cell. Bacteria that have a thick peptidoglycan (murein) layer stain purple or positive with the Gram stain. These cell walls contain teichoic acids. Organisms that have a thin peptidoglycan layer and outer lipopolysaccharide (LPS) stain negative on Gram stain. Gram-negative bacteria also have a periplasmic space. Part of the cell envelope surrounding the cytoplasm is the cytoplasmic membrane. It is an osmotic barrier that also houses enzymes and transports solutes into and out of the cell.

Bacteria have three basic shapes: coccus (round), bacillus (rod-shaped), and spirochete (helical). The grouping of cells is characteristic. Cocci can be in chains, clusters, pairs, or tetrads.

Cell appendages include capsules, fimbriae, and flagella. The capsule is a virulence factor; it protects the bacterium by allowing it to evade phagocytosis. Fimbriae (pili) are hairlike structures that aid in the attachment to surfaces. Common pili are adhesins for attachment. The sex pilus is involved in conjugation and gene exchange. Flagella are complex structures that give the bacterium motility. Flagella can be located at one end (monotrichous) of the cell, at both ends (lophotrichous), or around the cell (peritrichous).

Under adverse conditions, some bacteria can sporulate, that is, they form spores. They become metabolically dormant and increase the thickness of the cell envelope. The spore state is maintained until growth conditions become favorable.

KEY TERMS AND ABBREVIATIONS

Match the term in the left column with the definition on the right.

1. ____ base sequence
2. ____ flagellum
3. ____ transcription
4. ____ translation
5. ____ phenotype
6. ____ plasmid
7. ____ oxidation
8. ____ transposon
9. ____ DNA polymerase
10. ____ codon
11. ____ fimbriae
12. ____ spore
13. ____ nucleoid
14. ____ transformation
15. ____ transduction
16. ____ conjugation

A. base sequence for an amino acid
B. enzymes that adds nucleotides
C. cell-to-cell contact for transfer of a DNA strand
D. gene that can jump between chromosome and plasmid
E. genetic code
F. structure that allows survival in adverse conditions
G. metabolic pathway using oxygen as terminal electron acceptor
H. miniature chromosome
I. conversion of DNA into mRNA
J. DNA from two bacteria come together in one cell through the action of viruses
K. bacterial chromosome plus RNA and protein
L. the uptake of free DNA from the environment
M. protein synthesis
N. observable characteristics
O. hairlike structures for attachment
P. motility structure

TRUE OR FALSE

1. ____ Energy is transferred by translation processes.
2. ____ Plasmids can be passed to other bacterial species.
3. ____ Transcriptional regulation involves the repression of certain genes.
4. ____ Energy is stored in ATP.
5. ____ Under adverse conditions, bacteria thicken their cell envelope and form pili.

MULTIPLE CHOICE

1. ____ In an oxidation-reduction reaction when an electron is transferred to oxygen, the oxygen molecule is said to be
   A. oxidized.
   B. reduced.
   C. catabolized.
   D. none of the above.

2. ____ Facultative anaerobes
   A. cannot grow in the presence of oxygen.
   B. can switch chemical pathways depending on the availability of oxygen.
   C. require high levels of CO_2.
   D. are strict aerobes.

3. ____ tRNA is important
   A. in transcription.
   B. in translation.
   C. in regulating gene expression.
   D. in oxidative phosphorylation.

4. ____ The basis of the Gram stain is
   A. the cytoplasmic membrane.
   B. the periplasmic space.
   C. presence of a capsule.
   D. cell wall differences.

5. ____ Which statement is false?
   A. Prokaryotic cells contain organelles.
   B. Prokaryotes have a cell wall composed of peptidoglycan.
   C. Eukaryotic cells have a cytoskeleton.
   D. The nucleoid contains the chromosome.

ANSWERS

Key Terms and Abbreviations

1. E
2. P
3. I
4. M
5. N
6. H
7. G
8. D
9. B
10. A
11. O
12. F
13. K
14. L
15. J
16. C

True or False

1. F
2. T
3. T
4. T
5. F

Multiple Choice

1. B
2. B
3. B
4. D
5. A

3 Host-Microorganism Interactions

OBJECTIVES

Upon completion of this chapter, the reader should be able to:
1. Explain the spread of disease involving reservoirs, vectors, and hosts.
2. List host defense mechanisms.
3. List strategies employed by pathogens to evade the host's defenses.
4. Explain humoral immunity.
5. Explain cell-mediated immunity.
6. Compare active and passive immunity.

SUMMARY OF KEY POINTS

The variety of life on earth is constantly interacting. There are myriad complex relationships. Of importance is the fact that these relationships, which include the host-microorganism relationship, are always bidirectional. All organisms share the common goal of survival. There are sequential steps in the development of this host-microorganism relationship and the subsequent development of infection and disease.

In every infection there must be a source or reservoir. The reservoir can be a person, animal, or something in the environment. Person-to-person spread of disease is well documented (e.g., sexually transmitted diseases). Animals can be heavily infested with microorganisms and act as reservoirs. Zoonoses are diseases that result from contact with animals or animal products (e.g., anthrax and tularemia from contact with animal skins and carcasses). The soil and water of our environment harbor bacteria and fungi. The reservoir for *Sporothrix schenckii*, a fungus, is the environment; it is found on plants and soil. There must be a mode of transmission to bring the infectious agent from the reservoir to the host. If a living thing transmits infection, it is known as a *vector*. Arthropods are frequently vectors; humans can acquire disease by the bite of a mosquito or tick (e.g., malaria and Lyme disease). Nonliving things can be vectors as well; these are called *fomites*. An infection that is spread within a hospital setting (nosocomial) can be transferred by objects such as contaminated electronic thermometers or a saline flush solution.

Once the organism reaches its human host, it must establish residence. Colonization is the persistent survival of the organism in or on the body. In order to colonize, the microorganism must survive the body's defense mechanisms. Intact skin is our first line of defense. It is both a physical and chemical barrier; the sweat and oils produced limit bacterial growth. The mucous membranes of the respiratory and genitourinary tract are protective.

Mucus traps bacteria before they can reach the cells. Mucus also contains substances, such as lysozyme and lactoperoxidase, that are harmful to bacteria. The mechanical process of saliva flow and the flushing action of urination physically carry microorganisms away from the cell surface. The low pH of the stomach destroys bacteria on food before they reach the intestines. Ciliated cells that line the respiratory tract move mucus and trapped bacteria away from the lung.

Once the organism has bypassed these protective barriers, the organism must attach and adhere to host surfaces. This is accomplished by pili and adhesion substances. The formation of biofilms, a complex adhesive ecological community, enhances the attachment of other organisms. Successful completion of access and attachment allows the microorganism to become a colonizer or normal flora. Some of these organisms are transient and some become resident flora. Successful colonization also implies the ability to coexist with other microbes.

From the host's perspective, anything that disrupts host defenses allows microbe entry and invasion. Trauma from wounds or surgical procedures breaks the surface barriers and allows organisms access to deep tissue areas. Once inside the host, nonspecific host responses are activated. Phagocytes circulate through the body. When they happen upon foreign substances, they ingest and destroy the bacteria and foreign particles. The two types of phagocytes are macrophages and neutrophils (polymorphonuclear leukocytes). Phagocytes contain lysosomes that have toxic chemicals in them. Once ingested, the microorganisms are destroyed in the lysosome.

A complex series of events occurs at the cellular level once a microorganism attaches to a phagocyte. There are receptor molecules on the surface of all cells. Attachment of the microbe to a receptor on the phagocyte triggers a respiratory burst within the phagocyte and activation of the complement system. The complement system is a complex series of proteins that can produce a rapid response to a trigger stimulus. Chemical signals in the form of cytokines are released by the phagocyte. This attracts other neutrophils and phagocytes to the site. There is inflammation, characterized by redness, swelling, pain, and heat.

A more specific response to a microorganism involves the activation of the immune system. Components of the immune system include immunoglobulins (antibodies), antigens, and lymphocytes. There are three types of lymphocytes: B cells, T cells, and natural killer cells (NK cells). The B cells produce antibody in response to a particular antigen (protein on the invading microorganism that the body recognizes as foreign). T cells can act as regulators of the immune response or as killers. Virus-infected cells are recognized by both killer T cells and

NK cells. These cells function in the two arms of the immune system: antibody-mediated immunity (humoral immunity) and cell-mediated immunity (cellular immunity).

Antibody-mediated immunity centers on the function of the B cells and the production of antigen-specific antibodies. Antibodies (immunoglobulins) are produced in response to the presence of a specific antigen. There are five classes of immunoglobulins (IgG, IgM, IgA, IgD, IgE) but the first antibody produced in response to infection is IgM. When IgG and IgM circulate, they bind to those specific microorganisms and destroy them. Antibody also binds to virus particles and toxins; this inactivates them by blocking their attachment sites (receptors).

A distinction needs to be made between colonization and infection. Many organisms live in or on the body without causing damage and disease. Some microorganisms and the host have a mutually beneficial relationship (commensalism). An example of commensalism is the relationship between the little-known bacterium *Wigglesworthia* and the tsetse fly; the bacterium lives in the fly's gut and produces vitamins needed by the fly. Infection involves damage to the host that could be localized or system-wide. The ability of an organism to cause disease is its virulence (pathogenicity). Those organisms that cause disease are pathogens and the characteristics that contribute to the production of disease are virulence factors. The distinction between colonizer and pathogen is not always clear. If there are breaks in the host's defenses, a normally harmless colonizer can take advantage of the situation to enter new areas and proliferate. It becomes an opportunistic pathogen.

Some strategies and virulence factors used by microorganisms are listed below.
- Attachment
  - Pili are structures that extend out from the microbe to contact the host cell.
  - Adhesins promote the binding of bacteria to host cells.
- Invasion
  - Enzymes, such as hyaluronidase and collagenase, destroy host tissues.
  - After ingestion by phagocytes, bacteria are released unharmed.
- Survival against inflammation
  - Capsule formation is a way to avoid phagocytosis.
  - Microorganisms may survive within phagocytes by evading their killing mechanisms.
  - Some microbes kill phagocytes.
  - Some microorganisms may avoid complement activation.
- Survival against the immune system
  - Some microbes change their surface antigens.
- Microbial toxins
  - Exotoxins cause damage in surrounding or distant tissue.
  - Endotoxin is the lipopolysaccharide of gram-negative cells that activates the complement and coagulation cascades to cause systemic damage.

- Pathogenicity islands
  - Mobile genetic elements of virulence genes transfer virulence capabilities among bacteria.

Once the organism has established itself in the host, disease onset can be quick in an acute infection, or there can be a long delay before disease presentation (latent infection). The disease may also progress slowly and persist over years in a chronic infection. There are no cures for some diseases; the best treatment is prevention. Prevention can take the forms of immunization or prophylactic antimicrobial therapy. In active immunization the body's immune response is stimulated to produce antigen-specific antibodies. The childhood immunizations (e.g., DPT and Hib) use live attenuated organisms or capsular antigens to stimulate antibody production. In passive immunity, antibodies produced in one host are passed to another either naturally (e.g., mother to fetus) or by administration of immunoglobulins (e.g., tetanus immune globulin). If the risk of developing an infection is high, the patient can be treated prophylactically, before symptoms appear, with antimicrobials.

Epidemiology is the study of the occurrence, distribution, and causes of disease. This is the work of the public health sector. Epidemiologists and microbiologists work closely together to identify disease. The goal is to prevent or eliminate disease.

KEY TERMS AND ABBREVIATIONS

Match the term in the left column with the definition on the right.

1. _____ zoonoses
2. _____ vector
3. _____ fomite
4. _____ colonization
5. _____ commensal
6. _____ pathogen
7. _____ reservoir
8. _____ complement system
9. _____ humoral immunity
10. _____ cell-mediate immunity
11. _____ virulence
12. _____ endotoxin
13. _____ exotoxin
14. _____ prophylaxis
15. _____ epidemiology
16. _____ active immunity
17. _____ passive immunity

A. pathogen source
B. inanimate vector
C. mutually beneficial relationship
D. immunity mediated by T cells
E. disease resulting from contact with animals
F. LPS layer
G. transmits infection
H. study of disease distribution
I. persistent survival on host
J. cause of disease
K. immunity mediated by B cells
L. toxin causing damage at distant site
M. administration of immunoglobulins
N. pathogenicity
O. prevention
P. stimulating an immune response
Q. series of proteins that amplify an immune response

TRUE OR FALSE

1. _____ The first antibody produced in response to infection is IgG.
2. _____ NK cells recognize and kill virus-infected cells.
3. _____ A stethoscope can be a fomite and spread a nosocomial infection.
4. _____ IgG can bind to virus particles and inactivate them.
5. _____ The bacterium that lives in the gut of the medicinal leech and provides vitamins for the leech is a vector.

MULTIPLE CHOICE

1. _____ Cells that are part of the immune system and nonspecifically fight infection include all of the following except
   A. basophils.
   B. phagocytes.
   C. B cells.
   D. NK cells.

2. _____ Virulence factors include all of the following except
   A. hyaluronidase.
   B. complement cascade.
   C. exotoxin.
   D. endotoxin.

3. _____ Which is not a host defense mechanism?
   A. Changing surface antigens
   B. Mucous layer
   C. Ciliated cells
   D. Low pH

4. _____ The administration of the Hib vaccine to a child
   A. provides passive immunity.
   B. kills the invading *Haemophilus* organisms.
   C. may cause a latent infection.
   D. stimulates active immunity.

5. _____ The phagocytosis of a bacterium by a macrophage
   A. triggers the release of cytokines.
   B. activates the complement cascade.
   C. Neither A nor B
   D. Both A and B

ANSWERS

Key Terms and Abbreviations

1. E
2. G
3. B
4. I
5. C
6. J
7. A
8. Q
9. K
10. D
11. N
12. F
13. L
14. O
15. H
16. P
17. M

True or False

1. F
2. T
3. T
4. T
5. F

Multiple Choice

1. C
2. B
3. A
4. D
5. D

REFERENCES

Dale C, Welburn SC: The endosymbionts of tsetse flies: manipulating host-parasite interactions, *Int J Parasitol* 31:627, 2001.

4 Laboratory Safety

OBJECTIVES

Upon completion of this chapter, the reader should be able to:
1. List the elements of a comprehensive safety program.
2. Define a chemical hygiene plan and list its elements.
3. Differentiate between sterilization and disinfection.
4. Explain the acronym RACE.
5. Define MSDS.
6. Explain Standard Precautions.
7. Explain biosafety levels and how they pertain to microbiology.
8. Explain how to properly package an infectious substance.

SUMMARY OF KEY POINTS

Laboratory safety is of paramount importance to the medical technologist. Safety programs include elements for the safe handling of specimens and biological materials as well as fire, electrical, and chemical hazards. In addition to these elements, a comprehensive safety program for the laboratory addresses ergonomics, emergency preparedness, training, and education.

A key element in safety for the microbiologist involves sterilization and disinfection. Sterilization is the process whereby all forms of microbial life are killed. This includes the killing of bacterial spores. Disinfection is the process whereby pathogenic organisms are destroyed but not all microorganisms or spores may be killed. Physical methods of sterilization include:

- Incineration
- Moist heat
- Dry heat
- Filtration
- Ionizing (gamma) radiation.

Chemical sterilization can involve the use of gases such as ethylene oxide and formaldehyde vapor. Glutaraldehyde and peracetic acid are used to sterilize medical equipment in a cold sterilization process.

Disinfection involves physical and chemical methods. Boiling, pasteurization, and nonionizing radiation are methods of physical disinfection. Microbiologists are most familiar with chemical disinfection processes. The classes of chemicals that may be used to disinfect include alcohols, aldehydes, halogens, heavy metals, phenolics, and quaternary ammonium compounds.

Antiseptics are disinfectants used on skin. Typical disinfectants used in medicine include 70% alcohol, 1% to 10% povidone-iodine solution, and chlorhexidine gluconate. The efficacy of disinfectants and antiseptics depends on such factors as type of organisms present, concentration of disinfectant, length of contact time, and the amount of organics (e.g., blood or mucus) present.

The halogens include chlorine and iodine. The Centers for Disease Control and Prevention (CDC) recommends that tabletops be cleaned with a 1:10 dilution of bleach following blood spills. The Clinical and Laboratory Standards Institute (CLSI), formerly known as NCCLS, in document H3-A5 recommends the use of povidone-iodine or chlorhexidine gluconate to cleanse the skin before blood culture collection. In the laboratory, phenolics are commonly used to disinfect countertops.

In the 1980s, the Occupational Safety and Health Administration (OSHA) published a hazard communications standard. The purpose of this regulation is to ensure the safety of the worker by mandating education and the safe handling of hazardous chemicals in the workplace. Each laboratory must have a chemical hygiene plan. The College of American Pathologists has designated the following elements be included in a chemical hygiene plan:
- Designation of a qualified chemical hygiene officer
- Policies that involve hazardous chemicals
- Criteria for the use of personal protective equipment (PPE) and controlled devices
- Criteria for monitoring exposure levels
- Provision for medical consultation and examinations
- Provision for employee training
- A copy of the OSHA laboratory standard

Laboratories are also required to maintain a file of every chemical in use with its corresponding material safety data sheet (MSDS). The MSDS contains information on the physical and chemical properties, hazardous ingredients, fire and toxicity data, health effects and first aid, and storage and handling. The National Fire and Protection Agency (NFPA) has devised a coding system of symbols and colors to identify the hazards of chemicals; these labels must be on all chemicals. The MSDSs must be available to every employee at all times. It is the responsibility of every employee to be familiar with the chemical hygiene plan.

Fume hoods are used to prevent the inhalation of toxic fumes. Air is exhausted to the outside but is not filtered to trap pathogenic organisms. A biological safety cabinet (BSC) is used for handling infectious materials. Chemical spill kits must be available for use and every employee must be trained in spill cleanup procedures. Appropriate protective equipment must be included in the kits or be available.

Fire and electrical safety are important. Each laboratory must have evacuation routes posted and fire drills must be conducted periodically. Employees must be educated in the types of extinguishers available and remember the standard acronym RACE:

1. **R**escue and remove injured individuals.
2. **A**ctivate the fire alarm.
3. **C**ontain the fire.
4. **E**xtinguish the fire, if possible.

All electrical sockets should be grounded. Electrical cords should be checked for fraying. Extension cords should never be used in the laboratory.

Compressed gas cylinders containing CO_2 and anaerobic gas mixtures must be securely stored. To prevent the cylinders from falling, gas tanks must be chained. There should be a metal cap covering the regulator when the cylinder is not in use.

The biosafety of laboratory workers is a critical element of laboratory operation. Good laboratory practice will protect workers from infectious diseases encountered in the workplace. Laboratory practices that reduce the risk of infection include Standard Precautions, safety devices, PPE, and appropriate decontamination and disposal of biological hazards. Microbiologists must be aware of processes that can generate aerosols; these include centrifugation, vortexing, and "hot looping" (the common practice of quickly cooling an inoculating loop by stabbing it into agar). The five most frequently acquired infections in the clinical microbiology laboratory are shigellosis, salmonellosis, tuberculosis, brucellosis, and hepatitis. The employer must offer the hepatitis B vaccine to employees. Vaccines are not available for all infectious agents.

The CDC has published guidelines to reduce the transmission of infectious agents. These are known as Standard Precautions. The premise is to treat all blood and body fluids from every patient as potentially infectious. Assume all patients are potentially infectious for HIV and other blood-borne pathogens. Thorough and frequent hand washing is a simple but critical act than can prevent transmission of pathogens. There should be no mouth pipetting, eating, drinking, smoking, manipulating contact lenses, or application of cosmetics in the laboratory. Gloves and a laboratory coat should be worn in the laboratory when working with specimens; the laboratory coat must not be worn out of the laboratory or in "clean" areas, such as offices and lounge areas.

The laboratory must also have an Exposure Control Plan that identifies the hazards to employees and provides the means to protect the worker. Elements of the plan include education and orientation, Standard Precautions, engineering controls and safe work practices, PPE, and a postexposure plan that includes accident investigation and prevention of recurrence. The Environmental Protection Agency (EPA) publishes guidelines for the reduction of and proper disposal of hazardous waste. Infectious waste includes agar plates and tubes. These should be double-bagged in leak-proof plastic bags and clearly identified as a biohazard. Glass and sharps should be placed in puncture-resistant containers that are autoclaved or incinerated.

Engineering controls include the BSC, PPE, signage, protective barriers, and a postexposure control plan. Signage involves the placement of the biohazard symbol on refrigerators that contain infectious material and on laboratory doors. A high-risk activity for the microbiologist is the subculturing of positive blood cultures. This should be done in the BSC. A BSC is similar to a fume hood but infectious materials are removed from the air as it passes through a HEPA filter. Cabinets are graded by the degree of biological containment they can produce. Class II cabinets have vertical laminar flow that directs airflow into HEPA filters. Class III cabinets offer the most protection and sterilize both incoming and outgoing air. Most clinical microbiology laboratories have a class IIA cabinet; these require routine inspection and function checks. PPE includes gloves, laboratory coats, masks, goggles, and HEPA respirators. Respirators and N95 disposable masks should be fit tested.

All laboratory accidents and exposures must be reported to the supervisor and safety officer. Employees must be evaluated by a physician and given immediate medical care. In the event of an exposure incident, it may be determined that HBIG (hepatitis B virus immunoglobulin) or an HBV booster immunization should be given. Postexposure control may also involve the administration of antiretroviral therapy. Follow-up assessment and treatment are part of this plan. This is detailed in OSHA's Bloodborne Pathogen Standard.

Important information on biologic safety has been published by the CDC and is available on their website at *www.cdc.gov/od/ohs/biosfty/biosfty.htm.*

There are four biosafety levels that are identified by the combinations of laboratory practices and techniques, safety equipment, and laboratory facilities. Biosafety Level 1 represents a basic level of containment and is appropriate for undergraduate teaching laboratories. Biosafety Level 2 is appropriate for the handling of clinical specimens. Each microorganism is assigned a biosafety level based on the activities typically associated with the growth and manipulation of the infectious agent required to identify or type it. *Escherichia coli* and *Bacillus anthracis* are both listed as level 2 organisms. Biosafety Level 3 precautions must be in place when working with cultures of *Mycobacterium tuberculosis* or *Brucella*.

Microbiologists must be trained in the proper packaging and handling of infectious substances and understand the current federal shipping requirements. A substance can be categorized as a "diagnostic specimen" or "infectious substance." If a clinical specimen is being sent to a reference laboratory for initial workup, it would be a diagnostic specimen because it is not known what, if any, infectious agents may be present. An infectious substance would be a culture of *M. tuberculosis*. The shipper (sending person or institution) is responsible for safe and appropriate packaging. The shipper is responsible for any fines or penalties. Infectious substances should be wrapped with absorbent material and placed in a primary receptacle. This must go into a secondary receptacle, usually a hard plastic watertight container. This then goes into a tertiary container, usually a cardboard box that has met certain test standards. A Shipper's Declaration must accompany the package. Shipping and packaging regulations can be found at *www.cdc.gov/od/ohs/biosfty/shipregs.htm*.

KEY TERMS AND ABBREVIATIONS

Match the term in the left column with the definition on the right.

1. _____ MSDS
2. _____ PPE
3. _____ Standard Precautions
4. _____ antiseptic
5. _____ disinfectant
6. _____ chemical hygiene plan
7. _____ engineering control
8. _____ biosafety level

A. safety goggles
B. 1:10 bleach solution
C. procedures for safe handling based on degree of infectiousness
D. 70% isopropyl alcohol
E. sheet listing chemical toxicity and exposure treatment
F. protective barrier
G. comprehensive list of safety precautions for handling chemicals
H. handling all specimens as infectious

TRUE OR FALSE

1. _____ All chemicals must have an NFPA label on them.
2. _____ Chlorhexidine gluconate can be used to cleanse the skin before drawing a blood culture.
3. _____ Gas tanks must be chained to one another but not to the wall.
4. _____ Fume hoods filter air and remove pathogens before discharging it outside.
5. _____ An example of an engineering control is the biohazard symbol on the refrigerator.

MULTIPLE CHOICE

1. _____ Standard Precautions include all of the following except
   A. hand washing after removing gloves.
   B. using PPE when handling specimens.
   C. wearing the laboratory coat into the cafeteria.
   D. using an automatic pipettor.

2. _____ Routine clinical specimens should be handled with the precautions designated for
   A. biosafety level 1.
   B. biosafety level 2.
   C. biosafety level 3.
   D. biosafety level 4.

3. _____ The proper way to package a culture of *M. tuberculosis* for shipment to a reference laboratory includes all of the following except
   A. putting the label "diagnostic specimen" on the box.
   B. wrapping the culture with absorbent material.
   C. putting the culture in a plastic biohazard bag.
   D. putting the primary receptacle in a hard plastic container.

4. _____ Standard Precautions apply to all the substances listed except
   A. blood.
   B. semen.
   C. peritoneal fluid.
   D. sweat.

5. _____ Microbiologists must be especially careful not to generate infectious aerosols. Practices that can generate aerosols include all of the following except
   A. hot looping.
   B. vortexing.
   C. streaking a plate.
   D. grinding tissue.

ANSWERS

Key Terms and Abbreviations
1. E
2. A
3. H
4. D
5. B
6. G
7. F
8. C

True or False
1. T
2. T
3. F
4. F
5. T

Multiple Choice
1. C
2. B
3. A
4. D
5. C

REFERENCES

National Committee for Clinical Laboratory Standards: Procedures for the collection of diagnostic blood specimens by venipuncture; Approved standard H3-A5, fifth edition, Wayne, Pa, 2003, National Committee for Clinical Laboratory Standards.

National Committee for Clinical Laboratory Standards: Protection of laboratory workers from occupationally acquired infections; Approved standard, M29-A2, Wayne, Pa, 2001, National Committee for Clinical Laboratory Standards.

5 Specimen Management

OBJECTIVES

Upon completion of this chapter, the reader should be able to:
1. Explain basic specimen preservation and transport requirements.
2. List conditions for specimen rejection.
3. Explain the method for inoculating media for both quantitative and semiquantitative culture.
4. Explain the phrase "streaking for isolation."

SUMMARY OF KEY POINTS

The history of medical diagnosis and the clinical laboratory dates to 300 BC when Hippocrates advocated the examination of urine to diagnose disease. The nineteenth century in the United States saw the formation of laboratories and was the era of public health. Discoveries in bacteriology paved the way for milk pasteurization and water treatment practices. Laboratories were performing tests to detect tuberculosis, cholera, typhoid, and diphtheria. Microbiologists today perform a variety of diagnostic activities; these include microscopy, immunologic and molecular testing, cultivation, susceptibility testing, and antibody detection.

This work begins with the specimen itself. The microbiology laboratory should publish guidelines for the correct collection, handling, and transportation of specimens. Improper specimen collection affects the quality of the culture or test. Contaminating normal flora can mask the presence of pathogens. Improper skin cleansing before a blood culture collection can allow cutaneous organisms to contaminate the culture and perhaps lead to delayed or improper treatment.

Specimen transport, preservation, and storage are important so that the microbiology department will have viable organisms to work with. The optimal situation is the transport of the specimen to the laboratory within 2 hours of collection. If this cannot be done, the specimen may need to be preserved by the use of transport media, such as Cary-Blair for stool specimens or buffered formalin for ova and parasite specimens. Blood specimens should be anticoagulated; the anticoagulant for blood cultures is sodium polyethanol sulfonate (SPS). Specimens may need to be stored until they can be tested. Temperature, pH, and oxygen levels are crucial to organism viability. Specimens for anaerobic culture should never be refrigerated. Urine should be stored at refrigerator temperature.

Only properly labeled specimens should be accepted. This is a patient safety issue. Specimen labeling and type must match the information on the test requisition. There must be established criteria for specimen rejection.

Some unacceptable conditions include specimens received in a fixative such as formalin, the wrong swab type for the test requested (especially important for molecular methods), and insufficient quantity for test requested. When irretrievable specimens (e.g., surgical biopsy tissue) are involved, every effort should be made to communicate with the physician and to rectify the problem. If a specimen is received with multiple test requests, there may be insufficient material to perform all tests. Communication with the clinician is necessary to prioritize testing.

Steps in the culture process include: direct microscopic examination, specimen preparation, inoculation of media, incubation, identification, susceptibility testing, and result reporting. Specimens must be examined for suitability for the test. Some specimens will be examined microscopically, usually by Gram stain. Sputa must be screened; saliva should not be cultured. Deep respiratory specimens will not contain squamous epithelial cells. Direct microscopic examination will give information on the presence of leukocytes and other cell types and bacterial cell types.

Specimen preparation may involve homogenization (grinding) or mincing of the specimen, concentration by centrifugation, or decontamination. It is best to concentrate some liquid specimens by centrifugation before inoculation of media. A bronchoscopy specimen should be handled this way. Respiratory specimens for mycobacterial culture should be decontaminated to remove the normal respiratory flora.

Media is selected based on specimen type. In general, a nutritive medium should be included with differential and selective media. Nutritive media are nonselective and support the growth of a broad range of organisms. Blood and chocolate agars are examples. Differential media provide a visual differentiation of organisms based on metabolic differences. Selective media inhibit the growth of certain groups of organisms. MacConkey agar is both differential and selective. It selects gram-negative organisms by inhibiting the growth of gram-positive organisms, and it contains an indicator that turns lactose-fermenting colonies pink.

Specimens can be plated quantitatively or semiquantitatively. Urine cultures represent a quantitative culture because a known amount of material is put onto the plate. Inoculating loops can be in 1- or 10-μL sizes. Respiratory specimens and tissues from burn victims can also be cultured quantitatively. A semiquantitative culture involves a four-quadrant system. The specimen is placed in the first quadrant and then cross-struck into the third quadrant. The quantity of specimen and number of organisms decreases in each quadrant. This is referred to as

17

streaking for isolation. The goal is to have isolated colonies in the fourth quadrant. Growth is roughly quantitated; growth in all four quadrants is graded as 4+, or heavy growth, while growth in two quadrants would be graded as 2+.

The correct incubation conditions must be used. Fungi grow best at 28° C, but most bacteria, viruses, and mycobacteria grow best at 35° C. Atmospheric conditions are also important. Ambient air is atmospheric air with 21% oxygen and less than 1% CO_2. Anaerobes require 0% oxygen with 5% to 10% CO_2. Capnophiles, such as *Haemophilus influenzae*, require increased CO_2. Microaerophiles, such as *Campylobacter*, grow best in reduced oxygen (5% to 10%) and increased CO_2 (8% to 10%).

Certain results are termed *critical* in that they are either life-threatening or have serious impact. These must be communicated to the clinician immediately. Some critical values in microbiology are positive blood cultures, positive cerebrospinal fluid Gram stain or culture, *Streptococcus pyogenes* in a wound, positive acid-fast stain, and positive cryptococcal antigen test.

TRUE OR FALSE

1. _____ The anticoagulant of choice for blood cultures is EDTA.
2. _____ Specimens for anaerobic culture should be refrigerated if processing cannot be done immediately.
3. _____ Bronchoscopy specimens should be centrifuged and the sediment used to inoculate culture media.
4. _____ Urine cultures represent a semiquantitative technique.
5. _____ The presence of gram-negative diplococci in the Gram stain of a cerebrospinal fluid would be considered a critical result and should be immediately called to the attention of the clinician.

ANSWERS

True or False
1. F
2. F
3. T
4. F
5. T

6 Role of Microscopy

OBJECTIVES

Upon completion of this chapter, the reader should be able to:
1. List the four types of microscopy and give a clinical use for each type.
2. Explain magnification with a light microscope.
3. Explain the principle of fluorescence microscopy.
4. Explain the clinical use of the following stains and dyes: Gram stain, Ziehl-Neelsen, calcofluor white, acridine orange, auramine-rhodamine.

SUMMARY OF KEY POINTS

Microscopy is an integral part of laboratory science. The microbiologist uses microscopy to directly examine patient specimens as well as cultivated organisms. Microscopy is the use of a microscope to magnify objects too small to be seen with the naked eye. Bacteria cannot be seen with the naked eye. Use of the microscope combined with specific stains or dyes is a rapid, inexpensive way to detect organisms in clinical specimens.

There are four types of microscopy used in diagnostic microbiology. Bright-field (light microscopy) and fluorescence microscopy are the two methods most widely used in clinical laboratories. The basic principle is that visible light is passed through the object and through a series of lenses in such a way that the reflected light allows magnification of the object. There are three principles of light microscopy: magnification, resolution, and contrast. In light microscopy, magnification is the product of the objective lens and the ocular lens. The objective lens is closest to the specimen and the ocular lens is closest to the eye. The ocular lens magnifies 10 times (10×) and the objective lens can magnify 10 times (10×) or up to 100 times (100×). If a 40× objective lens is used, the total magnification is (10×) × (40×) = 400×. Simply enlarging an object is not sufficient to see detail. Two objects close together give overlapping images and may merge into one. Resolution is the extent at which the detail in a magnified object is defined. The resolving power is the closest distance between two objects that when magnified allows them to be distinguished as two separate objects. For light microscopes, resolving power

is greater when oil is put between the objective lens and the slide; this prevents the light rays from dispersing as they pass through the slide. Special sealed oil immersion lenses are designed for this purpose. This lens provides 100× magnification to give a total of 1000× magnification with oil immersion. Another element of light microscopy is contrast. This is the ability to differentiate the object from the background. Contrast is commonly achieved with the use of special dyes and stains.

To stain a patient specimen or material from culture media, the material must first be affixed to the slide. Gently warming the slide on a slide warmer (60° C) for 10 minutes will improve adherence so the material is not washed off during the staining process. Fixation with 95% methanol for 1 minute may also be done. The type of stain used is dependent on the microorganism being sought. The principle stain used is the Gram stain. The Gram stain divides bacteria into two broad groups: those that take up crystal violet (gram-positive bacteria) and those that decolorize with alcohol or acetone (gram-negative bacteria).

The Gram stain is a four-step process after the specimen has been fixed to the slide. The primary stain is crystal violet. Gram's iodine, a mordant, is applied next. The crucial step is the decolorization step. Decolorization distinguishes gram-positive organisms from gram-negative ones. After decolorization, gram-positive organisms retain the crystal violet; these cells appear purple. Gram-negative organisms are cleared of crystal violet. The last step is the counterstain of safranin. Gram-negative organisms appear pink or red due to the safranin.

Gram-positive organisms have a thick peptidoglycan layer with teichoic acid in their cell walls. The teichoic acid contributes to the ability to resist alcohol decolorization. Gram-negative organisms have a thinner peptidoglycan layer. Organisms that are old or have been treated with antibiotics stain gram-variable because of loss of cell wall integrity. If the procedure has been performed correctly, leukocytes and red blood cells will appear pink. Slides that have been under-decolorized retain the crystal violet. Fungi stain gram-positive.

A stained direct smear is examined at 1000× magnification for the presence of leukocytes, red blood cells, squamous epithelial cells, and the presence of bacteria or fungi. The Gram reaction, cell morphology, and cellular arrangement are noted. The relative amounts of bacteria (e.g., few, moderate, many) are also noted. The observation of intracellular bacteria is important; it is indicative of a true infective process.

Some bacteria stain poorly with the Gram stain. An acid-fast stain is specifically for bacteria whose cell walls contain mycolic acids that make them resistant to decolorization. These are called acid-fast bacteria (e.g., *Mycobacterium tuberculosis*). Staphylococci are non–acid-fast; they will be decolorized. This stain is useful in differentiating a few microorganisms with a degree of acid-fastness but are not mycobacteria. These include *Nocardia* spp. and the coccidian parasites (e.g., *Cyclospora*).

There are two acid-fast staining methods. The classic one, Ziehl-Neelsen, requires heat for carbolfuchsin uptake by the cell wall. A modification of this procedure that changed the phenol concentration is the Kinyoun stain; it is called the cold method because heat is not required. Acid-fast organisms appear red.

Rather than use stains, contrast can be achieved with phase contrast microscopy. In phase contrast microscopy, as light passes through the different thicknesses of the cell, its speed (phase) changes based on the thickness. The light is slowed or deflected with differing intensities. A thick nucleus will slow light and deflect it differently than the thinner cytoplasm. The advantage to phase contrast microscopy over light microscopy is that this method can be used with living cells. The staining process kills the organisms.

Fluorescent molecules absorb light at one wavelength and emit it at another wavelength. Fluorescent dyes (fluorochromes) absorb the energy of nonvisible, ultraviolet wavelengths of light, become excited, and emit the energy in the form of visible light at a higher wavelength. This is fluorescence. Each fluorochrome has characteristic wavelengths for absorption and emission. Fluorescent microscopy uses two filters between the light source and the eyepiece that allow light of only the emitted wavelength to pass through. The fluorescing object appears bright against a dark background. The color of the fluorescent light is dependent on the dye and light filters used. The dye used is dependent on the organism being sought. If a fluorescent dye alone is used, the process is called *fluorochroming*. If the fluorescent dye is coupled to specific antibodies, it is called *immunofluorescence*.

Fluorochroming is similar to the Gram stain because the dye interacts directly with the bacterial cell. Common fluorochrome stains used include acridine orange stain, auramine-rhodamine stain, and calcofluor white stain. Acridine orange is a nonspecific stain because it binds to nucleic acids and stains all nuclei. Auramine-rhodamine is used in mycobacterial cultures. And calcofluor white is used to enhance the visibility of fungal elements in clinical specimens.

Immunofluorescence is used to find certain types of microorganisms in clinical specimens. An antigen-specific antibody is conjugated (linked) to a fluorescent dye. This dye-antibody conjugate will only bind to its specific antigen. This method is used to scan patient specimens for certain bacteria that are difficult or slow to grow.

Dark-field microscopy has similarities to phase contrast microscopy; both alter microscopic technique to make objects visible rather than use stains. In dark-field microscopy, light is directed at the object at an angle. Only light that hits the object is deflected and directed up toward the eye. The cell appears illuminated and the background is dark. This method is used to find spirochetes in clinical specimens.

Electron microscopy is similar in principle to light microscopy. Electrons are focused at an object instead of a beam of light. Some of the electrons are scattered and some are focused to form an image. Magnification of 100,000× or more can be achieved with this method.

KEY TERMS AND ABBREVIATIONS

Match the term in the left column with the definition on the right.

1. ____ objective lens
2. ____ ocular lens
3. ____ resolution
4. ____ fluorescence
5. ____ contrast
6. ____ fluorochrome

A. maintaining detail
B. differentiation of object from the background
C. lens closest to the specimen
D. release of excitation energy in the form of light
E. lens closest to the eye
F. fluorescent dye

TRUE OR FALSE

1. ____ Old bacteria may stain gram-variable.
2. ____ Phase contrast microscopy can be used to view living cells.
3. ____ An organism being viewed with a 50× objective lens has a total magnification of 50×.
4. ____ Immersion oil helps increase resolution.
5. ____ Dark-field microscopy is used to scan clinical specimens for *Treponema pallidum*.

ANSWERS

Key Terms and Abbreviations

1. C
2. E
3. A
4. D
5. B
6. F

True or False

1. T
2. T
3. F
4. T
5. T

7 Traditional Cultivation and Identification

OBJECTIVES

Upon completion of this chapter, the reader should be able to:
1. List the four types of media and give examples of each type.
2. Explain how the different types of media can be used to detect and isolate pathogens.
3. Explain how to inoculate culture media.
4. List the incubation options with respect to temperature and atmosphere.
5. Explain how enzyme tests can be used to identify organisms and list the use of the following tests: catalase, oxidase, indole, PYR, hippurate hydrolysis.
6. Explain turbidity and how it is measured.

SUMMARY OF KEY POINTS

The initial information derived from a Gram stain of clinical material is important as a preliminary inspection of the specimen. Much useful information can be gotten from a good quality stained smear. But the essence of microbiology is cultivation of organisms to isolate all bacteria present in the clinical specimen, to determine which are true pathogens or contaminants, and to obtain sufficient growth for identification. Cultivation is the process of growing organisms in vitro (in an artificial environment) and not in their actual in vivo site.

When growing organisms in the laboratory, nutritional requirements must be considered. Some organisms are fastidious and cannot grow without a particular nutrient. Media can be in liquid (broth) or solid (agar) form. The indication of growth in broth is the development of turbidity or cloudiness. For bacteria to be visible to the naked eye, there need to be 10^6 bacteria per milliliter. One cell gives rise to a single colony. All cells in that colony have the same genetic and phenotypic characteristics. Cultures from this single colony are considered "pure."

There are four categories of media: enrichment, supportive (nutritive), selective, and differential. Enrichment media contain specific nutrients required for growth of a particular organism. Regan Lowe charcoal agar is enriched to support the growth of *Bordetella pertussis*. Supportive media, also called nutritive media, support most nonfastidious organisms. Selective media inhibit the growth of some organisms while allowing other groups to grow. CNA agar selects for gram-positive organisms by inhibiting the growth of gram-negative ones. Differential media contain a factor that can be used to distinguish certain characteristics. XLD agar differentiates *Salmonella* spp. and *Shigella* spp. from other enterics.

Below are some artificial media routinely used in microbiology. This list is not complete. Please refer to Table 7-1 in the text.
- Chocolate agar—similar to blood agar except that cells have been lysed to release hemin and NAD that will support the growth of *Haemophilus* and *Neisseria*
- Columbia CNA with blood—addition of colistin and nalidixic acid suppresses the growth of most gram-negative organisms
- Hektoen enteric (HE) agar—bile salts and dyes selectively slow the growth of nonpathogenic enterics and allow *Salmonella* spp. and *Shigella* spp. to grow
- MacConkey agar—most frequently used selective and differential medium for gram-negative bacilli
- Sheep blood agar—supports all but most fastidious organisms
- Thayer-Martin agar—enriched and selective medium for *N. meningitidis* and *N. gonorrhoeae*

These media will not support the growth of obligate intracellular parasites. Viable host cells are required for culture of chlamydia, rickettsiae, and rickettsiae-like organisms.

In addition to nutrients, environmental requirements for growth must be considered. These are oxygen and CO_2, temperature, pH, and moisture. Aerobic bacteria require oxygen to grow while anaerobic bacteria cannot grow in the presence of oxygen. Facultative anaerobes can grow either aerobically or anaerobically. Microaerophiles require low levels of oxygen. Capnophiles grow best with higher concentrations of CO_2. Most medically important bacteria grow at 35° to 37° C, but for some bacteria growth is enhanced at different temperatures. Commercially prepared media are in the neutral pH range of 6.5 to 7.5.

There are several methods of providing optimum incubation conditions that include incubators, candle jars, and various atmosphere-generating systems. Most bacteria will grow within 24 to 48 hours, but some require longer incubation times.

Proper inoculation of culture media is important to achieve isolation of individual colonies. A dilution streak technique for semiquantitative analysis is depicted in Figure 7-9 in the text. Putting a known amount of specimen on the plate allows quantitation of colony-forming units. This method is used for urine cultures and is depicted in Figure 7-10 in the text. The inoculating loop should be flamed for sterilization between streaking quadrants.

Colonies are evaluated for morphology to provide preliminary information and to determine the need for subculture and organism identification. Evaluation of colonies includes:
- Type of media (selective, differential, nutrient) that support growth

- Relative quantities of each colony type to determine the predominant organism
- Colony characteristics that include size, pigmentation, odor, surface appearance, and changes in the agar (e.g., pitting or hemolysis)
- Gram stain of suspect colonies with subculture for additional pure growth, if necessary

Once an organism has been isolated in culture, it must be identified. Two basic identification schemes are used. Identification is accomplished by genotypic characterization using one of the molecular methods available. Or identification is based on phenotypic observations of morphology and metabolic activities. Please refer to Figure 7-13 in the text for an example of a bacterial identification flowchart. Clinical laboratories typically rely on flowcharts such as this to identify medically significant isolates. The Clinical and Laboratory Standards Institute (CLSI), formerly known as NCCLS, has published a guideline of approved abbreviated identification schemes in NCCLS document M35-A.

Several enzyme tests measure the presence of a specific enzyme or a metabolic pathway. Some of these enzyme tests are:

- Catalase test—catalyzes hydrogen peroxide with the release of water and oxygen and useful in differentiating staphylococci from streptococci
- Oxidase test—detects the presence of cytochrome oxidase and useful in differentiating gram-negative bacteria
- Indole test—detects the presence of indole, an end product in the degradation of tryptophan and used in the presumptive identification of E. coli.
- Urease test—detects the presence of urease by the hydrolysis of urea and is indicated by a pH and color change
- PYR test—detects the hydrolysis of the substrate L-pyrrolidonyl-β-naphthylamide (PYR) and used to differentiate streptococci
- Hippurate hydrolysis—detects the hydrolysis of the substrate hippurate and used in the identification of Campylobacter jejuni

There are tests to determine the metabolic pathways for carbohydrate oxidation and fermentation, amino acid degradation, and single substrate utilization.

- In oxidation-fermentation reactions, acids will be produced in the presence of oxygen (oxidation) or with no oxygen (fermentation). A pH indicator is in the test system to show a color change if acid is produced. The oxidative-fermentation (O-F) test is used. Please refer to Figure 7-16 in the text. This information is useful in separating the gram-negative bacilli into major groups.
- The amino acids lysine, arginine, ornithine, and phenylalanine can be catalyzed into amines by decarboxylase enzymes. Decarboxylation is an anaerobic process that requires an acidic environment for activation; the end products are alkaline. Production of these end products can be detected by a pH-sensitive dye. This test is useful in differentiating fermentative and nonfermentative gram-negative bacteria.
- Focus can be on one single substrate and the ability of the organism to utilize it. An example of its use is in

differentiating the Enterobacteriaceae E. coli and Citrobacter spp. They look alike on MacConkey agar, but E. coli does not utilize citrate and Citrobacter spp. do. Inhibition of growth is another characteristic that can be used to identify organisms. With few exceptions, gram-positive bacteria are susceptible to the antimicrobial vancomycin. Most clinically relevant gram-negative bacteria are resistant. Growth in the presence of various salt concentrations is useful in the identification of enterococci and Vibrio spp. Other common uses of growth inhibition tests are the susceptibility to optochin, solubility in bile, and ethanol survival. To determine growth in the presence of inhibitors, turbidity can be measured. Turbidity is the ability of particles in suspension to deflect light rays; put simply, it refers to the cloudiness of the liquid. Optical density is a measurement of turbidity and is determined in a spectrophotometer.

To identify organisms to the species level, metabolic profiles are needed. Once the metabolic activities of the organisms are known, the information is compared to established profile databases. Please refer to Figure 7-17 in the text. Reference databases are maintained by the manufacturers of identification systems and are based on continuously updated taxonomic information. Identification systems (manual or automated) convert test results into a numeric code and use that code to determine the probability that a correct identification has been made. Please refer to Table 7-3 in the text. The more parameters tested for each organism, the better the probability of correct identification. This information is stored in computer databases for fast and easy access.

Commercially available identification systems are widely used and take various formats. Conventional biochemical reactions have been miniaturized from test tubes into microtitre tray format. Other identification systems are fully automated and have miniaturized this microtitre plate format into smaller "cards." Examples of some commercial identification systems can be found in Table 13-1.

KEY TERMS AND ABBREVIATIONS

Match the term in the left column with the definition on the right.

1. _____ turbidity
2. _____ selective media
3. _____ differential media
4. _____ enriched media
5. _____ microaerophile
6. _____ capnophile
7. _____ facultative anaerobe
8. _____ hemolysis

A. requires low levels of oxygen
B. media inhibits the growth of some organisms
C. lysis of red blood cells
D. media contains factors used to distinguish certain characteristics
E. can grow aerobically or anaerobically
F. grows best in 5% to 10% CO_2
G. cloudiness
H. media contains nutrients required for growth

TRUE OR FALSE

1. _____ CNA agar selects for gram-negative organisms and suppresses the growth of gram-positive ones.
2. _____ Turbidity is used as a measure of growth in a broth medium.
3. _____ Chlamydiae cannot be grown on agar media.
4. _____ The growth of *Campylobacter jejuni* can be enhanced at 20° C.
5. _____ The inoculating loop should be flamed for sterilization between streaking subsequent quadrants.

MULTIPLE CHOICE

1. _____ A 5% sheep blood agar plate is an example of which media type?
   A. Enriched
   B. Nutritive
   C. Selective
   D. Differential

2. _____ An enzyme test useful in differentiating staphylococci from streptococci is
   A. urease test.
   B. oxidase test.
   C. catalase test.
   D. hippurate hydrolysis test.

3. _____ A medium useful in differentiating *Salmonella* spp. from the other *Enterobacteriaceae* is
   A. hektoen enteric agar.
   B. Thayer-Martin agar.
   C. chocolate agar.
   D. Regan Lowe agar.

4. _____ *Vibrio* spp. can be detected by using the inhibition of other gram-negative organisms with
   A. vancomycin.
   B. salt.
   C. citrate.
   D. optochin.

5. _____ Greening around colonies on a blood agar plate is referred to as
   A. pitting.
   B. alpha hemolysis.
   C. beta hemolysis.
   D. gamma hemolysis.

ANSWERS

Key Terms and Abbreviations

1. G
2. B
3. D
4. H
5. A
6. F
7. E
8. C

True or False

1. F
2. T
3. T
4. F
5. T

Multiple Choice

1. B
2. C
3. A
4. B
5. B

REFERENCES

National Committee for Clinical Laboratory Standards: *Abbreviated identification of bacteria and yeast;* Approved Guideline M35-A, Wayne, Pa, 2002, National Committee for Clinical Laboratory Standards.

8 Nucleic Acid–Based Analytic Methods for Microbial Identification and Characterization

OBJECTIVES

Upon completion of this chapter, the reader should be able to:

1. Explain nucleic acid hybridization.
2. Explain the polymerase chain reaction.
3. Briefly explain PNA FISH and its clinical applications.
4. Explain how restriction endonucleases are used.
5. Explain the advantages of real-time PCR.
6. Explain how molecular methods are used for organism identification, susceptibility testing, and determining strain relatedness.

SUMMARY OF KEY POINTS

Up to this point the discussion has focused on phenotypic methods of bacterial cultivation and identification. Although these strategies make up the foundation of the work performed in the microbiology laboratory, there are limitations with these methods. Some organisms are fastidious and difficult to grow, causing delays in identification. Molecular methods offer a substantial tool to diagnose disease in a timely and effective manner. Molecular methods involve the direct analysis and manipulation of genes rather than the products of those genes. These methods can be applied to bacteria, fungi, viruses, and parasites.

Molecular methods can be divided into three categories: hybridization, amplification, and sequencing and enzymatic digestion of nucleic acids. Hybridization is based on base sequence homology or the relatedness of two strands of nucleic acids. Amplification methods multiply the target nucleic acid without actually having to cultivate the organism. Sequencing determines the organism's genetic blueprint.

Nucleic Acid Hybridization Methods

Nucleic acids consist of two strands (duplex) with complementary bases sequences. These strands are homologous or closely related to one another. The bases always bond in a particular way—adenine to thymine and guanine to cytosine. In hybridization assays, one strand (target) from the unknown organism is put with another strand (probe) from an organism of known identity. If the probe and target strands are complementary to one another, there is positive identification. Please refer to Figure 8-1 in the text. There are four basic steps in a hybridization assay.

1. Production and labeling of single-stranded probe nucleic acid
2. Preparation of single-stranded target nucleic acid

3. Mixture and hybridization of target and probe nucleic acid
4. Detection of hybridization

The selection and design of the probe depends on how the probe will be used. If the probe is to be used to recognize one specific organism, then the probe's nucleic acid sequence must be one that is unique to that organism. If the target is DNA, the DNA must be denatured to a single strand while maintaining its integrity. The ability of the probe to bind to its target depends on the base sequence homology between the two strands and the stringency (environmental conditions) set for the hybridization reaction. Greater stringency means there has to be a greater degree of complementarity between target and probe. There is less tolerance for deviations. As stringency increases, specificity increases. These assays must have a way to detect hybridization. This is done by a reporter molecule that chemically complexes with the probe DNA. Reporter molecules can be radioactive or chemiluminescent. Biotin-avidin and digoxigenin can also be used as reporter molecules. Please refer to Figure 8-2 in the text.

Hybridization can take place in a liquid or solid format. The reaction is faster in liquid than in solid format, but the nonhybridized, unlabeled probes (background noise) have to be separated from the labeled probe. After the unlabeled probes are removed, a detection method is used. Please refer to Figure 8-3 in the text.

Solid support can take various forms: filter hybridizations, sandwich hybridizations, and in situ hybridizations. In filter hybridization, the target is affixed to a membrane. The membrane is processed to release target DNA and denature it to a single strand. The labeled probed is added and incubation is allowed. Unbound probe is washed away and the membrane is processed for detection. Southern hybridization involves gel electrophoresis for separation of previously purified and digested nucleic acid fragments from the target. The fragments are stained to reveal banding patterns and the bands are transferred to a membrane, where they are exposed to the probe. Sandwich hybridization involves the use of two probes. One probe is attached to the solid support and captures the target. A second labeled probe sandwiches the target between the two probes. This double-probe method decreases nonspecific reactions. In situ hybridization uses patient tissues or cells as the solid support. The advantage of this method is the combination of molecular methods with histologic examination. Please refer to Figure 8-4 in the text.

Peptide nucleic acid (PNA) probes are synthetic pieces of DNA. The synthetic structure of the backbone gives these probes improved hybridization characteristics. PNA FISH is a fluorescence in situ hybridization technique that targets species-specific rRNA sequences. The probe penetrates the organism's cell wall and hybridizes to rRNA within the organism. The result is fluorescent microorganisms. This method can be used to directly probe positive blood cultures.

To increase the sensitivity of the hybridization assay, methods have been developed that amplify the signal. An example is the assay to detect the human papillomavirus in clinical specimens. Reporter molecules are layered on the antibody directed toward the DNA-RNA hybrid. This produces a greater signal (chemiluminescence) for each antibody bound to target.

Amplification Methods—PCR-Based

Hybridization reactions are highly specific for organism detection and identification but are limited in their sensitivity. The possibility of a false-negative result exists if there are few organisms present. One way to improve the test is to amplify the target without relying on organism multiplication. The polymerase chain reaction (PCR) utilizes the process of nucleic acid replication to make multiple copies of the target DNA. A single copy of the nucleic acid target is multiplied to 10^7 or more copies.

There are three steps in PCR: denaturation, annealing of primers, and primer extension. The nucleic acid target has to first be released or extracted from the organism or sample by heat, chemical, or enzymatic methods. Once extracted, the target nucleic acid is added to the reaction mix (primers, covalent ions, buffer, and enzyme). A thermal cycler is used for the process. The target nucleic acid is denatured to a single strand by heating to 94° C. Primers (short, single-stranded sequences of nucleic acid) are used to anneal (hybridize) to a nucleic acid target. Primers act like probes. They are designed to be used in pairs that flank the target sequence. The primer provides a starting point for DNA polymerase to add nucleotides and build a new strand. A heat-stable form of DNA polymerase, *Taq* polymerase, is used because the stringency of the reaction is increased at the higher temperature. Figure 8-7 in the text shows that for each target sequence originally present, two double-stranded fragments with the target sequence have been produced. These fragments are used to begin the process again. This cycle is repeated 30 to 40 more times to produce 10^7 target copies. These target copies are called *amplicons*. Amplicons are detected by using a labeled probe specific for the target sequence within the amplicon. This increases specificity.

PCR has provided a powerful tool for clinical diagnosis. Several modifications expand its utility in clinical settings. Some derivations of the PCR method include multiplex PCR, nested PCR, quantitative PCR, RT-PCR, arbitrary primed PCR, and PCR for nucleotide sequencing. Multiplex PCR uses more than one primer pair so that different targets can be amplified in the same reaction. This method has been used to detect several viral agents of encephalitis in a single reaction tube. Quantitative PCR both detects and quantitates the actual number of targets originally in the clinical specimen. This has been used to

determine the viral load in diseases such as HIV and hepatitis. This information is important to the clinician in determining response to therapy. Reverse transcription PCR (RT-PCR) amplifies an RNA target and is useful in detecting RNA viruses in clinical specimens.

Real-time PCR uses small, automated instruments that combine amplification with measurement of the amplified product. These instruments combine thermocycling (target DNA amplification) with the ability to detect hybrids as they are being formed. This is detection of amplicons in real time. They not only detect amplicons but also quantitate the amount of product, which allows a quantitation of the original number of target copies in the specimen. With some systems rapid thermal cycling can detect product in 30 minutes.

Some real-time PCR instruments perform a melting curve analysis. Every DNA fragment melts (becomes single-stranded) at a characteristic temperature called the melting temperature (Tm). This temperature is the point where 50% of the DNA is single-stranded. It is dependent on the base sequence, particularly the guanine and cytosine content. Light cyclers can monitor the fluorescence continuously while raising the temperature gradually. The Tm is used to distinguish base pair differences. It has been useful in detecting mutations or polymorphisms in target DNA.

Amplification Methods: Non–PCR-Based

Two broad categories of amplification methods are not based on PCR. One strategy amplifies the signal used to detect the target nucleic acid. The other category directly amplifies the target nucleic acid. An example of a signal amplification method is the ligase chain reaction (LCR). LCR uses two pairs of probes. Each strand of DNA has two probes that span the target sequence. The space between the probes is closed using a DNA ligase. On heating the joined probes are released and used as templates for the next cycle. Probe DNA is amplified. Another approach is to amplify the signal used to detect hybridization between the target and the probe by increasing the number of reporter molecules per probe.

Sequencing and Enzymatic Digestion of Nucleic Acids

The first eukaryotic genomes to be entirely sequenced were the yeast *Saccharomyces cerevisiae* and the parasite *Plasmodium*. The nucleotide sequence of the genome is the blue print for the organism. The ability to sequence DNA is a remarkable tool that has many applications. If we can sequence the DNA of a pathogen, we can identify it. We can identify previously unknown organisms. And we can establish the relatedness between species. Organisms can be identified using PCR in conjunction with automated sequencing. This application is most useful in identifying mycobacteria, *Nocardia*, and organisms that commercial automated systems fail to identify.

High-density DNA probes rely on the hybridization of a fluorescent-labeled nucleic acid target to large sets of oligonucleotides that have been synthesized at precise locations on a glass substrate. The hybridization pattern of the probe is used to determine primary structure information about the target. This method has been used to determine drug resistance mutations for viruses and for pathogen identification.

Enzymatic digestion of DNA uses enzymes known as restriction endonucleases. Each enzyme recognizes a specific nucleotide sequence known as the restriction site. The endonuclease cleaves the nucleic acid strand at that restriction site. The number and size of fragments produced is dependent on the length and nucleotide sequence of the strand being digested and the enzyme being used. After digestion, the fragments are separated by size during gel electrophoresis. The nucleic acid bands in the gel are stained with fluorescent ethidium bromide. This produces a restriction pattern of bands unique for each region of DNA analyzed. The differences between restriction patterns is known as *restriction fragment length polymorphisms* (RFLPs). RFLPs reflect differences in nucleotide sequences and can be used to identify organisms and establish strain relatedness.

A variation of this method, called *ribotyping*, takes advantage of the fact that all bacteria contain ribosomal genes. It uses probes encoding for ribosomal RNA in Southern hybridization after enzymatic digestion of DNA.

Applications of Nucleic Acid–Based Methods

Molecular methods are used for the direct detection of organisms in patient specimens, identification of organisms grown in culture, and for the characterization of organisms. Direct detection of organisms in clinical specimens is most useful when identification methods are slow (e.g., *Mycobacterium tuberculosis*), when reliable identification methods do not exist (e.g., parasitic or viral agents), when specimens need to be screened for only one or two pathogens (e.g., *Chlamydia trachomatis* and *Neisseria gonorrhoeae*), when quantification of pathogens is needed for disease management (e.g., viral load for HIV), and when further testing, such as antimicrobial susceptibility testing, is not required.

Once organisms are grown in culture, molecular methods may be advantageous in identification over traditional phenotypic methods. It takes weeks for mycobacteria to grow. Once there is growth in a clinical specimen, it would take several more weeks to arrive at an identification by culture methods. A key use of molecular probes is the detection of *M. tuberculosis* in liquid culture systems. Because of cost and speed, traditional enzymatic methods are preferred for the rapid identification of *Staphylococcus aureus* and other common bacterial isolates.

PCR has been used to detect resistance genes among enterococci, staphylococci, and mycobacteria. And molecular methods have been used in epidemiologic investigations to determine strain relatedness.

The primary laboratory tool for epidemiology is pulsed-field gel electrophoresis (PFGE). In this method, intact bacterial chromosomal DNA is digested into large fragments. A restriction endonuclease enzyme is chosen that has few restriction sites on the DNA to limit the number of fragments. The digested DNA undergoes

electrophoresis. Because the fragments are so large, the electrical field has to be pulsed to resolve the banding patterns. The premise is that strains that have similar PFGE profiles, like RFLP profiles, have similarities in their nucleotide sequences.

KEY TERMS AND ABBREVIATIONS

Match the term in the left column with the definition on the right.

1. ____ homologous
2. ____ probe
3. ____ reporter molecule
4. ____ PNA probe
5. ____ PCR
6. ____ denaturation
7. ____ primer
8. ____ amplicon
9. ____ thermocycling
10. ____ restriction endonuclease

A. target copy
B. polymerase chain reaction
C. target DNA amplification
D. enzyme that cleaves DNA at specific sites
E. synthetic piece of DNA
F. complementary base sequences
G. DNA becomes single-stranded
H. molecules used for detection purposes
I. strand of DNA from known organism
J. short single-strand sequence of nucleic acid

TRUE OR FALSE

1. ____ Hybridization in a solution format must have nonhybridized probe removed to reduce background noise.
2. ____ Ethidium bromide is used to label reporter molecules.
3. ____ The sensitivity of the HPV hybridization test is increased by the amplification of the reporter signal.
4. ____ PCR produces large quantities of amplicon.
5. ____ Reverse transcription PCR is useful for detecting RNA viruses in clinical specimens.

MULTIPLE CHOICE

1. ____ The method preferred in epidemiologic investigations is
   A. multiplex PCR.
   B. PFGE.
   C. LCR.
   D. RT-PCR.

2. ____ Which method allows the pathogen to be identified within the tissue?
   A. In situ hybridization
   B. PFGE
   C. PCR
   D. LCR

3. _____ A method useful in detecting DNA mutations or polymorphisms is
   A. in situ hybridization.
   B. quantitative PCR.
   C. real-time PCR.
   D. PNA probes.

4. _____ Which statement about stringency is not true?
   A. As stringency increases, the specificity of hybridization increases.
   B. With greater stringency, there is a higher degree of base-pair complementarity.
   C. Hybridization stringency is not affected by temperature.
   D. Under low stringency the same probe may bind targets from different species.

5. _____ Which statement about hybridization is not true?
   A. Hybridization is detected by using reporter molecules.
   B. One strand of nucleic acid must originate from a known organism.
   C. Biotin-avidin can be used to label reporter molecules.
   D. The target nucleic acid must not be denatured.

ANSWERS

Key Terms and Abbreviations
1. F
2. I
3. H
4. E
5. B
6. G
7. J
8. A
9. C
10. D

True or False
1. T
2. F
3. T
4. T
5. T

Multiple Choice
1. B
2. A
3. C
4. C
5. D

9 Immunochemical Methods Used for Organism Detection

Chapter 9 Immunochemical Methods Used for Organism Detection

OBJECTIVES

Upon completion of this chapter, the reader should be able to:
1. Explain the difference between polyclonal and mono-clonal antibodies.
2. Explain precipitin tests.
3. Describe latex agglutination.
4. Explain immunofluorescence.
5. Explain the ELISA assay.

SUMMARY OF KEY POINTS

The traditional approach to the diagnosis of infectious disease has been to isolate and identify the infecting organism in cultures. There are, however, fastidious organisms that either do not grow well in culture or require long periods of incubation (e.g., *Bartonella*). Sometimes organisms do not survive the transport to the laboratory or fail to grow on artificial media (e.g., *Treponema pallidum*). In these instances, important diagnostic information can be gained by simply detecting the presence of the organism in a clinical specimen. Immunochemical methods can be used to detect the presence of organisms without the requirement of viability.

The basis of immunochemical methods is the antigen-antibody reaction. Antigens are foreign substances, usually proteins or carbohydrates, that stimulate the production of antibodies in an animal host. Antibodies are proteins that attach to these antigens in a process designed to rid the body of these foreign antigens. An antigen can be a surface molecule on a bacterium, a physical structure such as the cell wall, or a chemical produced by the pathogen, such as a toxin. The chemically unique area of the antigen that contacts the antibody molecule is the epitope. A large antigen molecule can have several epitopes.

Direct microbial antigen detection began in the early 1900s when it was discovered that the serum and urine of patients with typhoid fever contained a soluble substance that would precipitate when mixed with rabbit anti-*Salmonella* antiserum. Antibodies used in immunodiagnosis are produced by immunizing animals, such as rabbits or sheep, with an infectious agent and then isolating and purifying the antibody produced by the animal. Because there are many antigens on the bacterial cell, these antibodies will be heterogeneous and what is called *polyclonal*. Polyclonal antibodies do not give uniform results because they lack specificity. They will react with several different antigens. It was discovered that patients with multiple myeloma have cells that make one particular immunoglobulin and that these cells divide uncontrollably like cancer cells. These identical cells all make the same immunoglobulin. This aberrant process was put to use to make monoclonal antibodies. Myeloma cells are immortal in culture. A malignant antibody-producing myeloma cell was fused with an antibody-producing B cell to form a hybridoma cell. Clones of this cell continuously produce specific antibody. Please refer to Figure 9-2.

There are many immunologic methods used for the detection of microorganisms. The following categories of tests are reviewed:
- Precipitin tests
- Particle agglutination
- Immunofluorescent assays
- Enzyme immunoassays
- Other immunoassays

There are two precipitin tests, double immunodiffusion and counterimmunoelectrophoresis (CIE). These tests are based on the classic Ouchterlony method of detecting soluble antigen. In double immunodiffusion, small wells are cut out of agar in Petri dishes. The patient specimen is put into one well and antigen-specific antibody is put in the other well. As the liquids diffuse toward one another, a visible line forms where antigen meets antibody. This visible band is the zone of equivalence. This method is used to detect fungal exoantigens. But this method is slow (18 to 24 hours). To hasten the migration process, electric current is applied. This is known as *counterimmunoelectrophoresis*. This method can be used for any antigen with available antiserum.

Particle agglutination tests have replaced CIE. In agglutination tests, agglutination or clumping is used as a visual indicator of the antigen-antibody reaction. An artificial carrier molecule, such as a latex bead, has antibody bound to its surface. Antigen found in the patient specimen will bind to the antibody on the beads. One antibody molecule has two antigen-binding sites, so there is cross-linking of particles and agglutination. Please refer to Figures 9-5 and 9-6 in the text. Latex agglutination tests are commonly used in the microbiology laboratory for a variety of tests, such as the cryptococcal antigen test and the *Escherichia coli* O157 antigen test used for rapid screening of suspect colonies of *E. coli*. Controls must be run with every latex agglutination test. Coagglutination is similar to latex agglutination, but the antibody is bound to a particle to enhance the visibility of the reaction. The particles are killed, treated *S. aureus* organisms that contain a large amount of protein A, an antibody-binding protein. Commercial test kits using this method have been prepared for grouping of streptococci and detection of *Neisseria gonorrhoeae*. Another agglutination test uses liposomes as agglutinating particles. This makes the reaction more visible and easier to read.

Immunofluorescent assays use monoclonal or polyclonal antibodies conjugated to fluorescent dyes. The patient specimen is fixed onto a glass slide. The fluorescent antibody is put on the specimen, incubated, washed, and counterstained to color the background with a nonspecific stain. Using a fluorescent microscope, the antigen appears bright against a dark background. These tests can be done using a direct (DFA) or indirect technique (IFA). In DFA, the fluorescent dye is attached directly to the antibody. In IFA, the fluorescent dye is attached to a second antibody that sandwiches the antigen-specific antibody between it and the patient specimen. These tests are widely used to detect *Bordetella pertussis*, *Legionella pneumophila*, and other pathogens.

Enzyme immunoassays (EIAs) or enzyme-linked immunoassays (ELISAs) have been in use for almost 50 years. These tests use the catalytic properties of enzymes to detect immunological reactions. In general, enzyme-labeled antibodies are allowed to react with the antigen. Once the antigen-antibody complexes form, enzyme substrates are added. Measurement of the decrease of substrate concentration or increase in product concentration is used to detect the antigen-antibody reaction. Detection methods vary, but one strategy is to produce a colored endpoint. This is the basis for tests such as those for HIV and RSV. There are two variations of this test method. One has the antibody directed against the specific antigen bound to a solid matrix that can be inside a well or on beads. These are solid-phase immunosorbent assays (SPIAs). A very popular variation of SPIA is to use a flow-through membrane as the solid support. Nitrocellulose and nylon are used as membranes with absorbent material below the membrane to pull the liquid reactants through the membrane. This system improves the speed and sensitivity of ELISA reactions by allowing nonreacted components to flow through and away from the antigen-antibody complexes bound to the membrane. This is the basis for many rapid antigen tests used to directly test patient specimens. Examples of these tests are the group A streptococcus test using throat swabs and the influenza viruses A and B test using nasal washes.

Other immunoassays use radionucleotides (RIA) or fluorochromes (FIA) for the detection system. RIA procedures have been replaced by other methods that do not require the use of radioactive substances. Another variation is the optical immunoassay (OIA) that utilizes changes in light reflection to detect antigen-antibody complexes.

KEY TERMS AND ABBREVIATIONS

Match the term in the left column with the definition on the right.

1. _____ antigens
2. _____ antibodies
3. _____ polyclonal
4. _____ monoclonal
5. _____ agglutination

A. from the same cell line
B. cross-linking of particles to form visible clumping
C. foreign proteins
D. from different cell lines
E. immunoglobulins

TRUE OR FALSE

1. _____ Precipitin tests detect soluble antigen.
2. _____ The latex agglutination test for *Cryptococcus neoformans* uses antigen-coated latex beads.
3. _____ A popular test for *Bordetella pertussis* is the DFA test.
4. _____ Membrane-bound SPIA assays have the advantage of speed and sensitivity over conventional ELISA tests.
5. _____ Use of polyclonal antibodies increases the specificity of immunoassays.

ANSWERS

Key Terms and Abbreviations
1. C
2. E
3. D
4. A
5. B

True or False
1. T
2. F
3. T
4. T
5. F

10 Serologic Diagnosis of Infectious Diseases

OBJECTIVES

Upon completion of this chapter, the reader should be able to:
1. Explain the humoral response and the production of antibody.
2. Explain syphilis testing on both serum and CSF.
3. Explain the Western blot test and how it is used.
4. Describe ELISA.
5. Explain the complement fixation test.

SUMMARY OF KEY POINTS

Serology is the study of disease through the measurement of antibody levels in serum. To understand serology, one must understand immunology. Immunology is the study of the immune system. The immune system is a defense system that must recognize "self" from "nonself." Markers of nonself include antigens. Key players in the immune system are T and B lymphocytes; these cells mediate the two types of specific immune responses. The B cells make antibodies directed against the foreign antigen. This is the humoral response directed against free-floating substances in blood or lymph. T cells function in the cell-mediated immune response. They can be cytotoxic by killing virus-infected cells on contact or can be regulators (helpers) in cell-to-cell communication. Other cells of the immune system work nonspecifically against foreign substances; these are the phagocytic cells (neutrophils and macrophages), natural killer cells (NK cells), and basophils and eosinophils.

In humoral immunity, antibody molecules are produced that are specific for the antigens encountered. Antigens can be various proteins on a cell surface or within the cell or they can be products made by the foreign cells (e.g., exotoxins). One pathogen typically produces many antigens (e.g., the hepatitis B virus presents a surface antigen, a Be antigen, and a core antigen) that can elicit an antibody response. Different antibodies may be produced at different times during the course of a disease. Antibodies can function in several ways:

■ Opsonizing antibodies attach to the surface of pathogens and act as opsonins. Opsonins are substances capable of enhancing phagocytosis.
■ Neutralizing antibodies bind to and block surface receptors on the toxin. This can directly inactivate them. Antibodies directed against insect or snake venom bind these antigens and directly inactivate them by steric effects.
■ Complement-fixing antibodies attach to antigens and activate the complement pathway.

Although there are five classes of antibodies (immunoglobulins), routine serology methods focus on IgG and IgM. IgA is found in secretions such as saliva and tears. IgE rises in response to parasitic infections and is the trigger for the release of histamine from mast cells. IgG is the prototype antibody molecule. It is the most abundant immunoglobulin in serum and can leave the blood to go to tissues (e.g., cross the placenta and be found in fetal circulation). IgM is a pentameric molecule. It is the first class of immunoglobulin produced in response to infection. It is a large molecule that cannot leave the bloodstream. It is used to diagnose infection in newborns; any IgM in the serum of newborns is diagnostic because it was produced by the baby itself. Please refer to Figures 10-1 and 10-2 for the basic structure of IgG and IgM.

To use these antibodies to help diagnose and manage disease, an understanding of the primary and secondary immune responses is necessary. A primary response occurs when a host first encounters a particular antigen. Stimulated by the antigen, B cells undergo clonal expansion and develop into antibody-secreting plasma cells. IgM is produced in the primary response. Memory cells are generated. This is a self-limiting response. A second encounter with the same pathogen stimulates IgG production. Cells that originally made IgM switch to produce IgG. This response happens quickly and is called an *anamnestic response*. Not only the detection of but also the rise and fall of these antibody levels is used in disease management. Please refer to Figure 10-3.

The concentration of these antibodies in serum is measured and expressed as the titer. The titer is the reciprocal of the highest dilution of patient's serum in which the antibody is still detectable. Serum is serially diluted and tested for the presence of antibody. Patients with large amounts of antibody (i.e., a high concentration in serum) will have antibody detectable at high dilutions. Titers are expressed as ratios (e.g., 1:8, 1:16, 1:32). The optimal situation is to test paired acute and convalescent sera in the same test run to determine changes in concentration. A fourfold rise in titer is considered diagnostic of infection. Because there frequently is no convalescent serum or it arrives too late for therapy, IgM testing becomes a useful serologic tool.

Another use of antibody testing is the determination of immunity. People previously immunized have protective immunity if there are detectable levels of antibody in serum. One use is the screening of new employees at health care facilities for detectable antibody to rubella and measles viruses.

A single serum sample can be used to measure both antigen-specific IgM and IgG. Several options can be used to separate these two immunoglobulins. They can be separated by physical means. IgM is larger and heavier than IgG; centrifugation through a sucrose gradient can be used. Labeled antibody specific for IgM or the IgM capture sandwich assays may be used. Removal of IgM from the test system is beneficial because certain nonspecific and interfering results can be eliminated. Many patients produce IgM antibodies against their own IgG; this is rheumatoid factor. Test systems that remove IgM also separate the rheumatoid factor.

The following is a list of methods for antibody detection:
■ Direct whole pathogen agglutination assays
■ Particle agglutination tests
■ Flocculation tests
■ Counterimmunoelectrophoresis
■ Immunodiffusion assays
■ Hemagglutination inhibition assays
■ Neutralization assays
■ Complement fixation assays
■ Enzyme-linked immunosorbent assays
■ Indirect fluorescent antibody tests and other immunomicroscopic methods
■ Radio immunoassays
■ Fluorescent immunoassays
■ Western blot immunoassays

In direct whole pathogen assays, specific antibodies bind to surface antigens of the bacteria and cause the bacteria to clump together to form visible agglutinins. This bacterial agglutination test is used to detect antibodies to *Francisella tularensis* and *Brucella* spp. as part of the febrile agglutinin panel. These tests are useful when the bacteria are difficult to cultivate in vitro. Whole cells of parasites, such as *Plasmodium* and *Leishmania*, have been used for direct detection of antibody. Sometimes there is cross-reactivity between species; the Weil-Felix test detects cross-reacting antibodies against rickettsiae that also agglutinate *Proteus.*

Particle agglutination tests are discussed in Chapter 9. A variation of this test is the hemagglutination test. Treated red blood cells from animals can be used as carriers of antigen. A widely used microhemagglutination test is the one for detecting antibody to *Treponema pallidum* (MHA-TP). This is a passive or indirect test because the antibody target is not the blood cells but rather the antigen passively bound to them.

Flocculation tests are variations of the precipitin tests discussed in Chapter 9. In these tests the precipitin forms visible clumps. The most widely used flocculation test is the VDRL (Venereal Disease Research Laboratory test) directed against *T. pallidum;* this test is performed on cerebrospinal fluid (CSF). Patients infected with *T. pallidum* produce an antibody-like protein called *reagin* that binds to the test antigen and causes the particles to flocculate. Reagin is not a specific antibody directed against *T. pallidum.* Its use is as a screening tool. The rapid plasma reagin, or RPR, test has come into widespread use as a comparable screening tool for syphilis. Charcoal particles have been added to this to make flocculation more visible. The RPR is not recommended for testing CSF. Because certain diseases, such as infectious mononucleosis and autoimmune diseases, can cause false-positive results, a positive RPR test result is considered presumptive until it is confirmed by a specific treponemal test.

Immunodiffusion assays are used to detect antibody to pathogenic fungi. These tests are discussed in Chapter 9.

Hemagglutination inhibition assays are usually performed only at reference laboratories. These tests make use of the fact that many viruses can bind to the red blood cells from different species. Serum from the patient is treated to remove nonspecific inhibitors of red cell agglutination and nonspecific agglutinins. Patient serum is added to the test system that contains the virus. If patient antibodies are present, they will bind to the virus particles and block those binding sites. When red cells are added, virus particles cannot bind to the cells because they have already bound to the antibody. There is no agglutination (it is inhibited) with the red cells and the test is interpreted as positive for hemagglutination-inhibiting antibodies.

Neutralizing antibody blocks the host cell receptor site on the pathogen (virus). The patient's serum is mixed with a suspension of viral particles. If there is antibody, these viruses will have their binding sites blocked. A control suspension is also made that contains normal serum and viruses. Both suspensions are put into a cell culture system. Antibody present in the patient's serum blocks the virus and prevents it from invading the culture cells. The antibody neutralizes the virus so that there is no cytopathic effect seen. The control suspension is not blocked or neutralized; these cells show evidence of infection. This method has been used to test for streptococcal disease with *S. pyogenes.* This bacterium produces the hemolysin streptolysin O and the enzyme deoxyribonuclease B (DNase B). If antibodies are present in the patient's serum, neutralization tests will be positive.

The fixation of complement occurs during antigen-antibody reactions. The complement fixation test (CF) is a classic test to demonstrate the presence of antibody in serum. It is, however, a cumbersome test that is used chiefly by reference laboratories for the diagnosis of unusual infections. The complement fixation test depends on a two-stage reaction system. In the first (test system) stage, antigen, patient's serum, and a known amount of complement are added. If antibody is present, an antigen-antibody complex will form and complement will be consumed (fixed). In the next step, hemolytic complement activity is measured using sheep red blood cells. Only if complement had not been bound in the first stage will it be available to lyse the sheep cells in the second stage. A positive result is the failure of the red cells to lyse.

Enzyme-linked immunosorbent assays (ELISAs) are discussed in Chapter 9. These tests are commonly used because many serum samples can be tested at one time and the colored or fluorescent products can be detected by instruments. Commercial systems are available to detect antibody to the hepatitis viruses, herpes viruses, HIV, and

31

Chapter **10** Serologic Diagnosis of Infectious Diseases

many other pathogenic agents. Membrane-bound ELISA components have improved sensitivity. Antibody capture assays are useful for detecting IgM in the presence of IgG. Anti-IgM antibodies are fixed to the solid phase; only IgM in the patient's serum will be bound.

A widely used test method is the indirect fluorescent antibody determination (IFA) that is discussed in Chapter 9. There are commercially available kits for the detection of antibody to *Legionella* spp., *Toxoplasma gondii*, rubella virus, and *T. pallidum* (FTA-ABS).

Other immunoassays are the radioimmunoassay (RIA) and the fluorescent immunoassay (FIA) mentioned in Chapter 9. In the FIA the antigen is labeled with a compound that fluoresces. Binding of patient antibody to this labeled antigen can cause fluorescence. Measurement of fluorescence is a direct measurement of antigen-antibody binding.

The Western blot has become the test of choice for confirmation of presumptive results in many assays. It is recommended to confirm a positive Lyme test by ELISA and to confirm antibody testing for HIV. This method uses polyacrylamide gel electrophoresis to separate proteins from the target organism. A sheet of nitrocellulose paper is placed on the gel and electrophoretically blotted from the gel to the paper. The sheet is cut into strips that contain bands of target fragments. This is the solid phase. Serum and nitrocellulose strips are incubated. Antibody, if present, will bind to the specific antigens on the strip. After incubation the strips are washed and incubated with goat antihuman antibodies and an enzyme. The strips are washed again and an enzyme substrate is added. Colored bands occur where there has been an antibody-antigen reaction.

KEY TERMS AND ABBREVIATIONS

Match the term in the left column with the definition on the right.

1. _____ humoral response
2. _____ opsonin
3. _____ anamnestic response
4. _____ titer
5. _____ rheumatoid factor
6. _____ hemagglutination
7. _____ flocculation
8. _____ reagin

A. proteins that enhance phagocytosis
B. aggregation or clumping
C. IgM directed against one's own IgG
D. agglutination of RBCs
E. rapid appearance of antibodies in a secondary response
F. mediates antibody production
G. protein in blood produced during syphilis
H. measure of concentration expressed as a ratio

TRUE OR FALSE

1. _____ Any amount of IgG in the serum of newborns is diagnostic of infection.
2. _____ A fourfold rise in titer between acute and convalescent sera is considered diagnostic of infection.
3. _____ A popular hemagglutination test is the one used to detect antibody to *T. pallidum*.
4. _____ The confirmatory test for Lyme disease is the hemagglutination inhibition assay.
5. _____ Infection with *Francisella tularensis* can be diagnosed with a febrile agglutinin test.

ANSWERS

Key Terms and Abbreviations

1. F
2. A
3. E
4. H
5. C
6. D
7. B
8. G

True or False

1. F
2. T
3. T
4. F
5. T

11 Principles of Antimicrobial Action and Resistance

OBJECTIVES

Upon completion of this chapter, the reader should be able to:
1. Explain the action of the aminoglycosides.
2. Explain the action of beta-lactamases.
3. Explain antimicrobial action with respect to DNA synthesis and cell membrane function.
4. Explain resistance mechanisms developed by bacteria against the beta-lactam antibiotics and the quinolones.

SUMMARY OF KEY POINTS

Antibiotics are chemical compounds that are used to kill or inhibit the growth of infectious microorganisms. The word comes from the Greek words *anti* and *bios* and literally means "against life." Although our current age of antibiotic manufacture and use did not begin until 1928 with the discovery of penicillin by Fleming, crude plant extracts have been used for centuries to treat infections. Antibiotics were mass produced during World War II and came into general use in the 1950s. For antimicrobials to be effective, they must first be in an active form (pharmacodynamics). The route of administration (oral, intramuscular, intravenous) and the intended site must be considered. If the infection is in the urinary tract, the drug chosen needs to achieve therapeutic levels in urine. If there is a wound infection, the drug needs tissue penetration capabilities. Once the drug reaches the bacterium, it has to interact with the cell and either kill it (bactericidal action) or inhibit its growth (bacteriostatic action).

Antimicrobial agents are categorized by the mode of action on the bacterial cell target. The basic pathways or structures generally targeted are cell wall (peptidoglycan) synthesis, the cell membrane, protein synthesis, and DNA and RNA synthesis.

INHIBITORS OF CELL WALL SYNTHESIS

The bacterial cell wall confers structural rigidity, shape, and forms a physical barrier against the outside environment. The rigid component of the cell wall of all bacteria (except for mycoplasmas and ureaplasmas, which lack a cell wall) is peptidoglycan. This fact, plus the lack of a cell wall in humans, has made the cell wall a focus for drug development. The final stage of peptidoglycan synthesis requires enzymes called *transpeptidases*. The transpeptidases are one of the family of penicillin-binding proteins (PBPs).

- Beta-lactam antibiotics interrupt the synthesis of the cell wall by binding to these transpeptidases, or PBPs. Bacteria have developed resistance to this group of drugs by producing enzymes (beta-lactamases) that disrupt the antibiotic. Three beta-lactamase inhibitors (clavulanic acid, sulbactam, and tazobactam) can bind the beta-lactamase and tie it up. These are most effective combined with other beta-lactam antibiotics. In the combination amoxicillin/clavulanic acid, the clavulanate binds the beta-lactamase and allows the amoxicillin to work on the cell wall. Resistance can also be mediated by alterations in the PBPs.
- Another class of drugs that interferes with cell wall synthesis is the glycopeptides. This group is represented by vancomycin and teicoplanin. These drugs bind to the precursors of cell wall synthesis and block access of the building blocks to the transpeptidases. This stops cell wall synthesis and cell growth. Because of its large size, vancomycin cannot penetrate the membrane of most gram-negative bacteria and is, therefore, most effective against gram-positive organisms.
- Bacitracin also affects cell wall synthesis but, because of its toxicity, is limited to use in topical ointments.

INHIBITORS OF CELL MEMBRANE FUNCTION

The cytoplasm of all bacterial cells is surrounded by a cytoplasmic membrane that lies immediately within the cell wall peptidoglycan layer. The membrane functions in the synthesis and secretion of enzymes and bacterial toxins, acts as an insulating barrier across which an energy gradient can be built, retains metabolites, and excludes external compounds.

- The polymyxins (polymyxin B and colistin) act on the cell membrane and cause the intracellular materials to leak out. They have limited antimicrobial activity and are toxic to humans.
- Daptomycin is a new lipopeptide that works by binding and disrupting the cell membrane of gram-positive bacteria. It has activity against those organisms resistant

to the beta-lactams and glycopeptides, such as MRSA, VRE, and VRSA.

INHIBITORS OF PROTEIN SYNTHESIS

Protein synthesis can be disrupted at the ribosomal level by antibiotic binding either to the 50s or 30s subunit. To be effective, these antimicrobials must reach the inside of the bacterial cell. They are especially effective when used in combination with beta-lactam drugs (affect cell wall).

- Aminoglycosides bind the 30s ribosomal subunit, which interferes with translation of mRNA. Aminoglycosides include gentamicin, tobramycin, amikacin, and streptomycin. These are often used in combination with beta-lactams to achieve rapid killing by targeting both cell wall and membrane.
- The macrolide-lincosamide-streptogramin (MLS) group includes erythromycin, azithromycin, and clindamycin. These bind receptors on the 50s ribosomal subunit and disrupt the growing peptide chain. These are most effective against gram-positive bacteria.
- Ketolides have one available drug—telithromycin—and are derivatives of the macrolides.
- Oxazolidinones are represented by linezolid, which inhibits protein synthesis by a unique mechanism.
- Tetracyclines halt peptide chain elongation. They have a broad range of activity and are effective against intracellular pathogens, such as chlamydia, rickettsia, and rickettsia-like organisms.
- Chloramphenicol inhibits the addition of new amino acids and is effective against of wide range of both gram-positive and gram-negative bacteria. It is not often used because of its toxicity.
- Glycylglycine is a tetracycline derivative and has activity against both gram-positive and gram-negative organisms.

Inhibitors of DNA and RNA Synthesis

- The fluoroquinolones are derivatives of nalidixic acid; these include ciprofloxacin, levofloxacin, and ofloxacin. These interfere with DNA gyrase. These drugs have a broad spectrum of activity.
- Rifampin interferes with production of mRNA. It does not effectively penetrate the outer membrane of gram-negative bacteria. Because RNA polymerases mutate so frequently and cause resistance, rifampin is usually used in combination with other drugs.
- Metronidazole is believed to disrupt the DNA strands. It is not active until it is reduced and incorporated into DNA. It is most active against anaerobic bacteria.

Inhibitors of Other Metabolic Processes

Bacteria require folic acid to synthesize their DNA. They must make their own folic acid; anything that interferes with this synthesis affects bacterial survival.

- Sulfonamides inhibit this pathway. Synergism is achieved when a sulfonamide is used in combination with trimethoprim (e.g., trimethoprim-sulfamethoxazole).
- Trimethoprim targets the folic acid pathway but inhibits the enzyme dihydrofolate reductase. This drug

is active against both gram-negative and gram-positive species.

- It is not completely understood how nitrofurantoin works. This drug is only used to treat urinary tract infections.

Soon after antimicrobials were put into use, bacteria began to develop resistance to them. The changes that the cell undergoes to develop that resistance is referred to as *biologic resistance*. When the antimicrobial is no longer effective therapy, then there is clinical resistance. Biologic and clinical resistance do not necessarily coincide.

Antimicrobial resistance is the result of complex interactions among the organism, the drug, and the environment. We measure the susceptibility of the organism in an artificial environment and cannot exactly duplicate the conditions that would exist in a human host. But certain environmental factors can mediate resistance by either directly altering the drug or altering the organism's physiologic response to the drug. These factors include pH, anaerobic atmosphere, cation (e.g., Ca^{++}) concentrations, and thymine-thymidine content. An example of this is the decrease in erythromycin activity with decreasing pH. If we know the environmental requirements, then testing methods can be standardized.

Resistance mediated by the organism can either be intrinsic or acquired. Intrinsic resistance is natural resistance associated with the species or larger group. This is predictable resistance. Acquired resistance is unpredictable because it represents the acquisition of a new trait. Resistance may be acquired by a spontaneous genetic mutation, the transfer of resistance genes from another organism, or the combination of both these events. Some common pathways for antimicrobial resistance are listed below.

Resistance to Beta-Lactam Antibiotics

Several bacterial strategies mediate resistance to the beta-lactam antibiotics: enzymatic destruction of the drug, altered targets for the antibiotic, and decreased cellular uptake of the drug. Drug derivatives have been developed to resist destruction by the beta-lactamases; methicillin is a derivative of penicillin. Two drugs have been combined into a beta-lactamase inhibitor (e.g., ampicillin/sulbactam). Organisms can alter their PBPs and thereby alter drug action.

Resistance to Glycopeptides

Vancomycin is the only cell wall–inhibiting agent for use against gram-positive organisms that are resistant to the beta-lactams. High-level vancomycin resistance has been encountered among enterococci, rarely among staphylococci, and not encountered among streptococci. The mechanism involves altered cell wall precursors that do not bind vancomycin.

Resistance to Aminoglycosides

The primary mechanism for resistance to aminoglycosides is modifying enzymes. There are three types of modification processes: phosphorylation, acetylation, and adenylation.

Resistance to Quinolones

Resistance is most frequently mediated by decreased uptake or by production of an altered target. The gram-negative cell can limit quinolone access to the cell's interior site of DNA. Staphylococci have developed an active transport process to pump quinolones out of the cell; this is a decreased accumulation process rather than a decreased uptake change. The quinolones interfere with DNA gyrase, but mutational changes in the gyrases alter the drugs' target.

Antimicrobial resistance is not a new phenomenon. It is a survival tool that has been used by these microbes throughout evolution. Our widespread use of antibiotics is exerting selective pressure for the continuing emergence of resistance and the transfer of resistance genes among organisms.

KEY TERMS AND ABBREVIATIONS

Match the term in the left column with the definition on the right.

1. _____ bactericidal
2. _____ bacteriostatic
3. _____ beta-lactamase
4. _____ intrinsic resistance
5. _____ penicillin-binding proteins

A. enzyme that disrupts penicillins
B. transpeptidase
C. inhibits growth
D. natural resistance
E. kills bacteria

TRUE OR FALSE

1. _____ Vancomycin is most effective against the gram-negative organisms because it penetrates their cell membrane.
2. _____ The combination drug amoxicillin/clavulanic acid is effective against the beta-lactamases because one drug inhibits the enzyme and the other disrupts the cell wall.
3. _____ DNA synthesis can be inhibited by affecting DNA gyrase or production of mRNA.
4. _____ Metronidazole is most effective against the anaerobes because it is not active until it is reduced.
5. _____ A mechanism of drug action is to target the bacterial folic acid pathway.

ANSWERS

Key Terms and Abbreviations
1. E
2. C
3. A
4. D
5. B

True or False
1. F
2. T
3. T
4. T
5. T

Laboratory Methods and Strategies for Antimicrobial Susceptibility Testing

OBJECTIVES

Upon completion of this chapter, the reader should be able to:
1. Explain how to prepare a standard inoculum.
2. Explain the broth dilution method.
3. Explain the disk diffusion method.
4. Give several examples of situations that require supplemental testing.
5. Explain the serum bactericidal test and the clinical indication for its use.
6. Explain synergy and antagonism.

SUMMARY OF KEY POINTS

The microbiology laboratory assists clinicians in making treatment decisions by providing information on the infecting organism's antimicrobial susceptibility profile. For these results to be reliable and reproducible, it is important that there be standardization. Standard conditions for testing have been published by the Clinical and Laboratory Standards Institute (CLSI), Subcommittee on Antimicrobial Susceptibility Testing. The elements of the testing process that must be controlled and standardized include:
- Bacterial inoculum size
- Growth medium
- pH
- Cation concentration
- Blood and serum components
- Thymidine content
- Incubation atmosphere
- Incubation duration
- Antimicrobial concentrations tested

Although testing should be standardized, these conditions cannot replicate the environment within the human host. Variables that play an important role in patient outcome but cannot be addressed by susceptibility testing include antibiotic diffusion into tissues and cells, status of the patient's immune system, drug interactions, and serum protein binding of antimicrobial agents.

General considerations that apply to any test method used include the following:
- Inoculum preparation: Inconsistencies in inoculum preparation will affect test results. The two most important requirements are to use a pure culture and to use a standardized inoculum. The standard inoculum is a bacterial suspension of 1.5×10^8 colony-forming units (CFU)/mL. This is the equivalent optical density of the 0.5 McFarland standard. The turbidity of the test inoculum should be measured either by an instrument or visually comparing the test suspension to the McFarland standard.

- Selection of antimicrobial agents for testing: The antimicrobial panel should include drugs suitable for the organism being tested. This information should be derived by input from medical staff and pharmacy and the CLSI tables on suggested groupings of antimicrobial agents.

There are several conventional testing methods:
- Broth dilution
- Agar dilution
- Disk diffusion
- Commercial susceptibility testing systems

These methods are briefly discussed here. For more information, please refer to the text.

Broth Dilution

This was one of the first test methods developed. The test medium is broth. The drug to be tested is serially diluted in each tube (macrodilution) or microtitre well (microdilution) and a standardized bacterial suspension is added in each well. The trays are incubated at 35° C in air for 16 to 20 hours. Following incubation, the trays are examined for growth. Each tray should have two controls, a growth control and a sterility control. The growth control well should contain no antimicrobial. The sterility well should not be inoculated with bacterial suspension. The lowest antimicrobial concentration that completely inhibits visible growth is the minimal inhibitory concentration (MIC). The concentrations of drugs tested will vary for each drug. Once the MIC value has been determined, the result is interpreted using CLSI documents and tables. Interpretation categories are susceptible, intermediate, and resistant. Resistance indicates that the drug tested may not be an appropriate choice for treatment because the test result highly correlates with a resistance mechanism that leads to treatment failure or because the organism is not inhibited by serum-achievable levels.

Agar Dilution

The medium for this test is agar rather than broth. The antimicrobial dilutions are incorporated into the agar. This means that if there are four serial dilutions, then there would be four plates. Each plate is inoculated with 1×10^4 CFU. Results are interpreted the same way for broth dilution.

Disk Diffusion

The disk diffusion method puts the antimicrobial onto paper disks. The paper disk is placed on agar that has been inoculated with a standardized suspension of bacteria to match the 0.5 McFarland turbidity standard. As water is absorbed into the paper, the antimicrobial diffuses out into the agar. As the distance from the disk increases, the concentration of antimicrobial in the agar decreases. The plates are incubated at 35° C in air for 16 hours. The diameter of the zone of inhibition is measured and CLSI tables are used to interpret results. Unlike MICs, a numerical value has no clinical utility by itself. Only the category interpretation of sensitive, intermediate, and resistant is reported. This method is frequently referred to as the Kirby Bauer method after the developers of the test. The standard agar base for the test is Mueller Hinton agar, but certain fastidious organisms may require supplemented media.

Commercial Susceptibility Testing Systems

Several systems have developed microdilution panels that are already prepared. All that is added is the bacterial suspension. Overnight incubation is still required with these systems.

A diffusion in agar derivative is the E-test. This system uses plastic strips that contain the antimicrobial agent laid on the strip in a such a way as to produce a concentration gradient that allows the determination of MIC values.

There are several automated systems that vary in the degree of automation. Microbroth dilution is used.

It is sometimes necessary to do supplemental testing because it is known that conventional and commercial systems have difficulty detecting resistance to certain drugs. To ensure accuracy in resistance detection, the following approaches may be used.

- When testing staphylococci, oxacillin screen agar should be used when other methods provide equivocal results. Growth on the screen correlates highly with the presence of oxacillin resistance. Strains that are classified as resistant are considered resistant to all other beta-lactam antibiotics. A 30-µg cefoxitin disk for disk diffusion can be used to assist in detecting oxacillin-resistant staphylococci. Refer to CLSI guidelines. Staphylococci may have reduced susceptibility to vancomycin that is difficult to detect by some commercial methods and disk diffusion. Vancomycin screen agar may be used; strains that grow on the screen should be tested by broth microdilution to obtain definitive MIC values.
- Enterococcal resistance to vancomycin can be detected using a combined agar screen method and broth microdilution.
- Enterococcal high-level resistance to the aminoglycosides cannot be detected by conventional methods. Screens that use high concentrations of aminoglycosides have been developed specifically for this determination.
- Penicillin resistance among *Staphylococcus pneumoniae* has emerged. The penicillin disk diffusion test was not sensitive enough to detect subtle changes in susceptibility. The oxacillin disk screen may be helpful, but if the organism produces a zone less than 20 mm, additional testing must be done that produces a MIC value.
- Staphylococci can show inducible resistance to clindamycin and need to be differentiated from truly susceptible strains. If an isolate produces a profile that shows resistance to a macrolide (e.g., erythromycin)

and susceptibility to clindamycin, the "D" test must be done to differentiate the two resistance mechanisms.
- The most sensitive antimicrobial agent from a group may be used to predict resistance to other drugs. For example, staphylococcal resistance to oxacillin determines resistance to all beta-lactams, including penicillins, cephalosporins, and carbapenems.

Another strategy to detect resistance is to detect the presence of the resistance mechanism. Some tests of this nature are listed below.

- Beta-lactamases act on the beta-lactam agents by disrupting their structure. The cefinase disk (BD Microbiology Systems, Cockeysville, Md) is used to detect the presence of this enzyme. Beta-lactamase testing should be done on isolates of *Haemophilus influenzae*, *Neisseria gonorrhoeae*, *Bacteroides* spp., and *Moraxella catarrhalis*.
- There is an assay to detect the presence of chloramphenicol acetyltransferase (CAT). The presence of this enzyme establishes chloramphenicol resistance, but a negative test does not rule out chloramphenicol resistance.
- Molecular methods have been developed to detect the genes that encode for resistance. This method has been applied to the mycobacteria.

Bactericidal tests are special methods that help determine the complex interactions between drug, microbe, and host. These tests are difficult to perform and interpret. Some tests have been developed to explore drug-drug interactions (e.g., synergy or antagonism). These tests are described below.

- The minimal bactericidal concentration (MBC) test may be performed in serious life-threatening infections. The MBC is the lowest concentration of a drug that results in 99.9% killing of the bacteria being tested. The MBC involves a continuation of the conventional broth dilution procedure. A large difference exists between the concentration required to inhibit growth and the concentration required to kill. Treatment failure may be occurring because the MBC exceeds the achievable serum level of the drug or because the organism has become tolerant to the drug.
- In time-kill studies, the rate of killing over time is measured. Bacteria are inoculated into tubes of broth containing different concentrations of antibiotic. An aliquot is removed from each tube at specified time intervals, cultured, and CFU counts are performed. The results are plotted to provide a time-kill curve. Because of the technical specifications of this test, it is usually just a research tool.
- The serum bactericidal test is similar to the MIC-MBC test. In patients who have severe infections or in whom the activity of the drug cannot be predicted, it may be necessary to test for antibacterial activity in vivo. This is done by using the patient's own serum. Both trough and peak serum samples are tested.
- It may be necessary to use multiple therapies simultaneously and to test the effectiveness of drug combinations. Synergy testing is done to evaluate drug interactions. The time kill assay is one way to do this. If two drugs

have synergy together, the activity of the drug combination is significantly greater than the activity of the single most active drug alone. Antagonism results when the combined activity is significantly less than the activity of the single most active antimicrobial alone.

All laboratory analyses should be evaluated for relevance and accuracy. When should susceptibility testing be performed? Some aspects to consider in answering this question include the clinical significance of the isolate, the predictability of its susceptibility to the drugs of choice, and the availability of standardized testing methods. Performing testing on clinically insignificant isolates wastes resources but, more importantly, may provide misleading information to the clinician. Table 12-5 in the text offers some guidelines on the routine performance of susceptibility testing. It may happen, however, that after communication between the laboratory, infectious disease specialist, and clinician, it is decided that susceptibility testing is needed but there are no standardized methods. The microbiology laboratory should perform the test to the best of its ability and report the result with a comment that testing was performed by a nonstandardized method and that results should be interpreted with caution.

If susceptibility testing is performed, what antimicrobial agents are included for testing? There is published information available from CLSI regarding the inclusion of drugs in testing panels. Please see Table 12-6 in the text for a summary of this information.

It is incumbent on the laboratory to produce accurate results. Standardized methods remove some of the variability. Microbiologists must also be aware of the strengths and weaknesses of their primary susceptibility testing methods. It may be necessary to utilize more than one method to obtain accurate results. For example, after reviewing the susceptibility profile of an isolate, it may be necessary to do additional testing to detect the presence of extended-spectrum beta-lactamases (ESBLs) in the *Enterobacteriaceae*. One method employs a double disk diffusion technique using the beta-lactamase inhibitor clavulanic acid with ceftazidime and another disk with ceftazidime alone. Measurement of the zone of inhibition is used to determine presence or absence of these enzymes.

Review of susceptibility data can be greatly facilitated by automated expert data review. Automated systems have features that do this by following a series of expert rules. Examples of unusual susceptibility profiles for both gram-negative and gram-positive bacteria are listed in Table 12-7 in the text. Data review also involves tracking of susceptibility profiles within a particular institution. This information is useful for monitoring the emergence of resistance trends and for establishing empiric therapy guidelines. Empiric therapy is begun before an organism has been identified.

In some cases it is not sufficient to merely perform the testing and report the numbers. Microbiologists can provide useful information to the clinician that can be used to achieve successful treatment outcome. An example of a comment that can guide therapy would be the inclusion of the comment "serious enterococcal infections may require dual therapy with an aminoglycoside and a cell-wall active agent" when a culture yields an enterococcal isolate from a sterile site.

KEY TERMS AND ABBREVIATIONS

Match the term in the left column with the definition on the right.

1. _____ zone of inhibition
2. _____ MIC
3. _____ MBC
4. _____ synergy
5. _____ antagonism

A. lowest concentration of drug that achieves 99.9% killing
B. combined activity is less than the activity of a single drug
C. lowest concentration that inhibits growth
D. activity of drug combination is greater than the activity of a single drug
E. area of no growth around a disk

TRUE OR FALSE

1. _____ The bacterial suspension for testing must be comparable to the 0.5 McFarland turbidity standard.
2. _____ In broth microdilution methods, the sterility control should contain only broth.
3. _____ The relationship between MIC and zone size is as follows: as the zone size increases, the MIC increases.
4. _____ Mueller-Hinton is the standard agar base for testing.
5. _____ An organism that appears resistant to erythromycin and susceptible to clindamycin should be tested for inducible resistance by the "D" test.

ANSWERS

Key Terms and Abbreviations
1. E
2. C
3. A
4. D
5. B

True or False
1. T
2. T
3. F
4. T
5. T

REFERENCES

Bradford PA: Extended-spectrum β-lactamases in the 21st century: characterization, epidemiology, and detection of this important resistance threat, *Clin Microbiol Rev* 14:933, 2001.

16 *Staphylococcus, Micrococcus,* and Similar Organisms

OBJECTIVES

Upon completion of this chapter, the reader should be able to:
1. Name at least three types of infections caused by *S. aureus.*
2. Describe how to identify *S. saprophyticus* and its clinical significance.
3. Describe how to differentiate *S. epidermidis* and *S. saprophyticus.*
4. Describe how to differentiate between staphylococci and micrococci.
5. Explain the difference between colonization and infection.
6. Explain the clinical and epidemiologic significance of MRSA isolation.

SUMMARY OF KEY POINTS

In the family *Micrococcaceae* are the genera *Staphylococcus* and *Micrococcus.* These are gram-positive cocci that align in pairs, tetrads, or clusters. The name "staph" comes from *staphyle,* which means bunch of grapes.

The genus *Micrococcus* has two species, *M. luteus* and *M. lylae.* These are considered to be harmless saprophytes that inhabit the skin, mucosa, and oropharynx. *M. luteus* produces a yellow pigment and is susceptible to bacitracin. Both micrococci and staphylococci contain cytochrome enzymes. Catalase detects the presence of cytochrome oxidase; both genera are catalase-positive.

The staphylococci are nonmotile, non–spore-forming, facultative anaerobes that are resistant to bacitracin. Staphylococci are able to grow in the presence of salt; this characteristic is used to isolate staphylococci from clinical material. Mannitol salt agar contains 10% salt, mannitol, and phenol red as an indicator. Staphylococci produce colonies surrounded by a yellow halo. The clinically significant species include *S. aureus, S. saprophyticus, S. lugdunensis, S. epidermidis, S. haemolyticus,* and *S. schleiferi. S. aureus* is differentiated from other clinically significant species by its production of coagulase, positive Voges-Proskauer test, and negative PYR test.

INTEREST POINT

At the 2005 general meeting of the American Society for Microbiology, Drs. Proctor, Peters, and Kahl presented a workshop on staphylococcal small colony variants (SCVs). It is thought that SCVs may be responsible for the clinical syndrome defined by persistent, recurrent, and antibiotic-resistant staphylococcal infection. These patients may initially present with an acute *S. aureus* infection that produces the typical large colony morphology with hemolysis. One of several mutations may take place to change electron transport, which can then affect multiple phenotypic characteristics. The genetically same strain of *S. aureus* that presented with acute infection and characteristic morphology changes into a chronic infection that can persist for weeks to months. The colonies are small, nonhemolytic, and nonpigmented. In Gram stain the cocci are large, but in culture the colonies are one-tenth normal size and produce only weak catalase and coagulase reactions. The tube test requires 24 hours of incubation. SCVs can hide within host cells, proliferate there, and evade destruction. Look for SCVs in persistent, recurring infections if there are cocci in the Gram stain but no growth on plates, if there are two colony types in positive blood cultures (normal *S. aureus* and small colonies), or if in vitro antibiotic activity shows susceptibility but therapy fails. Oxacillin kills extracellular organisms but cannot penetrate host cells. Daptomycin is the only negatively charged antibiotic in use. Combined therapy of vancomycin with rifampin has produced good results. These microbiologists suggested the following result report: "Small colony variant suspected. Susceptibility testing results questionable."

S. aureus is the most virulent species encountered. Nearly all strains secrete enzymes and cytotoxins that include one of the four hemolysins, nucleases, proteases, lipases, hyaluronidase, and collagenase. These enzymes and toxins convert host tissues into nutrients required for growth. Some strains also produce exoproteins that include toxic shock syndrome toxin-1 (TSST-1), the staphylococcal enterotoxins, exfoliative toxin, and the Panton-Valentine leukocidin. TSST-1 and the enterotoxins are pyrogenic superantigens. The toxins damage the membrane of eukaryotic cells, some target erythrocytes while some affect neutrophils and macrophages. Certain clinical conditions predispose a person to *S. aureus* infection; these include diabetes mellitus, intravascular devices and prosthetic materials, chemotaxis defects such as Chediak-Higashi syndrome, neutrophil defects, and complement defects.

Staphylococcal food poisoning is probably the most common cause of food poisoning in the United States. It results from ingestion of one or more preformed enterotoxins on food that has been contaminated with *S. aureus*. Food contamination is usually related to improper handling by a worker who is colonized with *S. aureus*. Symptoms appear quickly (2 to 8 hours after eating) and resolve quickly. All of the enterotoxins cause vomiting.

Toxic shock syndrome (TSS) was first described in 1978; the syndrome was seen in a group of children 8 to 17 years of age who presented with high temperature, diarrhea, hypotension, diffuse rash, and renal failure. In the 1980s this multisystem disease was frequently observed in menstruating women who were using hyperabsorbable tampons. *S. aureus* was isolated from cervical and vaginal cultures. TSST-1 was the first toxin identified for TSS. It is a superantigen that activates T cells to produce cytokines, which have major systemic effects. TSS is characterized by rash with desquamation of skin and involvement of several organ systems.

The desquamation in TSS is not the same as that in scalded skin syndrome (SSS) seen in neonates. In SSS there are large watery blisters that appear and then the shedding of large areas of skin. The exfoliatin toxins cause extensive sloughing of skin.

Although the skin is a barrier to infection, if this barrier is breached by trauma or surgery, *S. aureus* can gain entry and cause the characteristic lesion of necrotic tissue, fibrin, and large numbers of live and dead neutrophils. Skin infections may be localized (folliculitis) or cause deeper infections. Toxins may cause skin rashes and fever. Septicemia may result from this local infection. During disseminated infection, other organs may become involved. *S. aureus* can cause a severe necrotizing pneumonia, septic arthritis, osteomyelitis, and endocarditis.

S. aureus is a well-documented opportunistic pathogen that has been a major cause of morbidity and mortality as a nosocomial infection. Nasal carriage may be a risk factor for infection. Some strategies employed to reduce or eliminate colonization include repeated applications of nasal mupirocin and chlorhexidine showers.

In the United States, most *S. aureus* strains are resistant to penicillin but susceptible to the penicillinase-stable penicillins, such as oxacillin and methicillin. Historically, methicillin was the representative drug for this group. There are very few strains that do not produce a beta-lactamase. This extracellular enzyme works by opening the beta-lactam ring in the antibiotic before the antibiotic can act on the organism. The cephalosporins are also susceptible to this beta-lactamase degradation. This intrinsic resistance to beta-lactam antibiotics is due

to a penicillin-binding protein (PBP) encoded by the *mec A* gene. An altered PBP now makes all beta-lactam antibiotics ineffective. We are seeing increasing numbers of *S. aureus* isolates that are resistant to oxacillin and methicillin. These methicillin-resistant *S. aureus* (MRSA) are a serious public health issue. There are limited treatment options leaving vancomycin as the drug of choice for severe MRSA infections. Unfortunately, there are now descriptions of a few isolates that show high-level resistance to vancomycin. Two relatively new antibiotics that may be useful are linezolid and daptomycin.

INTEREST POINT

Although vancomycin is considered to be the "gold standard" for the treatment of MRSA infections, treatment failure with vancomycin is not uncommon. One published report looked at 30 isolates from 30 patients with MRSA bacteremia (Sakoulas et al, 2004). The authors found a relationship between vancomycin MIC and clinical failure. Although all organisms were susceptible (vancomycin MIC $\leq$ 2 μg/mL) by standard methods of testing and criteria, vancomycin was only clinically effective in 9.5% of the cases where the MIC was 1 to 2 μg/mL. The treatment success rate increased to 55.6% when the vancomycin MIC was $\leq$ 0.5 μg/mL. Other drugs that test inhibitory to MRSA include linezolid and daptomycin. There is published literature describing treatment strategies that show in vivo synergy when rifampin is combined with vancomycin, trimethoprim-sulfamethoxazole, minocycline, or ciprofloxacin.

S. epidermidis and other coagulase-negative staphylococci (CoNS) have previously been dismissed as culture contaminants, but many times may be pathogens. Infections caused by these organisms usually involve indwelling catheters and artificial devices (prostheses). CoNS are now recognized as nosocomial pathogens. *S. epidermidis* is found on human skin and mucous membranes. It produces an exopolysaccharide ("slime") that can be seen by electron microscopy on catheters colonized with this organism. Its role in pathogenesis is not clear, but the slime seems to allow the staphylococci to persist on the catheter by impairing host defense mechanisms and antimicrobial killing. Other factors that may allow adherence to plastic surfaces include other surface polysaccharides, proteins, and hemagglutinin. *S. epidermidis* is a recognized pathogen in infections involving peritoneal dialysis catheters and valve endocarditis.

S. saprophyticus is a true urinary tract pathogen causing both upper and lower urinary tract disease in young, sexually active females. Several proteins may be responsible for its pathogenicity. A protein hemagglutinin may play a role in its attachment to uroepithelial cells as does a surface fibrillar protein. A urease has been implicated in the invasion of the organism into the urinary bladder. *S. saprophyticus* is differentiated from other nonhemolytic CoNS by its resistance to novobiocin (5-μg disk).

Other CoNS isolated from colonized shunts, catheters, and prosthetic devices are *S. lugdunensis* and *S. schleiferi*. Soft tissue infections and endocarditis have been associated with *S. lugdunensis* and *S. haemolyticus*.

KEY TERMS AND ABBREVIATIONS

Match the term in the left column with the definition on the right.

1. _____ impetigo
2. _____ scalded-skin syndrome
3. _____ toxic shock syndrome
4. _____ catalase
5. _____ beta-lactamase
6. _____ bacitracin
7. _____ novobiocin
8. _____ MRSA

A. life-threatening infection involving several organ systems
B. multidrug-resistant strain
C. extracellular enzyme that inactivates several classes of antibiotics
D. sloughing of epidermis usually seen in neonates
E. antibiotic used to differentiate staphylococci from micrococci
F. test that detects cytochrome oxidase
G. antibiotic used to differentiate the coagulase-negative staphylococci
H. superficial skin infection

TRUE OR FALSE

1. _____ Although it is common practice not to identify coagulase-negative staphylococci to the species level, an exception may be made if it is a repeated isolate from blood cultures.
2. _____ Chlorhexidine showers may be used to reduce colonization with *S. aureus*.
3. _____ Staphylococci will grow on 5% sheep blood agar and chocolate agars but not mannitol salt agar.
4. _____ One way to confirm oxacillin resistance in *S. aureus* isolates is to test for the presence of PBP 2a.
5. _____ The tube coagulase test should be read at 2 hours.

MULTIPLE CHOICE

1. _____ *S. saprophyticus* isolated from a female patient is a recognized cause of
   A. impetigo.
   B. toxic shock syndrome.
   C. urinary tract infection.
   D. folliculitis.

2. _____ One test used to differentiate *S. aureus* from *S. lugdunensis* is
   A. PYR.
   B. catalase.
   C. bacitracin sensitivity.
   D. novobiocin sensitivity.

3. _____ A hand wound culture produced a creamy white growth that is catalase- and coagulase-positive. The physician reported that the wound was caused by a dog bite. To prevent misidentification of the staphylococcal species, what additional test(s) should be performed?
   A. Novobiocin susceptibility
   B. PYR and VP
   C. Tube coagulase
   D. PYR and ornithine decarboxylase

4. _____ Selective media that can be used to isolate staphylococci includes
   A. 5% sheep blood agar.
   B. MacConkey agar.
   C. chocolate agar.
   D. mannitol salt agar.

5. _____ A gram-positive coccus that is catalase-positive, coagulase-negative, and resistant to novobiocin is
   A. *S. aureus*.
   B. *S. epidermidis*.
   C. *S. saprophyticus*.
   D. *S. lugdunensis*.

CASE STUDY

A 24-year-old woman presented to the emergency department complaining of fever, sore throat, and abdominal pain. A throat swab was collected and rapid streptococcal antigen test was done. It was positive. Urine was also collected for urinalysis. The urine was amber and cloudy and the microscopic examination showed many bacteria, 10 to 25 RBC/HPF, and WBCs that were too numerous to count. A urine culture was also done. After overnight incubation there was no growth on the MacConkey plate and greater than 100 colonies on the sheep blood agar plate. The colonies were white and nonhemolytic.

1. What are the first tests that should be done at this point to identify the isolate?
2. The isolate was a gram-positive, catalase-positive coccus. Explain all additional testing that should be done on this isolate.

ANSWERS

Key Terms and Abbreviations

1. H
2. D
3. A
4. F
5. C
6. E
7. G
8. B

True or False

1. T
2. T
3. F
4. T
5. F

Multiple Choice

1. C
2. A
3. B
4. D
5. C

Case Study

1. The colonies should be Gram stained to determine the Gram reaction and cell type (bacillus or coccus). After the Gram stain, a catalase test would provide useful information.
2. Gram positive cocci are staphylococci. The fact that the colonies are nonhemolytic would indicate the organism is not *S. aureus*, but a coagulase test should be done. If the organism is coagulase-negative, further testing needs to be done to determine if it is *S. saprophyticus*. The patient is a young woman who could be sexually active. *S. saprophyticus* is a common urinary pathogen in this patient population. To differentiate *S. saprophyticus* from other coagulase-negative staphylococci, sensitivity to novobiocin should be checked. *S. saprophyticus* is resistant to novobiocin. Susceptibility testing should also be performed.

REFERENCES

Boubaker K, Diebold P, Blanc DS, et al: Panton-Valentine leukocidin and staphylococcal skin infections in schoolchildren, *Emerg Infect Dis* 10:121, 2004.

Dinges MM, Orwin PM, Schlievert PM: Exotoxins of *Staphylococcus aureus, Clin Microbiol Rev* 13:16, 2000.

Proctor RA, Peters G: Small colony variants in staphylococcal infections: diagnostic and therapeutic implications, *Clin Infect Dis* 27:419, 1998.

Proctor RA, van Langevelde P, Kristjansson N, et al: Persistent and relapsing infections associated with small-colony variants of *Staphylococcus aureus, Clin Infect Dis* 20:95, 1995.

Sakoulas G, et al: Relationship of MIC and bactericidal activity to efficacy of vancomycin for treatment of methicillin-resistant *Staphylococcus aureus* bacteremia, *J Clin Microbiol* 42:2398, 2004.

Wegner DL: No mercy for MRSA, *MLO* 37:26, 2005.

17 *Streptococcus, Enterococcus, and Similar Organisms*

OBJECTIVES

Upon completion of this chapter, the reader should be able to:
1. Differentiate streptococci from staphylococci.
2. Differentiate the types of beta-hemolytic streptococci.
3. Differentiate the types of alpha-hemolytic streptococci.
4. Name at least two diseases associated with *S. pyogenes* and *S. agalactiae*.
5. Explain how to definitively identify *S. pneumoniae*.
6. Explain how to identify the enterococci.
7. Explain how to test for vancomycin resistance in enterococci and its significance.
8. Explain some of the basic tests used to identify streptococci. These should include NaCl tube or plate media, bile esculin hydrolysis, optochin disk testing, LAP testing, PYR, and bile solubility.

SUMMARY OF KEY POINTS

In 1985, the genus *Streptococcus* was split into several genera; this distinction was based on molecular typing that included DNA homology and 16s rRNA sequence analysis. These organisms are all facultative anaerobes that do not contain cytochrome enzymes or catalase. All are gram-positive but the arrangement of the cells helps differentiate the genera. Streptococci, enterococci, and *Leuconostoc* spp. divide in plane to form chains. Bacteria that divide in two planes to form pairs or tetrads include *Pediococcus* and *Gemella*. It is best to use growth from broth to determine cellular morphology in a Gram stain.

Streptococci are facultative anaerobes and are nutritionally fastidious; growth can be enhanced by adding blood or serum. *S. pneumoniae* and certain viridans streptococci require elevated levels of CO_2 for growth. Streptococci are catalase- and oxidase-negative. Many of these organisms are considered normal flora of the alimentary, respiratory, and genital tracts. Hemolytic reactions and Lancefield serologic tests based on cell wall polysaccharides are used to divide the streptococci into broad categories. There are the beta-hemolytic strains including *S. pyogenes* (group A) and *S. agalactiae* (group B) as well as groups C, F, and G. There is a broad group referred to as *viridans streptococci* that produce alpha-hemolysis (greening of blood agar).

There is another group, known as nutritionally variant streptococci, that was once thought to be forms of viridans streptococci; these are fastidious organisms that grow as satellite colonies around other bacteria. Viridans streptococci are not part of the Lancefield system because they lack the C carbohydrate.

Clinically significant streptococcal species that are beta-hemolytic include *S. pyogenes, S. agalactiae,* and groups C, F, and G. *S. pyogenes* produces extracellular products that include streptococcal pyrogenic exotoxin (SPE), hemolysins streptolysin O and streptolysin S, enzymes that degrade DNA, hyaluronidase, and streptokinase. Streptokinase dissolves clots by converting plasminogen to plasmin. Bacterial pharyngitis is most commonly due to *S. pyogenes,* but groups C and G have also been associated with pharyngitis. Scarlet fever results from strains that produce SPE. *S. pyogenes* is also associated with impetigo, cellulitis, necrotizing fasciitis, and streptococcal toxic shock syndrome. Important poststreptococcal sequelae include glomerulonephritis and rheumatic fever. The incidence of these problems has decreased dramatically in the United States with the advent of "rapid strep" tests and treatment with penicillin. Poststreptococcal rheumatic fever, however, is still a problem in some countries.

Group B streptococcus (GBS) was first recognized as a human pathogen in 1935 in several cases of fatal puerperal sepsis. By the 1970s, its importance as the cause of infection in postpartum women and neonates was recognized. About 30% of American women are colonized with GBS in the genital and gastrointestinal tract. Neonates are exposed at birth and may develop early-onset meningitis (within first 5 days of life) or late-onset infection (7 days to 3 months). The Centers for Disease Control and Prevention (CDC) has published guidelines for the control and prevention of perinatal group B streptococcal disease. GBS also causes skin and soft tissue infections; cellulitis, foot ulcers, abscess, and infection of decubitus ulcers are common. Diabetes usually predisposes patients to this type of infection, as well as to GBS arthritis and osteomyelitis. Although there are reports of isolates resistant to penicillin, penicillin is still the drug of choice. Ampicillin plus an aminoglycoside for neonatal bacteremia or meningitis produces synergistic killing.

43

S. pneumoniae causes disease because it escapes ingestion and killing by phagocytic cells; this resistance is due to the polysaccharide capsule it produces. *S. pneumoniae* is the leading cause of community-acquired bacterial pneumonia, meningitis, sinusitis, otitis media, and bacteremia. It colonizes the nasopharynx. Pneumococcal infection is most prevalent in the extremes of life and in patients with underlying disease. Viral infection predisposes to pneumococcal infection. Two types of vaccines are available to prevent infection by the most prevalent serotypes. One vaccine recommended for people older than 65 years of age or with certain underlying diseases contains a mixture of 23 pneumococcal capsular polysaccharides. The other vaccine approved in 2000 for infants and children is a 7-valent vaccine that includes all the serotypes that are drug-resistant. *S. pneumoniae* is susceptible to optochin, and is bile-soluble and bile esculin–negative.

Streptococci that are not beta-hemolytic, do not belong to Lancefield groups B or D, are not *S. pneumoniae*, and cannot grow in 6.5% NaCl broth are considered part of the large category called the viridans streptococci. Viridans means "green" and is derived from the Latin *viridis*. Most of these species are alpha-hemolytic and produce a greening on 5% sheep blood agar but they can also be nonhemolytic. Many species in this category grow better under anaerobic conditions; microaerophilic streptococci require a reduced level of oxygen to grow. Viridans streptococci are normal flora of the oral, respiratory, and gastrointestinal mucosa. Most are opportunistic pathogens. Their ability to adhere to epithelial and endothelial cells is a key factor in their ability to cause disease. They are a major agent of dental caries. This may be a predisposing factor in the development of endocarditis. The most common species of this group to cause endocarditis include *S. sanguis, S. mitis, S. mutans,* and *S. oralis*. Recent studies indicate that these viridans streptococci are showing increased rates of resistance to penicillin, levofloxacin, erythromycin, and azithromycin. For serious infections (i.e., multiple positive blood cultures and cultures from cerebrospinal fluid and sterile body sites), it is good practice to identify the organism to the species level and perform susceptibility testing.

The group of organisms that used to be called the nutritionally variant streptococci were thought to be viridans streptococci. These organisms grow as satellite colonies around organisms that produce pyridoxal, such as around staphylococci. These organisms require vitamin B_6 (pyridoxal) for growth. Standard 5% sheep blood plates do not support growth of these organisms. After 16s rRNA sequence analysis of this group of organisms, it was determined that they were not streptococci. Two new genera were proposed; *Abiotrophia* and *Granulicatella.* These organisms are part of the normal oral and intestinal flora but are known to cause sepsis and endocarditis. Little is known about susceptibility patterns for these organisms, but recent studies indicate there may be beta-lactam and macrolide resistance.

The genus *Enterococcus* used to be classified as group D enterococci. Little is known about the pathogenicity of these organisms. These organisms are normal flora of the gastrointestinal tract and vaginal vault. Two species are responsible for the majority of enterococcal infections; *E. faecalis* accounts for 80% to 90% of clinical isolates and *E. faecium* accounts for 5% to 15% of isolates. Their resistance to multiple antibiotics allows them to survive during courses of antimicrobial therapy. This is why they can cause superinfections in patients receiving broad-spectrum antibiotics. They can adhere to heart valves and renal epithelial cells, causing endocarditis and urinary tract infections. Although they inhabit the gastrointestinal tract, they are not known to cause gastroenteritis, but they are often isolated from intraabdominal and pelvic sites. They cause nosocomial infections and have been cultured from the hands of medical personnel and environmental sites, such as windowsills. Electronic thermometers have been implicated in the spread of resistant organisms.

The enterococci are intrinsically resistant to low levels of aminoglycosides, beta-lactams, trimethoprim-sulfamethoxazole, and low levels of lincosamides. They can acquire resistance to fluoroquinolones, macrolides, rifampin, vancomycin, tetracycline, and high levels of aminoglycosides. None of the cephalosporins have clinical activity against the enterococci. Intrinsic resistance to the aminoglycosides is due to their inability to penetrate the outer cell envelope. But when used with cell-wall active agents (ampicillin, penicillin, or vancomycin), there is synergistic killing.

Enterococci can transfer resistance genes among themselves by transferring plasmids or transposons. Plasmids can be transferred among enterococci and some streptococci, *S. aureus,* lactobacilli, *B. subtilis, L. monocytogenes,* and others. In the late 1980s, vancomycin resistance began to be noted. There are five recognized genes encoding vancomycin resistance. The vancomycin-resistant enterococci (VRE) have become important in infection control and in therapy failures. Hospital outbreaks have been reported for both *vanA* and *vanB* isolates. Patients may be colonized with more than one strain of VRE, but colonization of healthy individuals with VRE does not indicate a risk for infection. Unfortunately, recent reports have documented horizontal transfer of the *vanA* gene from vancomycin-resistant *E. faecalis* to methicillin-resistant *S. aureus.* Most strains (90% to 96%) remain susceptible to nitrofurantoin, which has been successfully used to treat urinary tract infections. Linezolid has been used but there is emerging resistance with therapeutic failure when linezolid was used alone.

KEY TERMS AND ABBREVIATIONS

Match the term in the left column with the definition on the right.

1. _____ streptolysin O	A. selective media for gram-positive organisms
2. _____ SPE	
3. _____ rheumatic fever	
4. _____ group B strep	B. pyrogenic toxin associated with scarlet fever
5. _____ CNA	
6. _____ *Leuconostoc*	C. large cocci in tetrads
7. _____ viridans streptococci	D. hemolysin

8. _____ LAP
9. _____ LIM broth
10. _____ *Pediococcus*

E. complication of *S. pyogenes* infection
F. mutans and anginosus group
G. *S. agalactiae*
H. usually only pathogenic in severely compromised patients
I. used to enhance detection of genital carriage of group B streptococci
J. used to differentiate *Leuconostoc* from *Enterococcus*

TRUE OR FALSE

1. _____ *S. agalactiae* is the only species of beta-hemolytic streptococci that will give a positive PYR reaction.
2. _____ *S. pneumoniae* can positively be identified by the optochin test.
3. _____ The viridans streptococci grow best under microaerophilic conditions.
4. _____ Nitrofurantoin is currently the drug of choice for treating uncomplicated VRE urinary tract infections.
5. _____ Nosocomial VRE outbreaks have been associated with hospital thermometers.

MULTIPLE CHOICE

1. _____ These organisms will not grow on sheep blood agar without the addition of vitamin B_6.
   A. *S. mutans*
   B. *Abiotrophia*
   C. *S. agalactiae*
   D. *E. faecalis*

2. _____ A rapid strep test was done using a throat swab collected from a 10-year-old boy. The result was negative. The best laboratory practice would be to
   A. use that swab to inoculate a sheep blood agar plate.
   B. use that swab to inoculate a sheep blood agar plate and place a bacitracin disk.
   C. report the result with no confirmatory testing.
   D. use the second swab collected to inoculate a sheep blood agar plate.

3. _____ The organisms that colonize 30% of American women and frequently cause meningitis in neonates are
   A. viridans streptococci.
   B. *S. pyogenes* sp.
   C. enterococci.
   D. *S. agalactiae* sp.

4. _____ All streptococci are negative for this test.
   A. Catalase
   B. Coagulase
   C. PYR
   D. Bile esculin

5. _____ A patient tested positive for anti-DNase B and negative for antistreptolysin O. These results would be consistent with the disease process of
   A. strep throat.
   B. *S. pneumoniae* bacteremia.
   C. pyoderma.
   D. *S. urinalis* infection.

CASE STUDY

A middle-aged man with diabetes presented to the emergency department complaining of progressive pain and swelling in his right lower leg. The pain and swelling came on suddenly. He denied any injury or mosquito bites to his leg. The skin on the leg appeared to be intact, but it was quickly obvious to the clinician that the inflammation was spreading up the leg. The skin was becoming purplish. A surgeon was called in. It was determined that the overlying skin was becoming loosened from the fascia. It was decided to take the man to surgery for debridement and possible amputation. By the time the surgeon and patient had prepared for surgery, the inflammation had spread up into the thigh area. The surgeon admitted he had never seen tissue necrosis spread this quickly. The leg was amputated at the hip. Biopsy tissue was taken for culture. Gram positive cocci were seen in the Gram stain. The next day beta-hemolysis around small white colonies in pure culture on the 5% sheep blood agar plate was observed. The growth was catalase-negative.
1. What tests could be done at this point to identify the organism?
2. What is the most likely clinical condition this patient is experiencing and what is the most likely cause?
3. The patient recovered with no sequelae. If the patient's leg had not been amputated, what might have happened?

ANSWERS

Key Terms and Abbreviations
1. D
2. B
3. E
4. G
5. A
6. H
7. F
8. J
9. I
10. C

True or False
1. F
2. F
3. T
4. T
5. T

Multiple Choice

1. B
2. D
3. D
4. A
5. C

Case Study

1. There are several commercially available kits for typing the polysaccharide antigen of the cell wall. However, there are several organisms that type positive for group A—*S. pyogenes* and the anginosus group, as well as different groups that type positive for groups C and G. These organisms can be sorted by using susceptibility to bacitracin and the PYR, Voges-Proskauer, and CAMP tests. There are also commercially available identification systems that utilize biochemical reactions.

2. The description fits that for necrotizing fasciitis. This is an inflammatory infection located deep in the fascia. There can be secondary necrosis of subcutaneous tissue. Because the infection is in the fascia, the pathogen has almost unrestricted ability to spread quickly horizontally along the fascia. *Streptococcus pyogenes* is the most probable etiologic agent.

3. Invasive group A streptococcal (GAS) infection can lead to rapidly progressive disease syndromes that include necrotizing fasciitis and streptococcal toxic shock syndrome (STSS). The morbidity and mortality for this type of infection is very high. In 1999, 9500 cases of invasive GAS disease were reported; there were 1100 deaths. The overall case fatality rate is estimated to be between 10% to 15%, but the rate for STSS can be as high as 60%. STSS is not the same as toxic shock syndrome associated with *S. aureus*.

Complications of GAS infection can include bacteremia associated with aggressive soft tissue infection, shock, respiratory distress syndrome, and renal failure. A high percentage of patients die even with aggressive modern treatments.

REFERENCES

Bourbeau PP: Role of the microbiology laboratory in diagnosis and management of pharyngitis, *J Clin Microbiol* 41:3467, 2003.

Cetinkaya Y, Falk P, Mayhall CG: Vancomycin-resistant enterococci, *Clin Microbiol Rev* 13:686, 2000.

Doern GV, Ferraro MJ, Brueggemann AB, et al: Emergence of high rates of antimicrobial resistance among viridans group streptococci in the United States, *Antimicrob Agents Chemother* 40:891, 1996.

Factor SH, Levine OS, Schwartz B, et al: Invasive group A streptococcal disease: risk factors for adults, *Emerg Infect Dis* 9:970, 2003.

Gilbert DN, Moellering RC, editors: *The Sanford guide to antimicrobial therapy 2006,* ed 37, Sperryville, Va, 2006, Antimicrobial Therapy, Inc.

Prabhu RM, Piper KE, Baddour LM, et al: Antimicrobial susceptibility patterns among viridans group streptococcal isolates from infective endocarditis patients from 1972 to 1986 and 1994 to 2002, *Antimicrob Agents Chemother* 48:4463, 2004.

Stevens DL: Streptococcal toxic-shock syndrome: spectrum of disease, pathogenesis, and new concepts in treatment, *Emerg Infect Dis* 1:69, 1995.

Willems RJL, Top J, van Santen M, et al: Global spread of vancomycin-resistant *Enterococcus faecium* from distinct nosocomial genetic complex, *Emerg Infect Dis* 11:821, 2005.

Zheng X, Freeman AF, Villafranca J, et al: Anitmicrobial susceptibilities of invasive pediatric *Abiotrophia* and *Granulicatella* isolates, *J Clin Micobiol* 42:4323, 2004.

18 *Bacillus* and Similar Organisms

OBJECTIVES

Upon completion of this chapter, the reader should be able to:
1. Describe general characteristics of the genus *Bacillus* and how to differentiate *B. anthracis* from other species.
2. Describe the three disease forms of anthrax.
3. Describe the clinical significance of *B. cereus*.

SUMMARY OF KEY POINTS

The genus *Bacillus* is composed of aerobic gram-positive bacilli that produce spores under aerobic conditions and are catalase-positive. They are ubiquitous in nature, inhabiting soils of all kinds and bottom deposits of fresh and salt water. They are thermophilic and psychrophilic; this means they can grow at temperatures between 75° C and 3° C. The defining feature of this genus is the production of spores in the presence of oxygen. The spores allow their survival and distribution. The spores are resistant to heat, desiccation, radiation, and disinfectants. Because of this, they have caused contamination of pharmaceutical products and foods. Intravenous drug users are at risk both from the injection paraphernalia and from the heroin itself, which contains several contaminating organisms that may include *B. cereus* and *B. anthracis*.

Bacillus anthracis is one of the most highly pathogenic organisms known. It is a large, nonmotile, gram-positive bacillus. It is the agent of anthrax. Anthrax disease in cattle and humans was reported in the literature for hundreds of years. Outbreaks associated with occupational exposure occurred in Europe in the 1800s. Woolsorter's disease was associated with the handling of animal hides, wool, and hair. In the 1930s, a vaccine was developed that is still in use for the vaccination of livestock. There are sporadic anthrax outbreaks among livestock and wildlife in North America; but anthrax is more of a risk in Africa, Asia, South and Central America, Eastern Europe, and the Middle East. From 1981 to 1989 in the United States, there were only four cases reported to the CDC.

Anthrax in humans has three forms: cutaneous, pulmonary, and gastrointestinal. Cutaneous anthrax occurs when spores get into cuts or abrasions and produce a very slow-healing ulcer that is covered with a black eschar (scab).

Swabs of the exudate of early lesions can be collected for culture. Intestinal anthrax occurs from eating contaminated meat; it has not been reported in the United States. There is rapid onset of abdominal pain, fever, vomiting, and bloody diarrhea. Gram-positive rods may be seen in paracentesis fluid. In pulmonary anthrax (woolsorter's disease), spores are inhaled and travel via macrophages from the lungs to the lymphatic system, where they germinate and multiply. In untreated cutaneous anthrax, approximately 20% of the cases are fatal compared to almost 100% fatality for inhalational anthrax.

Bacillus cereus is another medically significant species. *B. cereus* food poisoning is a toxin-mediated disease rather than an infection. Food becomes environmentally exposed; these spores can resist pasteurization and radiation. There were 24 outbreaks of *B. cereus* food poisoning in the United States between 1982 and 1987. Toxin-forming strains cause an acute but self-limited gastroenteritis. *B. cereus* has also been implicated in serious eye infections. Other species, such as *B. subtilis*, may cause opportunistic infections.

Because of the intentional release of anthrax spores in the United States in 2001, it is incumbent on the microbiology laboratory to be vigilant when processing clinical specimens. There is no person-to-person spread of disease; the risk factors are the inhalation or ingestion of spores and the ingestion of preformed toxin. To protect the laboratory worker, all clinical specimens and work with suspect colonies should be performed in a biosafety cabinet. If a large gram-positive rod is observed in a blood culture, the laboratory must rule out the possibility of anthrax.

All *Bacillus* species grow on 5% sheep blood agar and chocolate agar. Selective media such as PEA and MacConkey agar can be added to isolate the organisms. In Gram stains, *B. anthracis* appears as a large gram-positive rod. On sheep blood agar, *B. anthracis* colonies have a ground-glass appearance with irregular edges; they are nonhemolytic and tenacious. Hemolysis and motility are used to differentiate *B. anthracis* from other species. Motility can be observed by inoculating a few drops of trypticase soy broth with the suspect colony and examining the suspension microscopically. Motile bacteria tend to form chains of rods and move with a snakelike motion. Brownian movement should not be confused with motility.

47

Motility test media can also be used. If the isolate is catalase-positive, nonhemolytic, and nonmotile, then sentinel clinical laboratories should report the isolation of a *Bacillus* species but send the isolate to a reference laboratory to rule out *B. anthracis*.

KEY TERMS AND ABBREVIATIONS

Match the term in the left column with the definition on the right.

1. _____ eschar
2. _____ woolsorter's disease
3. _____ food poisoning
4. _____ opportunistic pathogen
5. _____ thermophilic
6. _____ psychrophilic

A. pulmonary anthrax
B. *B. subtilis*
C. *B. cereus*
D. can grow at 3° C
E. can grow at 75° C
F. scab

TRUE OR FALSE

1. _____ Anthrax cannot be acquired by direct contact with an infected person.
2. _____ Prophylaxis with ciprofloxacin is recommended following aerosol exposure to *B. anthracis*.
3. _____ *B. anthracis* has been isolated from the heroin used by intravenous drug users.
4. _____ No blood culture isolate of a large gram-positive rod should be dismissed as a contaminant without first ruling out anthrax.
5. _____ On Gram stain, spores appear clear because they do not take up the crystal violet.

MULTIPLE CHOICE

1. _____ Acute gastroenteritis is caused by
   A. *B. subtilis.*
   B. *B. cereus.*
   C. *Paenibacillus* spp.
   D. *Brevibacillus* brevis.

2. _____ *B. anthracis* can be quickly differentiated from the other *Bacillus* species by
   A. lecithinase zone.
   B. catalase.
   C. spore size.
   D. motility.

3. _____ A cause of serious eye infections is
   A. *B. subtilis.*
   B. *B. cereus.*
   C. *B. thuringiensis.*
   D. *B. megaterium.*

4. _____ A black eschar is indicative of
   A. cutaneous anthrax.
   B. woolsorter's disease.
   C. enterotoxin production.
   D. encapsulation.

5. _____ Which statement is false?
   A. Young bacilli stain gram-variable.
   B. *Bacillus* spp. do not grow on MacConkey.
   C. A unique feature of *Bacillus* spp. is their ability to produce spores in the presence of oxygen.
   D. There is an anthrax vaccine available for public health workers and military personnel.

CASE STUDY

A 38-year-old man who works in a federal building in Washington, D.C., complained of fever and chills with a nonproductive cough for 2 days. The emergency department physician ordered a chest x-ray, CBC, and two blood cultures. The patient's white count was slightly elevated and the chest x-ray showed infiltrates. The patient was given azithromycin and was sent home. The next day the laboratory reported that one (aerobic) of four blood culture bottles was positive with gram-positive bacilli.

1. After seeing the gram-positive rods in the blood smear, what should the microbiology technologist do next?
2. The growth next day showed dull irregularly shaped colonies on the sheep blood agar plate with no hemolysis. The technologist Gram stained these colonies and saw large gram-positive rods. What should she do next to get a presumptive identification?
3. The colonies were catalase-positive. There was difficulty interpreting the motility test. This clinical microbiology laboratory has a Class II biosafety cabinet, no autoclave, and no walls/door separating it from the rest of the laboratory. What should be done next?

ANSWERS

Key Terms and Abbreviations
1. F
2. A
3. C
4. B
5. E
6. D

True or False
1. T
2. T
3. T
4. T
5. T

Multiple Choice
1. B
2. D
3. B
4. A
5. A

Case Study

1. When the Gram reaction has been confirmed by making and staining another blood-broth smear, the ordering physician needs to be informed. There are several genera of gram-positive bacilli that are commonly seen in clinical specimens. But when these organisms are seen in a blood culture, *Bacillus anthracis* must be considered and ruled out. Extra precautions should be taken to protect workers. Once the positive blood culture is plated to at least sheep blood, chocolate, and MacConkey agars, the plates should be taped shut. Precautions should be taken not to generate aerosols and to work in a biological safety cabinet. *B. anthracis* in pure culture is highly infectious, more so than clinical specimens.

2. Working in a biosafety cabinet, a catalase test should be performed. If the organism is catalase-positive, motility should be checked. The wet mount motility test using trypticase soy broth works well. *B. anthracis* is nonmotile, as is *B. mycoides.* True motility should not be confused with erratic Brownian motion. Bacilli may move slower than the positive control organism.

3. The reference laboratory or state health department laboratory may be consulted. If *B. anthracis* cannot be ruled out, confirmatory testing should be made by a laboratory in the next level of the Laboratory Response Network.

REFERENCES

Cleary T, Miller N, Martinez OV: Evaluation of wet-prep motility test for presumptive identification of *Bacillus* species, *J Clin Microbiol* 40:730, 2002.

Dib EG, Dib SA, Korkmaz DA, et al: Nonhemolytic, nonmotile gram-positive rods indicative of *Bacillus anthracis*, *Emerg Infect Dis* 9:1013, 2003.

Ringertz SA, Hoiby EA, Jensenius M, et al: Anthrax in a heroin skin-popper, *Lancet* 356:1574, 2000.

19 Listeria, Corynebacterium, and Similar Organisms

OBJECTIVES

Upon completion of this chapter, the reader should be able to:

1. Explain the clinical significance of the isolation of *Listeria*.
2. List the tests that can be performed to do a rapid presumptive identification of *Listeria*.
3. Explain how to identify *Corynebacterium diphtheriae*.
4. Explain the clinical significance of *C. jeikeium*, *C. urealyticum*, and *C. pseudodiphtheriticum*.

SUMMARY OF KEY POINTS

Another group of aerobic, gram-positive, non–spore-forming bacilli include the genera *Listeria* and *Corynebacterium*. In the genus *Listeria*, the only human pathogen is *L. monocytogenes*. This organism has been found in freshwater, saltwater, sewage, soil, dust, meat products, dairy products, ice cream, fruits, and vegetables. Because it is so widespread, it frequently contaminates foods during processing. *L. monocytogenes* can cause acute self-limited febrile gastroenteritis in otherwise healthy adults. In nonpregnant adults who are immunocompromised, it causes meningitis, encephalitis, or septicemia. In pregnant women, it causes an influenza-like illness that, if untreated, may lead to amnionitis, fetal infection, abortion, stillbirth, or premature birth. Listeriosis can occur sporadically or epidemically; contaminated foods are the means of transmission.

L. monocytogenes is beta-hemolytic on sheep blood agar, shows "tumbling motility" in a wet prep and "umbrella" pattern in motility media, is catalase-positive, oxidase-positive, and esculin-positive. These organisms can escape the action of antibiotics by surviving and multiplying within phagocytes. The hemolysin, listeriolysin O, is the major virulence factor. The drug of choice is ampicillin but trimethoprim-sulfamethoxazole may also be used.

The genus *Corynebacterium* includes gram-positive rods that form "Chinese letter" arrangements; these cell formations have come to be described as *coryneform*. Clinical microbiologists also use the term *diphtheroids*. Most coryneform bacteria ferment glucose, are catalase-positive, and nonmotile. They are widely distributed in nature and can be found on skin and mucous membranes of humans.

Historically, diphtheria is the most important infectious disease caused by coryneform bacteria. Diphtheria is an acute, febrile, contagious illness spread by the respiratory route. In the nasopharynx, *C. diphtheriae* infection results in the production of a potent exotoxin that causes necrosis and inflammation (pseudomembrane).

This pseudomembrane formation in the oropharynx is characteristic and may lead to respiratory obstruction. In addition, the exotoxin may damage heart muscle and nerve tissue. Respiratory diphtheria is now rare in the United States with the last culture-confirmed case of diphtheria in 1996. The disease rate has dropped significantly due to immunization practices; sporadic cases can be prevented by booster vaccination.

Throat swabs and nasopharyngeal specimens should be collected for culture. Sheep blood agar, CNA agar, and either Tinsdale media or cystine-tellurite blood agar (CTBA) should be used. Nontoxigenic strains of *C. diphtheriae* may be carried in a person's throat or nasopharynx. Therefore tests for toxigenicity need to be done by one of several methods that include the use of live guinea pigs, immunodiffusion in the Elek test, and toxin gene detection by PCR. Drugs of choice are erythromycin and clindamycin but rifampin and penicillin have also been reported to be effective to eliminate the carrier state of the organism from the upper respiratory tract. The clinical management of diphtheria may also involve the use of diphtheria antitoxin.

One of the most commonly isolated species is *C. jeikeium*. It is lipophilic and most frequently isolated from blood and other sterile body fluids and wounds. Although not usually found on the skin of healthy people, it is common cutaneous flora in hospitalized patients and those treated with antibiotics. In Gram stains, they are pleomorphic and usually arranged in V forms or palisades. Growth can be enhanced on sheep blood agar by the addition of 1% Tween 80. *C. jeikeium* is multiply drug resistant but usually susceptible to the glycopeptides (e.g., vancomycin).

C. urealyticum is also multiply antibiotic resistant. It is frequently found on the skin of hospitalized patients. *C. urealyticum* is a well-documented cause of alkaline-encrusted cystitis and may play a role in renal stone formation.

KEY TERMS AND ABBREVIATIONS

Match the term in the left column with the definition on the right.

1. _____	lipophilic	A. hemolysin
2. _____	listeriolysin O	B. growth enhancer in agar
3. _____	alkaline-encrusted cystitis	C. cystine-tellurite medium
		D. having an affinity for lipids
4. _____	CTBA	E. chronic condition where crystals form on the bladder wall
5. _____	Tween 80	
6. _____	pseudomembrane	F. accumulation of bacteria, fibrin, and neutrophils

TRUE OR FALSE

1. _____ *C. diphtheriae* is only found in humans.
2. _____ Corynebacteria form spores.
3. _____ A virulence factor for *L. monocytogenes* is its hemolysin.
4. _____ The incidence of diphtheria in the United States has declined as a result of the use of antitoxin.
5. _____ *C. jeikeium* shows V forms on Gram stain.

MULTIPLE CHOICE

1. _____ *L. monocytogenes* can be presumptively identified by its
   A. Gram reaction.
   B. catalase reaction.
   C. motility.
   D. esculin reaction.

2. _____ Which statement about corynebacteria is false?
   A. The lipophilic species grow well on blood agar with Tween 80.
   B. *C. jeikeium* is associated with stone formation in the bladder.
   C. The corynebacteria are gram-positive.
   D. *C. diphtheriae* colonies appear black on Tinsdale agar.

3. _____ Which organism is a well-documented cause of alkaline-encrusted cystitis?
   A. *C. urealyticum.*
   B. *C. pseudodiphtheriticum.*
   C. *C. ulcerans.*
   D. *C. jeikeium.*

4. _____ A diabetic woman developed an ulcer on her toe. A culture grew tiny colonies of coryneform bacteria that were very resistant to antibiotics. Over several months additional cultures of the wound grew the same organism. The patient was not responding to treatment and eventually the toe had to be amputated. This organism was probably
   A. *C. urealyticum.*
   B. *C. pseudodiphtheriticum.*
   C. *C. ulcerans.*
   D. *C. jeikeium*

5. _____ One way to differentiate *Listeria* from *Bacillus* spp. is
   A. Gram reaction.
   C. catalase reaction.
   B. motility.
   D. spore formation.

CASE STUDY

A 73-year-old man was brought to the emergency department with complaints of fever, altered mental status, and possible urinary tract infection. He had a history of cardiac disease and chronic obstructive pulmonary disease (COPD). The man had recently been placed on methotrexate in an effort to control his COPD. Blood tests were done on admission. He had an elevated white count, creatine kinase, and troponin. A urine specimen was collected for urinalysis and culture and two blood cultures were drawn. The man developed respiratory failure and had to be intubated. The next day there was no growth on the urine culture but both blood cultures became positive; gram-positive bacilli were seen in the Gram stain. On day 3 of his admission, the blood cultures grew beta-hemolytic colonies that were catalase-positive.

1. What gram-positive bacilli are catalase positive?
2. What tests could be done quickly to get a presumptive identification of this organism?
3. The blood culture isolate was reported as *Listeria monocytogenes.* This was an unexpected finding. How could the patient have acquired this pathogen?

ANSWERS

Key Terms and Abbreviations

1. D
2. A
3. E
4. C
5. B
6. F

True or False

1. T
2. F
3. T
4. F
5. T

Multiple Choice

1. C
2. B
3. A
4. D
5. D

Case Study

1. *Bacillus* spp., *L. monocytogenes, Corynebacterium* spp.
2. Gram stain morphology can quickly differentiate coryneform bacteria from filamentous types *(Nocardia)* and regular rods *(Bacillus)* as well as spore formers from non–spore formers. If no spores are seen, motility could be done next to differentiate *Listeria* (motile) from *Corynebacterium* (nonmotile). Bile esculin agar should be inoculated since *Listeria* is bile esculin–positive.
3. *Listeria* is acquired by ingesting contaminated foods such as processed meat products, ice cream, and dairy products. The situation was compounded by this patient's underlying medical conditions and his immunosuppression with methotrexate used here as an antiinflammatory medication.

REFERENCES

Centers for Disease Control and Prevention: Preventing tetanus, diptheria, and pertussis among adolescents: use of tetanus toxoid, reduced diptheria toxoid and acellular pertussis vaccines. Recommendations of the Advisory Committee on Immunization Practices (ACIP), *Morb Mortal Wkly Rep* 55(RR03):1, 2006.

Centers for Disease Control and Prevention: Toxigenic *Corynebacterium diphtheriae*—Northern Plains Indian Community, August-October 1996, *Morb Mortal Wkly Rep* 46(22):506, 1997.

Funke G, von Graevenitz A, Clarridge JE, et al: Clinical microbiology of coryneform bacteria, *Clin Microbiol Rev* 10:125, 1997.

20 *Erysipelothrix, Lactobacillus,* and Similar Organisms

OBJECTIVES

Upon completion of this chapter, the reader should be able to:
1. Differentiate streptococci from *Arcanobacterium haemolyticum.*
2. Explain how to diagnose and identify *Gardnerella vaginalis.*
3. Differentiate between *Listeria, Erysipelothrix,* and *Lactobacillus.*
4. Explain the difference between erysipeloid and erysipelas.

SUMMARY OF KEY POINTS

The group of regular, non–spore-forming, gram-positive bacilli that have clinical significance are *Erysipelothrix rhusiopathiae, Arcanobacterium haemolyticum, Gardnerella vaginalis,* and *Lactobacillus* spp. These organisms are all catalase-negative. *Lactobacillus* spp. and *G. vaginalis* are part of the normal genital flora in women. *A. haemolyticum* and *E. rhusiopathiae,* however, are not components of the human commensal flora.

The genus *Erysipelothrix* was first described by Loeffler in 1886 as the cause of swine erysipelas. In 1909, the organism was isolated from cutaneous lesions in humans and the term *erysipeloid* was used to differentiate these lesions from those of human erysipelas caused by streptococci. *E. rhusiopathiae* is found worldwide and can be a commensal or pathogen in a variety of species from swine and sheep to crustaceans and fish. Most human cases are related to occupational exposure; persons at greatest risk of infection are butchers, fishermen, veterinarians, and abattoir workers. The usual route of infection is through cuts or scratches on the skin. During World War II there were outbreaks of disease in Norway in plants where fish was processed. The cause of these outbreaks was linked to the time delay experienced by fishing fleets that had to sail in convoy. The delay in processing allowed the microorganisms to multiply in the fish.

In patients with erysipeloid, skin biopsy is cultured. The organism grows on routine media. It is nonmotile, catalase- and oxidase-negative, produces either alpha-hemolysis or no hemolysis on sheep blood agar, and produces H_2S in TSI. Abbreviated identification schemes that do not include H_2S production could lead to misidentification as *Lactobacillus* spp. *E. rhusiopathiae* can also produce two colony types: small and moist or large with a serrated edge. Skin lesions tend to heal spontaneously but they can recur and persist for months. Healing is enhanced with antibiotic therapy. The drugs of choice are penicillin and cephalosporins.

Corynebacterium haemolyticum was first described in 1946 when it was isolated from U.S. servicemen and indigenous peoples in the South Pacific who were suffering from pharyngitis. Its classification was changed in 1982 to *Arcanobacterium. Arcanobacterium haemolyticum* has been isolated from young adults with pharyngitis, fever, and sometimes with pseudomembranes on the pharynx and tonsils that resemble diphtheria. About 25% of cases present with an erythematous rash on the trunk or extremities. A misdiagnosis as streptococcal infection can be made. *A. haemolyticum* is a facultative anaerobe that grows more slowly than streptococci and shows less defined beta-hemolysis. It can be easily masked by normal throat flora. *A. haemolyticum* is catalase-negative and tends to pit the agar beneath colonies on blood agar plates. In vitro susceptibility testing shows *A. haemolyticum* to be sensitive to erythromycin, penicillin, gentamicin, clindamycin, and the cephalosporins, although susceptibility testing is not needed to guide therapy.

INTEREST POINT

There was a report from the International Society for Infectious Diseases distributed through ProMED-mail describing an outbreak of *Arcanobacterium haemolyticum* in 142 school students in the city of Guri, South Korea, from May through June 2005. The children presented with summer cold symptoms as well as fever and rashes resembling scarlet fever. The Korea Center for Disease Control and Prevention also announced that the organism was resistant to antibiotics.

More information on this outbreak can be accessed at *http://www.promedmail.org/pls/promed/f?p=2400: 1202:10444497573846873155::NO::F2400_P1202_ CHECK_DISPLAY,F2400_P1202_PUB_MAIL_ID:X, 29526*

The genus *Lactobacillus* is defined by its production of lactic acid from glucose. These organisms are part of the normal flora of the oropharynx, gastrointestinal tract, and vagina. Lactobacilli are also found in foods such as dairy products because of their ability to ferment. Identification is not usually taken to the species level because they have little clinical significance. Lactobacilli grow on sheep blood agar and chocolate agar. They are catalase- and oxidase-negative and are facultative anaerobes. Lactobacilli can produce long, slender rods that may form long chains and be seen in urine sediment from female patients. Lactobacilli are part of the normal vaginal flora and may play a role in preventing bacterial vaginosis and candidiasis by producing hydrogen peroxide.

These organisms produce rare opportunistic infection in immunocompromised patients. *Lactobacillus* bacteremia has been described in the literature. Treatment of choice is currently a penicillin combined with an aminoglycoside.

Gardnerella vaginalis is a gram-variable bacillus that is associated with bacterial vaginosis, but has also been isolated from women with no signs of infection. Bacterial vaginosis produces a discharge with an offensive odor but few WBCs. A wet mount of vaginal secretions shows "clue cells" (squamous epithelial cells heavily covered with bacilli) and a noted absence of the normal numbers of lactobacilli. Another nonculture method for diagnosis of bacterial vaginosis is the use of 10% KOH that is added to vaginal discharge; a fishlike odor (whiff test) is characteristic of vaginosis. Routine culture of vaginal specimens for *G. vaginalis* is not recommended. However, *G. vaginalis* can be recovered from clinical specimens using the semiselective medium human blood bilayer-Tween agar (HBT). Presumptive identification of *G. vaginalis* can be made based on Gram stain morphology (small, gram-variable coccobacilli), catalase and oxidase reactions (both negative), and small zones of beta-hemolysis on HBT agar. Metronidazole is the drug of choice for treating bacterial vaginosis.

KEY TERMS AND ABBREVIATIONS

Match the term in the left column with the definition on the right.

1. _____ clue cells
2. _____ CNA
3. _____ HBT
4. _____ SPS
5. _____ erysipeloid

A. anticoagulant used in blood cultures
B. Columbia colistin-nalidixic acid
C. localized skin infection
D. human blood bilayer Tween agar
E. epithelial cells covered with bacteria

TRUE OR FALSE

1. _____ An HBT plate should be included in the battery of media for routine genital cultures.
2. _____ *Arcanobacterium haemolyticum* is part of the normal oral flora of humans and an opportunistic pathogen.
3. _____ *Gardnerella* is inhibited by the SPS added to blood culture bottles.
4. _____ *Lactobacillus* spp. are usually identified based on Gram stain morphology and catalase reaction.
5. _____ Clue cells are squamous epithelial cells that are covered with streptococci.

MULTIPLE CHOICE

1. _____ The only catalase-negative, non–spore-forming bacillus that produces H_2S is
A. *Gardnerella vaginalis.*
B. *Lactobacillus* spp.
C. *Erysipelothrix rhusiopathiae.*
D. *Arcanobacterium haemolyticum*

2. _____ *A. haemolyticum* can be missed in throat cultures if it is not specifically sought. Which statement about *A. haemolyticum* is true?
A. It is catalase-positive.
B. It pits the agar under colonies growing on sheep blood agar.
C. It is alpha-hemolytic.
D. It is resistant to erythromycin.

3. _____ Which statement about erysipeloid is false?
A. It is common in fish handlers.
B. The drug of choice is metronidazole.
C. Diagnosis is made by skin culture.
D. *E. rhusiopathiae* can produce two distinct colony types.

4. _____ When gram-positive aerotolerant rods are encountered in a clinical specimen, several genera need to be considered. Which statement is true?
A. *Actinomyces israelii* and *Gardnerella vaginalis* can be differentiated by their catalase reactions.
B. *Actinomyces* spp. produce spores while *E. rhusiopathiae* does not.
C. *Propionibacterium acnes* can be differentiated from *E. rhusiopathiae* by its catalase reactions.
D. H_2S production is a distinguishing characteristic of *G. vaginalis.*

5. _____ Bacterial vaginosis
A. is associated with a predominance of *G. vaginalis.*
B. can be diagnosed by serology testing.
C. is associated with a predominance of lactobacilli.
D. is identified by growth of *Gardnerella* on MacConkey agar.

CASE STUDY

A 37-year-old woman complained of a burning sensation upon urination. The physician ordered a urinalysis and culture on a clean-catch specimen. The urinalysis was unremarkable; the dipstick reactions were negative. After overnight incubation of the culture, there were two pink colonies on the MacConkey plate and 50 small alpha-hemolytic colonies on the sheep blood agar. The Gram stain of these alpha-hemolytic colonies showed long, thin, gram-variable bacilli.

1. What testing should be done at this point?
2. The alpha-hemolytic colonies were catalase- and oxidase-negative. What additional steps, if any, does the technologist need to take to identify the growth?
3. What should be done with the two pink colonies?

ANSWERS

Key Terms and Abbreviations

1. E
2. B
3. D
4. A
5. C

True or False

1. F
2. F
3. T
4. T
5. F

Multiple Choice

1. C
2. B
3. B
4. C
5. A

Case Study

1. A catalase test should be done and presence or absence of spores noted.
2. Presumptive identification of *Lactobacillus* spp. can be made based on the Gram stain morphology and reaction and the negative catalase and oxidase tests. No further workup is required; these organisms are not differentiated to the species level nor is susceptibility testing routinely done.
3. The pink colonies represent a lactose fermenter that could be any number of gram-negative organisms including *E. coli, Klebsiella,* or *Citrobacter.* The lactobacilli have low pathogenicity and would be considered vaginal contamination. With so much vaginal contamination, it would seem that the two colonies of gram-negative growth are also contamination. The report can read "50,000 CFU/mL Mixed Growth. Probable contamination."

REFERENCES

Cummings LA, Wu W, Larson AM, et al: Effects of media, atmosphere, and incubation time on colonial morphology of *Arcanobacterium haemolyticum, J Clin Microbiol* 31:3223, 1993.

Dunbar SA, Clarridge JE: Potential errors in recognition of *Erysipelothrix rhusiopathiae, J Clin Microbiol* 38:1302, 2000.

Linder R: *Rhodococcus equi* and *Arcanobacterium haemolyticum:* two "coryneform" bacteria increasingly recognized as agents of human infection, *Emerg Infect Dis* 3:145, 1997.

ProMED-mail on *Arcanobacterium haemolyticum* outbreak in South Korea in 2005. Available at: *http://www.promedmail.org/pls/promed/f?p=2400:1202:104444975738 46873155::NO::F2400_P1202_CHECK_DISPLAY, F2400_P1202_PUB_MAIL_ID:X,29526*

Reboli AC, Farrar WE: *Erysipelothrix rhusiopathiae:* an occupational pathogen, *Clin Microbiol Rev* 2:354, 1989.

21 *Nocardia, Streptomyces, Rhodococcus,* and Similar Organisms

OBJECTIVES

Upon completion of this chapter, the reader should be able to:
1. Describe/define nocardiosis and mycetoma.
2. Explain how to isolate and identify *Nocardia* species.
3. Explain the clinical significance of *Rhodococcus equi.*

SUMMARY OF KEY POINTS

The aerobic actinomycetes are gram-positive bacteria that are more filamentous and branched than the other gram-positive bacilli. They produce a fungus-like mycelium that fragments or breaks up into rod or coccoid forms. These are true bacteria in the order Actinomycetales. These bacteria are divided into two broad groups: those with mycolic acid in the cell wall and those with no mycolic acid. The mycolic acid confers partial acid-fastness that is seen when a modified acid-fast stain is performed. These aerobic actinomycetes are widespread in nature; they are found in soil and decomposing plant matter. They are considered to be opportunistic pathogens and are not frequently isolated in the clinical laboratory. They are slow growers; colonies grow after incubation for 3 days to 2 weeks. Most routine bacterial cultures are only held for 48 hours, so these organisms are usually recovered in routine fungal cultures.

The aerobic actinomycetes are commonly termed *nocardioform* because of their branching form. *Nocardia* species are the most important pathogens and are the reference group.

Nocardiosis is an infectious disease most commonly caused by *N. asteroides.* These organisms are capable of growing within macrophages and show a tropism for neuronal tissue. There are approximately 1000 new cases per year in the United States. Infection occurs by inhaling the bacteria or by traumatic direct skin inoculation. *N. brasiliensis* has been associated with cutaneous infections primarily in tropical countries. Local infection, known as a mycetoma, presents as either a chronically draining ulcerative lesion or as pustules and abscesses. The foot is a frequent site of infection that is acquired by walking barefoot. Mycetomas are characterized by draining sinus tracts. If the mycetoma is caused by an actinomycete rather than a fungus, the infection is called an actinomycetoma. Pulmonary nocardiosis presents with fever and productive cough that progresses to pneumonia with complications such as pleural effusions and empyema. Disseminated nocardiosis usually originates from a pulmonary infection. It is potentially life-threatening and may result in brain and skin lesions. The mortality rate is high, particularly in immunocompromised patients. Serious infections occur in individuals who are immunosuppressed, such as renal transplant patients, HIV-infected individuals or those with neoplastic disease.

The aerobic actinomycetes grow on routine media such as sheep blood agar, chocolate agar, Sabouraud dextrose agar at 25° to 45° C, but may take a minimum incubation time of 48 to 72 hours. Colonies of *Nocardia* are dry and chalky with color ranging from yellow to gray-white. Gram stain shows delicate, branching filaments. *Nocardia* tends to stain gram-variable with a beaded pattern. To prevent overgrowth with normal flora, selective media such as Martin Lewis and colistin nalidixic acid agar (CNA) can be used.

Drugs of choice for nocardiosis are the sulfonamides but trimethoprim-sulfamethoxazole may be used.

Actinomadura spp. are soil organisms that most commonly cause infections in the lower legs. These infections are more prevalent in tropical countries.

The *Streptomyces* are environmental organisms found in soil that have significance in the industrial and pharmaceutical fields. The antibiotic streptomycin comes from *Streptomyces* spp. The most common form of infection with these organisms is a mycetoma; there are rare reports of invasive disease.

Rhodococcus equi was first isolated in 1923 from lung infections in young horses. The first human infection was not reported until 1967. *R. equi* is found in soil where livestock graze; human infections result from environmental exposure. In a review of 125 cases reported between 1967 and 1996, 74% of the cases were reported between 1987 and 1996. The majority of those infections were seen in HIV patients. Pulmonary infections may mimic tuberculosis. *R. equi* is a strict aerobe that grows on blood agar and develops salmon pink colonies after

2 to 3 days of incubation. Isolates are frequently resistant to penicillin but are susceptible to erythromycin, vancomycin, and rifampin.

KEY TERMS AND ABBREVIATIONS

Match the term in the left column with the definition on the right.

1. _____ mycolic acid
2. _____ mycetoma
3. _____ actinomycetoma
4. _____ hypersensitivity pneumonitis
5. _____ GMS stain

A. infection with draining sinus tracts
B. silver stain used in histology
C. chronic skin lesion caused by actinomycetes
D. allergic reaction to actinomycetes
E. makes cell walls acid-fast

TRUE OR FALSE

1. _____ The ability to grow at 50° C is a characteristic of all thermophilic actinomycetes.
2. _____ The organisms that may be seen on Gram stain as gram-variable, beaded, branching filaments are *Nocardia* spp.
3. _____ The actinomycetes may appear acid-fast when stained with the Ziehl-Neelsen stain because of the lipid content of their cell walls.
4. _____ The virulence of the actinomycetes is due to their ability to live inside macrophages and resist intracellular killing.
5. _____ Pus with granules from draining skin lesion may contain microcolonies of *Nocardia* spp.

CASE STUDY

While scanning the Gram stain from a routine sputum culture, the technologist noted a few long gram-positive filaments. She inquired into the patient's diagnosis and found that the patient was currently in hospital for pneumonia and that he had been on long-term corticosteroid therapy.

1. Because the Gram stain is suspicious for actinomycetes, what is the next step in the processing of this sputum specimen?
2. What selective media commonly found in hospital laboratories can be used to enhance the isolation of actinomycetes by preventing the overgrowth of normal flora?
3. Why is communication between the laboratory and clinician so important in a situation like this?

ANSWERS

Key Terms and Abbreviations

1. E
2. A
3. C
4. D
5. B

True or False

1. T
2. T
3. F
4. T
5. T

Case Study

1. Because the Gram stain is suggestive of possible actinomycetes, rapidly growing mycobacteria need to be ruled out. If the bacteria are not acid-fast, a modified acid-fast stain can be performed using a reduced strength acid decolorizer. If this modified stain is negative, actinomycetes cannot be ruled out because there is such variability in their acid-fastness. Appropriate media and incubation times should be considered to recover these slow-growing organisms.
2. The actinomycetes will grow on a variety of media including sheep blood agar, chocolate agar, and Sabouraud dextrose agar. But because they grow more slowly than normal flora in respiratory specimens, they may be overgrown and masked by the normal flora. Selective media with antimicrobials added will allow recovery of nocardiae. Gram-positive selective media such as CNA agar can be used, as can Thayer Martin or Martin Lewis agar.
3. Communication between the clinician and the laboratory is important because the presence of an actinomycete in culture may represent true infection or contamination. The clinical picture is important in interpreting the culture results. An astute technologist may discover something during testing that the physician had not considered in the differential diagnosis. Given this patient's clinical history and the fact that this small hospital laboratory does not perform fungal or mycobacterial testing, the specimen was sent to a reference laboratory for further workup.

REFERENCES

Carey J, Motyl M, Perlman DC: Catheter-related bacteremia due to *Streptomyces* in a patient receiving holistic infusions, *Emerg Infect Dis* 7:1043, 2001.
Linder R: *Rhodococcus equi* and *Arcanobacterium haemolyticum*: two "coryneform" bacteria increasingly recognized as agents of human infection, *Emerg Infect Dis* 3:145, 1997.

22 | *Enterobacteriaceae*

OBJECTIVES

Upon completion of this chapter, the reader should be able to:

1. List the distinguishing characteristics of the *Enterobacteriaceae*.
2. List the plating media for stool cultures.
3. List the key identifying biochemical reactions for *Escherichia coli* and the abbreviated identification scheme.
4. Describe the different enteric infections caused by *E. coli*.
5. Explain how to differentiate *K. oxytoca* from *K. pneumoniae*.
6. Explain how to differentiate *P. mirabilis* from *P. vulgaris*.
7. Explain how to isolate and differentiate *Salmonella* and *Shigella* in clinical specimens.
8. Describe the clinical presentations of *Salmonella* infection.
9. Explain how to differentiate *Citrobacter* from *E. coli*.
10. List the pathogenic species of *Yersinia* and the clinical syndromes they cause.

SUMMARY OF KEY POINTS

There are hundreds of species of *Enterobacteriaceae* that are widely distributed in nature, on plants, in soil, and in the intestines of humans and animals. Some species have limited ecologic niches (e.g., *Salmonella typhi* causes typhoid fever and is found only in humans). This is such a large, heterogeneous group of bacteria that a taxonomy scheme using tribes was proposed by Ewing in 1963. Because of their colonization in the human intestine, they are often referred to as *enteric bacteria*. Besides being opportunistic pathogens and causing a wide range of human infection, they are also the chief cause of nosocomial infections.

The *Enterobacteriaceae* have the general characteristics of all being gram-negative bacilli that do not form spores, that are oxidase-negative, and that are biochemically active with the ability to ferment sugars. Virulence factors include the production of toxins; endotoxin from gram-negative bacteria is capable of inducing septic shock. They also produce adhesins, capsules, and hemolysins.

Although the *Enterobacteriaceae* are considered normal intestinal flora, primary intestinal pathogens include *Salmonella, Shigella,* and *Yersinia enterocolitica.* These infections result from ingesting contaminated food and water. Stool specimens for culture should be obtained early in the course of illness when the largest numbers of organisms are likely to be recovered. Fresh stool is better than a rectal swab. Stool specimens for culture should not be refrigerated or contaminated with urine. It is best to plate specimens within 2 hours of collection, but Cary-Blair is a good transport media. Most *Enterobacteriaceae* will grow on routine media such as sheep blood, chocolate, and MacConkey agars. More selective differential media should also be included; Hektoen enteric agar (HE), xylose-lysine-deoxycholate (XLD) agar, or *Salmonella-Shigella* (SS) agar should also be inoculated. Cefsulodin-irgasan-novobiocin (CIN) agar is selective for *Yersinia enterocolitica,* and MacConkey-sorbitol agar is used to differentiate sorbitol-negative *E. coli* O157:H7 from other *E. coli.* Enrichment broths, such as GN or selenite, may also be used but are not required.

E. coli is the best studied and most significant species in its genus. This organism can be motile or nonmotile, can ferment lactose or not, but usually produces a dry, pink colony on MacConkey agar. Typical test reactions are indole-positive, methyl red–positive, Voges-Proskauer (VP)-negative, and citrate-negative (designated as IMViC reactions). *E. coli* is also urease negative. *E. coli* is a normal inhabitant of the large intestine, but can cause bacteremia, meningitis, urinary tract infections, diarrhea, and other infections including pneumonia. It possesses the O (somatic), H (flagellar), and K (capsular) antigens.

E. coli was first reported as a cause of infantile diarrhea in the 1920s. Enteric infections can be due to at least five different varieties that operate by different mechanisms: enteropathogenic (EPEC), enterotoxigenic (ETEC), entero-invasive (EIEC), enterohemorrhagic (EHEC) serotype O157:H7, and enteroaggregative (EAEC). ETEC is an important cause of traveler's diarrhea, which is characterized by abdominal cramps and frequent explosive bowel movements. Transmission is by the fecal-oral route; contamination is most likely through unbottled water and raw vegetables such as salads. EIEC are capable of cellular invasion and so are different from other *E. coli* that are limited to the mucosal surfaces. These strains produce dysentery with fever and bloody diarrhea and leukocytes in the stool. Enterohemorrhagic *E. coli* is sometimes referred to as Shiga toxin–producing *E. coli* (STEC). *E. coli* serotypes O157:H7 and O157:nonmotile (NM) produce one or more Shiga toxins and cause a broad spectrum of symptoms from mild nonbloody diarrhea to severe bloody diarrhea (hemorrhagic colitis) and hemolytic uremic syndrome (HUS). About 6% of the patients with O157 diarrhea develop HUS; symptoms include acute renal failure, thrombocytopenia, and hemolytic anemia. This is potentially fatal, especially in young children. Undercooked meats (e.g., hamburgers), unpasteurized milk, and apple cider have been implicated in O157 outbreaks. There are non-O157:H7 STEC that cause enteric infections. Shiga toxin testing by enzyme immunoassay methods can be done in lieu of culture for O157 strains.

E. coli is also the most common cause of gram-negative bacteremia as well as urinary tract and kidney infections. These bacteria must be able to adhere to the epithelial cells lining the urinary tract. It is also a common cause of septicemia and meningitis in neonates; the babies acquire the bacteria in the birth canal or from contaminated amniotic fluid.

There is an approved abbreviated identification scheme for *E. coli* and other select organisms (NCCLS document M35-A). If gram-negative lactose-fermenting bacilli produce colonies that are beta-hemolytic on blood agar and are spot indole–positive and oxidase-negative, they may be reported as *E. coli*. This is not a presumptive identification.

Klebsiella species are widespread throughout the environment and are found in the gastrointestinal tract of humans, in the nasopharynx, and on the skin as transient flora.

They are encapsulated; this polysaccharide capsule gives this genus its moist, mucoid appearance on agar and allows it to evade phagocytosis. It is nonmotile and a major nosocomial pathogen. *K. oxytoca* is similar to *K. pneumoniae* except for indole production (*K. pneumoniae* is indole-negative). Both species are Voges-Proskauer–positive and ONPG (*o*- Nitrophenol-β-D-Galactopyranoside)-positive.

The two most common *Enterobacter* isolates are *E. cloacae* and *E. aerogenes*. The lysine, arginine, and ornithine decarboxylase reactions are used to differentiate the species. *E. sakazakii* and some species of *E. agglomerans* complex (reclassified and placed in the genus *Pantoea*) produce a yellow pigment that may range from bright yellow to pale yellow. *E. sakazakii* infections occur in neonates; this organism has been isolated from powdered milk and infant formula. *Enterobacter* spp. have been implicated in nosocomial infection or colonization that is often associated with contaminated medical devices and instrumentation.

Serratia marcescens is an opportunistic pathogen implicated in nosocomial urinary tract, wound, and bloodstream infections. It has also been isolated from antiseptic solutions used for joint injections and solutions for contact lens cleaning and storage. Some strains produce a red pigment.

The genus *Proteus* got its name from a Greek polymorphic sea god. These organisms are ubiquitous in the environment and found in the intestines of healthy humans and animals. They are associated with urinary tract infections. Their presence promotes stone formation. It is thought that the process involves the alkalinization of urine due to urea hydrolysis with the production of ammonium hydroxide. These deposits act as foreign bodies that obstruct urinary flow. *Proteus* and *Providencia* urinary tract infections tend to become chronic and to destroy the renal parenchyma. Both *P. mirabilis* and *P. vulgaris* will swarm on nonselective media, such as blood agar. Both are human pathogens that produce clear, lactose-negative colonies on MacConkey agar. *P. vulgaris* is differentiated from *P. mirabilis* by the indole and ornithine reactions. The swarming characteristic along with nonlactose fermentation and positive indole reaction can be used to rapidly identify *P. vulgaris*.

Citrobacter species are widespread throughout the environment. These organisms look like *E. coli* on MacConkey agar but are citrate-positive. *Citrobacter* meningitis is almost exclusively associated with *C. koseri* and involves babies younger than 2 months old with the highest incidence in neonates. A large percentage of these infants develop brain abscesses; those that survive frequently have neurologic defects. Person-to-person spread from hospital personnel or from mother to infant is the most likely source.

Salmonella species are motile gram-negative bacilli that are ubiquitous in animal populations. Human illness is usually linked to foods of animal origin. An estimated 0.01% of all shell eggs contain *S. enteritidis*. Consequently, foods containing raw or undercooked eggs (e.g., mayonnaise, ice cream, Caesar dressing, eggnog) and contaminated poultry pose a risk of infection. The organism is transmitted by direct contact with animals, by water, and occasionally by human contact. Salmonellosis has also been associated with contact with reptiles (e.g., lizards, snakes, turtles). Yearly estimates in the United States are 1.4 million cases of illness with about 600 deaths caused by nontyphoidal salmonellosis that produces diarrhea, fever, and abdominal cramps. Serious sequelae that include sepsis and meningitis occur among infants, the elderly, and immunocompromised persons. Typhoid fever is a bloodstream infection common in the developing world but not in the United States. Cases in the United States are related to foreign travel. Typhoid fever symptoms are a sustained high temperature and headache without diarrhea. Humans are the only reservoir. Transmission is by person-to-person contact or fecal contamination of food and water. Food handlers are an important source of infection. Virulence factors include the presence of fimbriae (for adherence), the ability to cross the intestinal mucosa, and enterotoxin production. Antigenic structures include the Vi, O and H antigens.

There are four clinical pictures associated with *Salmonella*. Gastroenteritis is the most frequent clinical manifestation characterized by mild to fulminant diarrhea, low-grade fever, nausea, and vomiting. It is often referred to as "food poisoning." Bacteremia without gastrointestinal symptoms presents with high, spiking temperature and positive blood cultures. Enteric fever is the classic typhoid fever caused by *S. typhi*. *S. typhi* invades the small bowel and causes inflammation but no diarrhea. Monocytes phagocytize the bacteria but they are not killed. *S. typhi* survives inside the white blood cells and travels through the bloodstream to the gallbladder. The gallbladder is the site of chronic carriage. In mild illness, treatment is supportive; administration of antibiotics is thought to prolong the carrier state. In severe illness and sepsis, the fluoroquinolones are the drugs of choice. For enteric fever, ceftriaxone may also be used.

Shigella has been recognized since the late nineteenth century as the cause of bacillary dysentery. Classic dysentery is characterized by scant stools containing blood, mucus, and pus. Humans and other large primates are the only natural reservoirs for *Shigella*. Disease is transmitted by the fecal-oral route. It is the most communicable of the bacterial diarrheas with as few as 200 viable organisms needed to produce disease. Sexual transmission of *Shigella* among homosexual men has also been noted.

Salmonella and *Shigella* will grow on selective media. On MacConkey agar, they are colorless or transparent colonies. On HE agar, *Salmonella* is blue-green with a black center whereas *Shigella* is green. On XLD, *Salmonella* is red with a black center and *Shigella* is colorless; *Salmonella* produces H$_2$S, which produces the black centers on these selective media.

In the genus *Yersinia,* there are three human pathogens: *Y. pestis, Y. pseudotuberculosis, Y. enterocolitica.* These are zoonotic infections that affect rodents, pigs, and birds, with humans as accidental hosts. Cells are small gram-negative coccobacillary forms. *Yersinia enterocolitica* is widely distributed in lakes and streams; pigs are the natural animal reservoir. Human pathogenic strains have been isolated from tonsils and fecal samples from slaughtered pigs. *Y. enterocolitica* causes acute enterocolitis in humans with secondary symptoms of polyarthritis, septicemia, erythema nodosum, and endocarditis. *Y. enterocolitica* can best be recovered from stool specimens if the plates are incubated at room temperature. Cefsulodin-irgasan-novobiocin (CIN) agar is a special selective media that has had very good recovery rates.

Yersinia pestis causes plague, a disease of antiquity that persists today. The first pandemic was the Justinian plague (AD 541-544) that began in Egypt after arriving from Ethiopia. It quickly spread through the Middle East and Mediterranean basin. Death rates are uncertain due to lack of records, but the second pandemic that included the epidemic known as the "Black Plague" (AD 1347-1351) killed an estimated 17 to 28 million Europeans. During the Hong Kong epidemic in 1894, two independent researchers, Yersin and Kitasato, identified the cause of the plague. Yersin made the connection between rats and the plague, and in 1897 the role of the flea in transmission was discovered.

Because *Y. pestis* has special nutritional requirements, it is an obligate intracellular parasite. Specimen processing can be handled in biosafety level 2 (BSL 2) conditions, but if aerosols may be produced, BSL 3 precautions must be followed. Plague occurs worldwide with most cases reported in developing countries in Asia and Africa. Between 1981 and 1995, 25 countries reported more than 21,000 cases to the World Health Organization with a fatality rate of about 10%.

In the United States, plague cases are reported in the Southwest states mostly from May to October when people are outdoors and have contact with rodents and their fleas. Humans are accidental hosts; important reservoirs in the United States are squirrels, chipmunks, and prairie dogs. There are three clinical forms of the plague: bubonic, pneumonic, and septicemic. Diagnosis is made by Gram stain and culture of a bubo aspirate. The aspirate, blood, and other fluids should be inoculated onto blood and MacConkey agar and into an enrichment broth. Presumptive diagnosis can be made if bipolar staining is seen in ovoid gram-negative rods in the fluid from buboes, blood, sputum, or cerebrospinal fluid. The local health department should be contacted immediately. The drug of choice is still streptomycin, which has been used since 1948.

Yersinia pseudotuberculosis causes the rarest of the yersinioses. This is a zoonotic infection mostly seen in children. It causes mesenteric adenitis, which is an appendicitis-like syndrome.

KEY TERMS AND ABBREVIATIONS

Match the term in the left column with the definition on the right.

1. _____ HE agar
2. _____ XLD agar
3. _____ CIN agar
4. _____ enterohemor-rhagic *E. coli*
5. _____ enterotoxigenic *E. coli*
6. _____ enteroinvasive *E. coli*
7. _____ dysentery
8. _____ zoonosis
9. _____ bubo
10. _____ HUS

A. enlarged lymph node
B. produces blood and WBCs in stool
C. *Salmonella* produces black bull's eye colony
D. travelers' diarrhea
E. diarrhea with blood and mucus
F. selective media for *Yersinia*
G. disease transmitted by animals
H. selective agar where nonfermenters are green
I. acute renal failure
J. produces Shiga toxin

TRUE OR FALSE

1. _____ Typhoid fever does not produce diarrhea.
2. _____ *Salmonella* causes classic dysentery.
3. _____ All *Enterobacteriaceae* are oxidase-positive.
4. _____ *Salmonella enteritidis* causes "food poisoning."
5. _____ *Proteus* is motile and will swarm on MacConkey agar.

MULTIPLE CHOICE

1. _____ Carriers of *Salmonella* harbor the organism in their
   A. colon.
   B. gallbladder.
   C. small intestine.
   D. pancreas.

2. _____ A clear red colony with a black center on XLD agar is most likely
   A. *E. coli.*
   B. *Shigella.*
   C. *Salmonella.*
   D. *Yersinia.*

3. _____ The test that can differentiate *P. mirabilis* from *P. vulgaris* is
   A. PYR.
   B. indole.
   C. oxidase.
   D. ornithine.

4. _____ The optimal temperature for growth of *Yersinia* is
   A. 25° C.
   B. 42° C.
   C. 35° C.
   D. 8° C.

5. _____ *K. oxytoca* can be differentiated from *K. pneumoniae* by which test?
   A. PYR.
   B. Indole.
   C. Oxidase.
   D. Ornithine.

CASE STUDY

A 2-year-old girl had just returned home from India after a 2-week visit with family. On the flight home, the child developed a fever that persisted for 2 days. The family pediatrician was consulted. He ordered a CBC, blood cultures, and urine for urinalysis and culture. The child's WBC count was high but the urine results were unremarkable. She was given acetaminophen and the parent was instructed to keep the child hydrated. The next day, both blood cultures were positive with a gram-negative rod. Per protocol, the physician was notified by telephone. After overnight incubation, the blood cultures grew a non–lactose-fermenting organism that was oxidase- and indole-negative.

1. What test(s) should the technologist do next?
2. The automated system identified the organism as *Salmonella* spp. The child did not have diarrhea. Is it possible to have *Salmonella* bacteremia?
3. The isolate was susceptible to ampicillin, ceftazidime, ceftriaxone, levofloxacin, and trimethoprim-sulfamethoxazole and resistant to tobramycin. Should the pediatrician use one of these drugs to treat the child?
4. Before this culture workup can be considered complete, what additional documentation needs to be done?

ANSWERS

Key Terms and Abbreviations

1. H
2. C
3. F
4. J
5. D
6. B
7. E
8. G
9. A
10. I

True or False

1. T
2. F
3. F
4. T
5. F

Multiple Choice

1. B
2. C
3. B
4. A
5. B

Case Study

1. The indole and oxidase tests do not match the profile for *E. coli* and the approved abbreviated identification algorithm. An automated system was used to perform identification and susceptibility testing.
2. *Salmonella* can present with four clinical pictures:
   ■ Gastroenteritis
   ■ Bacteremia
   ■ Enteric fever
   ■ Carrier state

Gastroenteritis is the most frequent clinical manifestation characterized by diarrhea, low-grade fever, nausea, and vomiting. This is often referred to as "food poisoning." Bacteremia without gastrointestinal symptoms presents with high temperatures, positive blood cultures, and negative stool cultures. Enteric fever presents as mild fever without diarrhea. This is the classic typhoid fever. In the last presentation, people with previous infection may become chronic carriers and shed the organism in their feces for up to 1 year. The gallbladder is the site of carriage.

3. If the illness is mild, antimicrobial therapy is not indicated. Antibiotics are thought to prolong the carrier state. If the illness is severe or the patient is septic, ciprofloxacin or norfloxacin are the drugs of choice but azithromycin, trimethoprim-sulfamethoxazole, and ceftriaxone may also be used.
4. Salmonellosis is a reportable disease. The health department should be notified.

REFERENCES

Amersfoort ES, VanBerkel T, Kuiper J: Receptors, mediators, and mechanisms involved in bacterial sepsis and septic shock, *Clin Microbiol Rev* 16:379, 2003.

Bottone EJ: *Yersinia enterocolitica*: the charisma continues, *Clin Microbiol Rev* 10:257, 1997.

Centers for Disease Control and Prevention: Preliminary FoodNet data on the incidence of infection with pathogens transmitted commonly through food—10 States, United States, 2005, *Morb Mortal Wkly* 55:392, 2006.

Kehl SC: Role of the laboratory in the diagnosis of enterohemorrhagic *Escherichia coli* infections, *J Clin Microbiol* 40:2711, 2002.

Kennedy M, et al: Hospitalizations and deaths due to *Salmonella* infections, FoodNet, 1996-1999, *Clin Infect Dis* 38(Suppl 3):S142, 2004.

National Committee for Clinical Laboratory Standards: Abbreviated identification of bacteria and yeast; Approved guideline M35-A, Wayne, Pa, 2002, National Committee for Clinical Laboratory Standards.

Park CH, Kim HJ, Hixon DL: Importance of testing stool specimens for shiga toxins, *J Clin Microbiol* 40:3542, 2002.

Perry RD, Fetherston JD: *Yersinia pestis*—etiologic agent of plague, *Clin Microbiol Rev* 10:35, 1997.

23 Acinetobacter, Stenotrophomonas, and Similar Organisms

OBJECTIVES

Upon completion of this chapter, the reader should be able to:
1. Explain the difference between fermentation and oxidation.
2. Explain the clinical significance of isolation of *Acinetobacter* spp. and *Stenotrophomonas maltophilia*.
3. Describe certain key features that differentiate these organisms from the *Enterobacteriaceae*.
4. Describe the susceptibility patterns for each organism.

SUMMARY OF KEY POINTS

Acinetobacter and *Stenotrophomonas* species are oxidase-negative nonfermenters. Unlike the *Enterobacteriaceae* that ferment glucose, these organisms either utilize glucose and are termed *saccharolytic* or do not utilize glucose and are termed *asaccharolytic*. Fermentation is an anaerobic process, whereas oxidation (respiration) is a more energy-efficient process that uses oxygen as the final electron acceptor. Nonfermentative gram-negative bacilli and coccobacilli are ubiquitous in nature and hospital environments. They are not usually considered normal human flora, although hospitalized patients may become colonized with these organisms in their respiratory tracts and on skin. Cultures yielding these organisms should be interpreted carefully for clinical significance.

Stenotrophomonas maltophilia has undergone several taxonomic classification changes from *Pseudomonas* to *Xanthomonas* to *Stenotrophomonas*. *Stenotrophomonas* comes from the Greek words *stenos*, *trophos*, and *monas*, which means "one feeding on few substrates" to describe its comparative metabolic inactivity. It has been found in a wide variety of environments and has been isolated from water sources, sewage, plants, soil, and loofah sponges. *S. maltophilia* is an opportunistic pathogen and is emerging as an important nosocomial pathogen; it is also being recovered more frequently from cystic fibrosis patients. It is most often recovered from respiratory specimens, especially if the patient is on mechanical ventilation, has a tracheostomy, and had previous treatment with broad-spectrum antibiotics. This organism will grow on MacConkey agar and other standard media. *S. maltophilia* is inherently resistant to many broad-spectrum antibiotic classes including the aminoglycosides and beta-lactam agents. It remains susceptible to trimethoprim-sulfamethoxazole. Susceptibility testing with automated methods may be unreliable.

Acinetobacter species are strict aerobes that have a coccobacillary form that can cause them to be confused with *Neisseria* on Gram stain. They also tend to resist decolorization, which adds to this identification confusion.

These organisms are almost all resistant to penicillin and the beta-lactams. Combination drug therapy is recommended. There is concern about increasing isolation of these organisms in that they are able to acquire and express resistance to a variety of antimicrobial agents, including imipenem.

KEY TERMS AND ABBREVIATIONS

Match the term in the left column with the definition on the right.

1. _____ fermentation
2. _____ oxidative metabolism
3. _____ saccharolytic
4. _____ asaccharolytic

A. utilizes glucose
B. does not utilize glucose
C. anaerobic metabolism
D. respiration with O_2 as final electron receptor

TRUE OR FALSE

1. _____ Because *Acinetobacter* spp. tend to resist decolorization, they can be mistaken for *Neisseria* spp.
2. _____ *S. maltophilia* can be differentiated from *Burkholderia cepacia* by the fact that *S. maltophilia* is oxidase-positive.
3. _____ The drug of choice for *S. maltophilia* is penicillin.
4. _____ *Acinetobacter* spp. are clear, non–lactose-fermenting colonies on MacConkey agar.
5. _____ There is concern about *Acinetobacter* spp. acquiring resistance to imipenem.

CASE STUDY

A 73-year-old man with an endotracheal tube has been in the intensive care unit on mechanical ventilation for 7 days. Sputum was suctioned and sent for culture. The culture produced growth in one quadrant; the colonies on the MacConkey plate were clear and those on the blood agar plate were a grayish-green and non–beta-hemolytic. An oxidase test was done; it was negative. The laboratory has a Vitek II that it uses for identification and susceptibility testing. Identification and susceptibility cards were set up on this organism. The next day, the Vitek identification was *Stenotrophomonas maltophilia* with only a few drugs listed from the susceptibility panel.
1. Why was testing for so many antimicrobials suppressed?
2. Care should be exercised in interpreting this result given this patient's clinical history. Why?
3. What is the drug of choice?

ANSWERS

Key Terms and Abbreviations

1. C
2. D
3. A
4. B

True or False

1. T
2. F
3. F
4. T
5. T

Case Study

1. *S. maltophilia* is resistant to many of the broad-spectrum antibiotics. It is resistant to the penicillins, aminoglycosides, and cephalosporins.
2. Hospitalized patients can become colonized with *Stenotrophomonas*. The clinician needs to determine whether this is colonization or infection, particularly in a respiratory site with mechanical manipulation.
3. Trimethoprim-sulfamethoxazole

REFERENCE

Denton M, Kerr KG: Microbiological and clinical aspects of infection associated with *Stenotrophomonas maltophilia, Clin Microbiol Rev* 11:57, 1998.

24 *Pseudomonas, Burkholderia, and Similar Organisms*

OBJECTIVES

Upon completion of this chapter, the reader should be able to:
1. Describe the clinical impact of *P. aeruginosa* infection.
2. Describe colonial and biochemical features of *P. aeruginosa*.
3. Describe the clinical importance to isolation of *B. cepacia* from respiratory specimens.
4. Describe melioidosis and its etiologic agent.

SUMMARY OF KEY POINTS

Pseudomonas and *Burkholderia* species are aerobic, straight, gram-negative bacilli that are oxidase-positive and motile (except for *B. mallei*). Many of these organisms have a worldwide distribution in nature.

Pseudomonas spp. are found in moist environments, in soil, and on plants. *Pseudomonas* spp. have become problematic in the hospital environment and have been found in disinfectants, ointments, soaps, irrigation fluids, eye drops, respiratory therapy equipment, dialysis fluids, hydrotherapy baths, contact lens solutions, cosmetics, and hot tubs. *Pseudomonas aeruginosa* is the organism most frequently recovered from clinical specimens. It is considered a true pathogen when isolated from any sterile site. Infections are most prevalent among patients with cystic fibrosis (CF) or burn wounds, among intravenous drug abusers, and patients with leukemia. Infections tend to occur where moisture accumulates, such as the outer ear in otitis externa (swimmer's ear"), tracheostomies, at catheter sites, and in weeping wounds. All pseudomonads produce a water-soluble fluorescent pigment called *pyoverdin*, but only *P. aeruginosa* produces the additional blue-green pigment called *pyocyanin*. This characteristic can be used to help identify culture isolates. *P. aeruginosa* has a blue-green metallic sheen and a fruity odor. *P. aeruginosa* is the most common and clinically important pathogen in CF patients. By adulthood, at least 60% of CF patients are infected with this pathogen. Chronic infection is the main cause of impaired lung function. A mucoid morphotype of *P. aeruginosa* infects CF patients and contributes to the poor prognosis for these patients. Isolates from CF patients must have susceptibility testing done. There may be several different morphotypes of *P. aeruginosa* with different antibiograms in these clinical specimens. In the final stages of chronic CF lung infection, *P. aeruginosa* may be resistant to all available antibiotics.

P. fluorescens, P. putida, and *P. stutzeri* are ubiquitous in soil and water and may be found in the hospital environment. These species are considered to have low virulence but infections do occur.

P. aeruginosa is intrinsically resistant to many antibiotics. Oral antibiotics with activity against this organism for CF patients are limited to the quinolones; ciprofloxacin is frequently combined with an inhaled antibiotic such as tobramycin or colistin. Susceptibility testing should always be done on this organism.

The *Burkholderia* species are found in soil, in water, and on plants. The most commonly isolated species from humans is *B. cepacia.* It is an opportunistic pathogen, particularly in CF patients and those with chronic granulomatous disease. *P. aeruginosa* is the predominant pulmonary pathogen in CF patients, but *B. cepacia* is emerging as a pathogen as well. Some patients are co-infected with both organisms. *B. cepacia* is capable of invading airway epithelium, which is thought to explain its ability to cause disseminated bacteremia and its antibiotic resistance. *B. cepacia* grows slowly; specific selective media, such as PC agar or OFPBL agar, is recommended for cultures from CF patients. There is documented patient-to-patient transfer of this pathogen in both health care and non–health care settings. Infection control practices should be instituted to prevent transmission.

INTEREST POINT

In June 2006, there was a voluntary product recall of perineal care washcloths that were contaminated with *Burkholderia cepacia.* The product in question had been distributed to hospitals and medical facilities in the United States and Canada during the first half of 2006. For more information, access the FDA website at *www.fda.gov/oc/po/firmrecalls/sage06_06.html.*

B. mallei is a pathogen of animals; it causes glanders in horses but rarely infects humans. *B. pseudomallei* causes melioidosis. This disease is endemic to Southeast Asia and Northern Australia. The most common presentation of this disease is pneumonia, although three modes of acquisition (inhalation, ingestion, inoculation) have been recognized. The "gold standard" for diagnosis is isolation of *B. pseudomallei* from body fluids. It is a slender gram-negative rod that shows bipolar staining. It is capable of surviving harsh environmental conditions, acidic environments, dehydration, and a wide temperature range. It is resistant to the quinolones and macrolides, and the only treatment that has demonstrated a mortality benefit is ceftazidime. Approximately 7% of returning American troops that were stationed in Vietnam have positive antibody titers to this organism.

KEY TERMS AND ABBREVIATIONS

Match the term in the left column with the definition on the right.

1. _____ mesophilic
2. _____ melioidosis
3. _____ pyoverdin
4. _____ cystic fibrosis
5. _____ pyocyanin

A. water-soluble fluorescent pigment
B. disease endemic to Southeast Asia
C. blue-green pigment
D. grows best between 25° and 40° C
E. genetic syndrome characterized by chronic infection

TRUE OR FALSE

1. _____ *Pseudomonas aeruginosa* produces flat pink colonies on MacConkey agar.
2. _____ *B. cepacia* is motile and oxidase-negative.
3. _____ Because *P. aeruginosa* is intrinsically resistant to many antibiotics, susceptibility testing should be done whenever it is isolated from clinical specimens.
4. _____ *B. pseudomallei* infection is a major public health concern in northern Australia.
5. _____ *P. aeruginosa* is the predominant pulmonary pathogen in CF patients.

CASE STUDY

A policeman, who is also a diver for the police force, had been diving for several days in Chesapeake Bay. Several days after these series of dives, he noticed that he had some pain when he touched his face near his ear and he had a swollen lymph node on his neck. The pain continued for 2 days. At that time he noticed some drainage from his ear. Open water diving is part of his job; an ear infection would prevent him from diving. The man went to his physician, who cultured the ear drainage. There was a light growth of a non–lactose-fermenting isolate on MacConkey agar. On the blood agar there was a light growth of beta-hemolytic colonies that had a metallic sheen. The colonies were oxidase-positive and indole-negative. When first examined, the culture seemed to have a fruity smell.

1. NCCLS Document M35 outlines an abbreviated identification scheme for certain commonly isolated bacteria. Based on this scheme, the technologist has enough information to name the isolate. What is the ear pathogen?
2. What needs to be done to finish this culture?
3. When the patient saw his doctor, the physician gave the man a prescription for ciprofloxacin. Is this antibiotic a good choice for this pathogen?

ANSWERS

Key Terms and Abbreviations

1. D
2. B
3. A
4. E
5. C

True or False

1. F
2. F
3. T
4. T
5. T

Case Study

1. The key identifying characteristics are the following: oxidase-positive gram-negative rod, grapelike smell, metallic sheen, spot indole–negative. The isolate is *P. aeruginosa*. If this were a CF patient, the isolate would have to be evaluated carefully because atypical morphotypes of *P. aeruginosa* are common.
2. Susceptibility testing should always be done on *P. aeruginosa* isolates because of their intrinsic resistance.
3. Ciprofloxacin is listed as one of the recommended drugs in *The Sanford Guide to Antimicrobial Therapy*, Thirty-Sixth Edition. But the results of the susceptibility testing will determine whether the antibiotic regimen needs to be changed.

REFERENCES

Cheng AC, Currie BJ: Melioidosis: epidemiology, pathophysiology, and management, *Clin Microbiol Rev* 18:383, 2005.

Lyczak JB, Cannon CL, Pier GB: Lung infections associated with cystic fibrosis, *Clin Microbiol Rev* 15:194, 2002.

Saiman L, Siegel J: Infection control in cystic fibrosis, *Clin Microbiol Rev* 17:57, 2004.

25 Achromobacter, Rhizobium, Ochrobactrum, and Similar Organisms

OBJECTIVES

Upon completion of this chapter, the reader should be able to:
1. List several species of environmental bacteria that have been implicated in human infection.
2. Describe the identifying biochemical features of *A. xylosoxidans*.
3. Explain the clinical significance of isolation of *A. xylosoxidans*, particularly from respiratory specimens.
4. List the identifying features of *Rhizobium radiobacter* and *Ochrobactrum anthropi*.

SUMMARY OF KEY POINTS

The organisms in this chapter are considered to be environmental organisms that occasionally cause human infection. These are all gram-negative rods that are not pigmented and are oxidase-positive. The three most significant organisms in this group are *Rhizobium radiobacter*, *Ochrobactrum anthropi*, and *Achromobacter xylosoxidans*. When these organisms are encountered in a clinical setting, they are usually associated with contaminated medical devices or are isolated from immunocompromised patients.

INTEREST POINT

In 2002 there was an outbreak of *Alcaligenes xylosoxidans* reported in an outpatient hematology office located in Los Angeles County in California. There was a cluster of bloodstream infections with *A. xylosoxidans* that were all associated with outpatient chemotherapy at a single oncologist's office. The Los Angeles County Department of Health Services investigated and determined that the probable cause was the reuse of a contaminated vial of heparin or saline that led to the formation of an *Alcaligenes* biofilm on the central venous catheters in place in these affected patients. For the full report of the investigation, go to *www.lapublichealth.org/acd/reports/spclrpts/2002/Special_Reports_2002.pdf.*

Achromobacter xylosoxidans (formerly called *Alcaligenes*) is oxidase-positive, grows on MacConkey agar, and utilizes both glucose and xylose. The utilization of xylose can be used to differentiate it from the other saccharolytic *Achromobacter* spp. It has been isolated from a variety of specimen types, particularly respiratory specimens. It may be emerging as an additional potential pathogen in cystic fibrosis (CF) patients. Data collected from the U.S. Cystic Fibrosis Foundation's National Patient Registry showed isolation rates for *Achromobacter*

spp. of 1.9% and 2.7% in 1996 and 1997. Data collected from a phase III clinical trial of aerosolized tobramycin recovered *A. xylosoxidans* from 8.7% of the 520 patients in the trial. It is not clear whether this organism is merely colonizing the respiratory tract of these patients or whether it may play a role in infection.

Rhizobium radiobacter is a soil inhabitant and a plant pathogen but is not considered to be a true human pathogen. It is an opportunist that rarely causes bacteremia, endocarditis, and peritonitis in immunocompromised patients. There are two documented cases of endophthalmitis associated with cataract surgery. In both cases, however, the patients were exposed to soil in an outdoor setting following surgery and before the surgical wounds had healed. This organism will grow on MacConkey agar as a non–lactose fermenter, is oxidase-positive, hydrolyzes esculin, and oxidizes glucose and xylose. It can be identified using the API 20NE system (bioMérieux, Hazelwood, Mo).

Ochrobactrum anthropi is a gram-negative rod that is aerobic, motile, a nonfermenter on MacConkey agar, and oxidase- and urease-positive. Its name comes from the Greek word *ochros*, which means "pale." It can produce pale yellow colonies. The natural habitat of this organism is unknown, but it has been found in water and soil and has been isolated from indwelling catheters, retained foreign bodies, and contaminated pharmaceuticals. It is an opportunistic pathogen that seems to be able to adhere to synthetic materials such as silicone tubing. The optimal antimicrobial therapy is not known.

KEY TERMS AND ABBREVIATIONS

Match the term in the left column with the definition on the right.

1. _____ non–lactose fermenter
2. _____ nosocomial
3. _____ psychrophilic
4. _____ eugonic
5. _____ lactose fermenter

A. grows well on common media
B. grows well at 20° C
C. clear colonies on MacConkey agar
D. pink colonies on MacConkey
E. infection acquired during hospitalization

TRUE OR FALSE

1. _____ *A. xylosoxidans* oxidizes xylose.
2. _____ *Psychrobacter* spp. grow best at 35° C.
3. _____ Outdoor activities, such as gardening, immediately following cataract surgery is a risk factor for *R. radiobacter* infection.

67

4. _____ *A. xylosoxidans* isolation from respiratory cultures of CF patients should be listed in the final report.
5. _____ A clustered isolation from two or more patients of an environmental organism should be reported to the local health department.

CASE STUDY

A 75-year-old woman was admitted to the hospital through the emergency department with a complaint of fever and trouble breathing. She admitted having chronic respiratory problems. Blood cultures were collected upon admission and the next day a sputum was collected for culture. The sputum Gram stain showed greater than 25 WBCs/LPF and 1 to 5 epithelial cells/LPF. Preliminary reports on the blood cultures were "no growth." The sputum culture had a heavy growth of clear colonies on the MacConkey plate. There was heavy growth of mixed types on the blood agar plate with alpha-hemolysis only visible in the first two quadrants. Growth on the MacConkey plate was Gram stained and subcultured to blood agar. The isolate produced short straight rods that were oxidase-positive. The organism was identified as *Achromobacter xylosoxidans*.
1. What is the significance of this organism in the sputum culture?
2. What is a key biochemical feature in the identification of this organism?

ANSWERS

Key Terms and Abbreviations
1. C
2. E
3. B
4. A
5. D

True or False
1. T
2. F
3. T
4. T
5. T

Case Study
1. The Gram stain showed that the specimen was an acceptable sputum specimen not contaminated with saliva as shown by the low epithelial cell count and high WBC count. The predominant organism on the plates was the gram-negative rod. Alpha-hemolytic streptococci are considered to be normal respiratory flora; alpha-hemolysis was not present in all quadrants and did not predominate. *A. xylosoxidans* has been implicated in respiratory infections.
2. It is saccharolytic (uses glucose) and oxidizes xylose.

REFERENCES

Lyczak JB, Cannon CL, Pier GB: Lung infections associated with cystic fibrosis, *Clin Microbiol Rev* 15:194, 2002.

Mandari H, Hamzavi S, Peairs RR: *Rhizobium (Agrobacterium) radiobacter* identified as a cause of chronic endophthalmitis subsequent to cataract extraction, *J Clin Microbiol* 41:3998, 2003.

Saiman L, et al: Identification and antimicrobial susceptibility of *Alcaligenes xylosoxidans* isolated from patients with cystic fibrosis, *J Clin Microbiol* 39:3742, 2001.

Vaidya SA, Citron DM, Fine MB, et al: Pelvic abscess due to *Ochrobactrum anthropi* in an immunocompetent host: case report and review of the literature, *J Clin Microbiol* 44: 1184, 2006.

26 *Chryseobacterium, Sphingobacterium,* and Similar Organisms

OBJECTIVES

Upon completion of this chapter, the reader should be able to:
1. Recognize the potential significance of colonies with pale yellow pigmentation.
2. Recognize the need to interpret automated identification results with caution.
3. Utilize certain key biochemical reactions to make a presumptive identification.

SUMMARY OF KEY POINTS

The organisms in this chapter are environmental organisms that are rarely implicated in human disease. These are organisms that can survive in moist environments, thus contaminating water sources and pharmaceuticals. Debilitated and immunocompromised patients are more at risk for infection. Many of the organisms listed in this chapter produce a yellow pigment, are oxidase-positive, and grow on MacConkey. These organisms may be difficult to identify with commercial systems. Key biochemical reactions can give a presumptive identification.

Chryseobacterium meningosepticum is a gram-negative bacillus ubiquitous in nature. The most common reports of infection with this organism involve babies; meningitis among neonates is the most common presentation. These bacilli are straight rods that may appear thinner in the center than at the ends. They are nonmotile, oxidize glucose, and are indole-positive, they but do not hydrolyze urea. *Chryseobacterium* spp. are inherently resistant to many antimicrobials and have a high mortality rate among infants.

> ### INTEREST POINT
> There is a published case study in which *Sphingobacterium spiritivorum* was isolated in pure culture from the water reservoir of a steam iron. Repeated exposure to this bacterium while ironing caused a hypersensitivity pneumonitis in the woman who used this iron. When the woman used an iron with no liquid reservoir, she was free of symptoms. This woman could truly claim that she was allergic to ironing.

Sphingobacterium species are yellow-pigmented, oxidase-positive bacilli that will usually grow on MacConkey. They are indole-negative and urea-positive; these two reactions can be used to differentiate this genus from *Chryseobacterium* spp. and *Empedobacter brevis*. *Sphingobacterium* spp. have occasionally been isolated from human specimens, such as blood, urine, and respiratory secretions, but rarely are associated with serious infection.

Susceptibility data for these organisms is in the literature; however, there are no validated testing methods for these organisms.

TRUE OR FALSE

1. _____ The *Sphingobacterium* spp. produce pale yellow colonies on culture.
2. _____ *Chryseobacterium* spp. have been implicated in neonatal meningitis.
3. _____ Key biochemical reactions to differentiate these species include indole and urea reactions.
4. _____ Not all these environmental species will grow on MacConkey agar but they do grow on blood agar.
5. _____ A key identifier for *C. meningosepticum* is its ability to hydrolyze urea.

ANSWERS

True or False
1. T
2. T
3. T
4. T
5. F

REFERENCES

Chiu C, et al: Atypical *Chryseobacterium meningosepticum* and meningitis and sepsis in newborns and the immunocompromised, Taiwan, *Emerg Infect Dis* 6:481, 2000.

Kampfer P, Engelhart S, Rolke M, Sennekamp J: Extrinsic allergic alveolitis (hypersensitivity pneumonitis) caused by *Sphingobacterium spiritivorum* from the water reservoir of a steam iron, *J Clin Micobiol* 43:4908, 2005.

27 Alcaligenes, Bordetella (Non-pertussis), Comamonas, and Similar Organisms

OBJECTIVES

Upon completion of this chapter, the reader should be able to:
1. List the few organisms that produce pink colonies.
2. Explain the clinical significance of *B. bronchiseptica* and how to differentiate it from the other two agents of whooping cough.

SUMMARY OF KEY POINTS

The organisms in this chapter represent a diverse group of bacteria that are usually found in the environment but may also be found in the respiratory tract of animals. These organisms may be motile or nonmotile, usually grow on MacConkey agar, and are usually oxidase-positive.

The genus *Bordetella* consists of several species but only three of these are found in humans. *B. pertussis* and *B. parapertussis* are the agents of whooping cough. *B. bronchiseptica* causes "kennel cough" in dogs and respiratory disease in cats, rabbits, and other animals. Humans are occasionally infected when they have contact with animals. This organism is isolated more frequently from children and immunocompromised patients. *B. bronchiseptica* can be distinguished from the other two human pathogens by the fact it is motile and urease- and nitrate-positive. It is a straight gram-negative rod that grows well on standard media. The drug of choice for treating the whooping cough–like illness caused by this organism is erythromycin.

Roseomonas spp. are a group of aerobic gram-negative bacteria that produce pink colonies on blood agar and clear colonies on MacConkey agar. *Roseomonas* is resistant to vancomycin and may grow slowly. These are waterborne coccobacilli that are only rarely isolated from humans. They have been isolated from blood and wounds and from central venous catheters.

TRUE OR FALSE

1. _____ *B. bronchiseptica* is the only nonmotile member of this genus.
2. _____ One way to separate these genera is to do a flagella stain and note the placement and number of flagella.
3. _____ *B. bronchiseptica* can be differentiated from the other species by its motility and urease reactions.
4. _____ The *Comamonas* spp. may appear as curved rods.
5. _____ *Roseomonas* spp. have been isolated from catheter tips and blood cultures.

ANSWERS

True or False

1. F
2. T
3. T
4. T
5. T

REFERENCES

De I, Rolston KVI, Han XY. Clinical significance of *Roseomonas* species isolated from catheter and blood samples: analysis of 36 cases in patients with cancer, *Clin Infect Dis* 38:1579, 2004.

Lorenzo-Pajuelo B, et al: Cavitary pneumonia in an AIDS patient caused by an unusual *Bordetella bronchiseptica* variant producing reduced amounts of pertactin and other major antigens, *J Clin Microbiol* 40:3146, 2002.

28 Vibrio, Aeromonas, Plesiomonas, and Chromobacterium

OBJECTIVES

Upon completion of this chapter, the reader should be able to:

1. Describe key characteristics for the genus *Vibrio* and selective culture media.
2. Describe the spectrum of disease associated with *V. cholerae*, *V. parahaemolyticus*, and *V. vulnificus*.
3. List key biochemical characteristics of the genera *Aeromonas* and *Plesiomonas*.
4. Describe clinical presentation associated with *Aeromonas* and *Plesiomonas* infection.

SUMMARY OF KEY POINTS

Organisms in the family *Vibrionaceae* are facultative anaerobes with polar flagella; they are oxidase-positive, reduce nitrate to nitrite, and ferment glucose. *Vibrio* species have historical interest in that *V. cholerae* caused the first cholera pandemic in 1817. We are currently in the seventh pandemic, which began in 1961 when the El Tor biotype emerged in Indonesia. Pathogenic species are found in brackish and marine environments in temperate and tropical regions throughout the world. They are associated with mollusks and crustaceans. Human disease results from the ingestion of contaminated water, consumption of contaminated food, and exposure of wounds to contaminated water. All species are halophilic and require salt for growth, except *V. cholerae* and *V. mimicus*. Presumptive identification can be made based on this salt requirement. *Aeromonas* and *Plesiomonas* will grow in nutrient broth without salt and can be found in freshwater environments. These organisms are not considered normal human flora. Lysine, arginine, and ornithine reactions can be used to differentiate the *Vibrio* species. The somatic antigens 01 and 0139 are present on those organisms that cause diarrheal disease and epidemics; non-01 strains usually do not produce the toxin that causes this disease. These organisms will grow on MacConkey agar as nonlactose fermenters and on blood agar as smooth iridescent colonies. A selective medium is TCBS (thiosulfate citrate bile salts sucrose) agar.

The diarrhea caused by *V. cholerae* is toxin-mediated. The bacterium adheres to the intestinal cell and produces enterotoxin. The toxin stimulates cAMP production, which causes chloride to be secreted. Water is secreted as well. A hallmark of this diarrheal syndrome is a massive loss of water and salt from the body. The patient may produce 10 to 30 watery stools with flecks of mucus per day; this is the characteristic "rice water" stool. The patient suffers dehydration and an electrolyte imbalance that can lead to shock and death. Supportive therapy to replace fluid should be coupled with antimicrobials. Effective drugs against the *Vibrio* spp. include doxycycline, ceftazidime, fluoroquinolones, and aminoglycosides.

V. parahaemolyticus also causes gastroenteritis following ingestion of contaminated seafood. Eating raw or undercooked shellfish is a source of illness, but cooked seafood cross-contaminated with raw seafood can also cause illness. Symptoms include diarrhea, cramps, nausea, vomiting, fever, and chills. Illness is usually mild and self-limiting lasting 1 to 3 days. *V. parahaemolyticus* has also been isolated from wound infections where there has been exposure to salt or brackish water.

V. vulnificus is a particularly virulent species that causes wound infections that can lead to septicemia and death. Septicemia has a high fatality rate. Conditions that predispose a person to septicemia include chronic liver disease or immunocompromising conditions.

INTEREST POINT

Vibrio illness after Hurricane Katrina in August 2005 was monitored in the three states struck by the hurricane. From August 29 to September 11, there were 22 new cases of *Vibrio* illness that included 5 deaths. The organisms involved were *V. vulnificus*, *V. parahaemolyticus*, and nontoxigenic *V. cholerae*. No cases of toxigenic *V. cholerae* serogroups 01 or 0139 were identified. Of these 22 cases, 18 were wound infections caused by *V. vulnificus* and *V. parahaemolyticus*; 5 of these patients died. Refer to *www.cdc.gov/mmwr/preview/mmwrhtml/mm5437a5.htm*.

In the family *Aeromonadaceae* are the genera *Aeromonas* and *Plesiomonas*. The *Aeromonas* spp. are waterborne organisms that ferment glucose and are oxidase- and catalase-positive. They have been associated with a variety of diseases in both warm- and cold-blooded animals. They have been associated with gastroenteritis, septicemia in immunocompromised patients, and serious wound infections. The species most often implicated in human disease are *A. hydrophila* and *A. veronii*.

A. veronii biovar *sobria* has an interesting relationship with leeches. It is a free-living bacterium that is a symbiont in the gut of the medicinal leech, *Hirudo medicinalis*. In the 1980s, leeches began to be used after microvascular surgery to relieve venous congestion. The use of leeches improved the success rate of the operation but frequently caused infections with *Aeromonas*. The leech lacks proteolytic enzymes necessary to digest ingested blood, but the bacterium supplies those enzymes. Prophylactic antibiotics are given now whenever medicinal leeches are used.

The genus *Plesiomonas* has only one species, *P. shigelloides*. This organism is ubiquitous in water

71

and soil. Humans become infected by eating contaminated seafood or unwashed food. Risk factors for infection are foreign travel or underlying disease, such as cancer. These organisms are straight, motile gram-negative rods that grow on sheep blood agar and most enteric media. They are nonhemolytic, ferment glucose, are oxidase-positive, and appear as non–lactose fermenters on MacConkey agar. *P. shigelloides* has been associated with gastroenteritis, often with prolonged illness.

KEY TERMS AND ABBREVIATIONS

Match the term in the left column with the definition on the right.

1. _____ halophilic	A. selective agar for *Yersinia*
2. _____ pandemic	B. diarrhea producing blood and WBCs
3. _____ cholera	C. worldwide epidemic
4. _____ dysentery	D. toxin-mediated diarrheal disease
5. _____ Cary-Blair	E. selective agar for *Vibrio* isolation
6. _____ TCBS agar	F. salt-loving
7. _____ CIN agar	G. transport medium

TRUE OR FALSE

1. _____ *V. cholerae* does not require salt for growth.
2. _____ *V. cholerae* is the prototype for toxin-mediated diarrhea and causes rice-water stools and dehydration.
3. _____ *V. parahaemolyticus* has caused wound infections in saltwater fishermen.
4. _____ *P. shigelloides* has been isolated from postsurgical wound infections where medicinal leeches have been used.
5. _____ Skin infections with *V. vulnificus* often lead to septicemia.

CASE STUDY

A 37-year-old woman, who had been treated for irritable bowel syndrome (IBS) and was taking an acid-suppressing medication, developed severe diarrhea after arriving home from a trip to Florida with her husband. She had abdominal pain and developed a fever. She presented to the emergency department. Blood was drawn for cultures and for a CBC and chemistry panel. Stool was also collected for fecal WBCs, *C. difficile* toxin testing, and culture. The stool was negative for *C. difficile* toxin and positive for WBCs. Her blood work indicated she was slightly dehydrated. The woman was admitted. After overnight incubation, the MacConkey plate had both lactose-fermenting and non–lactose-fermenting colonies. The stool was tested for Shiga toxin; none was detected. The clear colonies on the MacConkey plate were investigated and identified as *Plesiomonas shigelloides*.

1. What tests will differentiate *Plesiomonas* from *Shigella*?
2. The gastroenterologist who had been following this patient for IBS thought she had acquired toxigenic *E. coli* during her stay in Florida. After seeing the culture results, the gastroenterologist again questioned the woman. She revealed that she ate raw oysters while in Florida, but her husband had eaten them as well and he did not become ill. How does this information help explain her current illness?

ANSWERS

Key Terms and Abbreviations

1. F
2. C
3. D
4. B
5. G
6. E
7. A

True or False

1. T
2. T
3. T
4. F
5. T

Case Study

1. The simplest way to differentiate the species is with an oxidase test. *Plesiomonas* is oxidase-positive; the *Enterobacteriaceae* are oxidase-negative.
2. The woman had an underlying condition of IBS and was taking an acid-suppressing medication. The acidic environment of the stomach actually helps sterilize food before it reaches the intestines. This situation increased her risks of infection with the waterborne *Plesiomonas* presumably gotten from the raw oysters.

REFERENCES

Abbott SL, Cheung WKW, Janda JM: The genus *Aeromonas*: biochemical characteristics, atypical reactions, and phenotypic identification schemes, *J Clin Microbiol* 41:2348, 2003.

Centers for Disease Control and Prevention: *Vibrio* illness after Hurricane Katrina—multiple states, August-September 2005, *Morb Mortal Wkly* 54:928, 2005.

Centers for Disease Control and Prevention: *Vibrio parahaemolyticus* infections associated with consumption of raw shellfish—three states, 2006, *Morb Mortal Wkly* 55:854, 2006.

Kain KC, Kelly MT: Clinical features, epidemiology, and treatment of *Plesiomonas shigelloides* diarrhea, *J Clin Microbiol* 27:998, 1989.

29 *Sphingomonas paucimobilis* and Similar Organisms

OBJECTIVES

Upon completion of this chapter, the reader should be able to:
1. Recognize the role of some environmental bacteria in the contamination of medical equipment.

SUMMARY OF KEY POINTS

There are a variety of environmental bacteria that are ubiquitous in nature and can survive in a broad range of environments. Many of these organisms are well studied for their roles in applied environmental microbiology. One such organism is *Sphingomonas paucimobilis*, formerly classified as *Pseudomonas paucimobilis*. This organism has been studied for its ability to degrade polycyclic aromatic hydrocarbons (e.g., creosote waste), a class of hazardous chemicals with the potential to be carcinogenic and mutagenic. *S. paucimobilis* has also been isolated from the hospital environment and clinical specimens. Isolation from humans does not necessarily mean infection. *S. paucimobilus* was isolated from sinus washings from four patients over a 5-week period. Upon investigation it was determined that the saline used for irrigation had been contaminated by tap water because of improper storage. There are rare reports of infection in humans that include bacteremia, meningitis, wound infection, and peritonitis in patients undergoing chronic ambulatory peritoneal dialysis. *S. paucimobilis* and other related environmental organisms will grow on blood and chocolate agars but may not grow on MacConkey agar. They will grow in thioglycollate broth and can be recovered in blood culture systems. *Sphingomonas* spp. may produce a yellow pigment on blood agar. Susceptibility studies have been limited by the number of clinical isolates, but all isolates in one study produced beta-lactamase and were susceptible to ceftriaxone, amikacin, and tetracycline.

TRUE OR FALSE

1. _____ Medical supplies should not be stored under sinks to avoid contamination with tap water leaking from the sink.
2. _____ Many environmental bacteria produce a yellow pigment.
3. _____ Microbiologists need to be alert to the clustered isolation of unusual organisms that may indicate hospital use of contaminated equipment.
4. _____ Vancomycin is the drug of choice for these gram-negative opportunists.
5. _____ These environmental organisms are grouped together because they are oxidase-positive and oxidize glucose.

ANSWERS

True or False
1. T
2. T
3. T
4. F
5. T

REFERENCES

Morrison AJ, Shulman JA: Community-acquired bloodstream infection caused by *Pseudomonas paucimobilis:* case report and review of the literature, *J Clin Microbiol* 24:853, 1986.
Mueller JG, Chapman PJ, Blattmann BO, Pritchard PH: Isolation and characterization of a fluoranthene-utilizing strain of *Pseudomonas paucimobilis, Appl Environ Microbiol* 56:1079, 1990.

OBJECTIVES

Upon completion of this chapter, the reader should be able to:

1. Differentiate the two forms (coccoid and bacillary) of *Moraxella.*
2. Determine the significance of these species of *Moraxella* and *Neisseria* if recovered in culture.

SUMMARY OF KEY POINTS

There are quite a few species within the genera *Moraxella* and *Neisseria*, but not all are typically human isolates. Some, such as *N. weaverii* and *M. canis,* are oropharyngeal flora in dogs and cats. These are usually seen in humans as a result of bite wounds. Other than the three frequently isolated pathogens *Moraxella (Branhamella) catarrhalis, N. gonorrhoeae,* and *N. meningitidis,* these organisms rarely cause infection and should be considered as potential contaminants. Many *Moraxella* spp. are considered to be normal mucosal flora with low virulence.

There is documentation in the literature that these rare isolates may also be a cause of infection. *Neisseria elongata* subsp. *nitroreducens* was renamed and reclassified in 1990. One fourth of the strains received at the Centers for Disease Control and Prevention for analysis were from cases of bacterial endocarditis. Data were collected over a 16-year period and found that most of these isolates originated from blood but were also recovered from wounds, respiratory secretions, and peritoneal fluid. Individuals at risk for infection had preexisting heart damage or had undergone dental manipulations. *Moraxella lacunata* has been well documented as a cause of eye infection, but it has also recently been implicated as the cause of a presumed endocarditis in a young child.

These organisms grow well on blood and chocolate agars as well as in commercial blood culture systems but do not grow well on MacConkey agar. These generally nonpathogenic strains are gram-negative coccobacilli, in contrast to *M. catarrhalis* and most *Neisseria* spp., which are true cocci. These coccoid and bacillary forms of *Moraxella* can be differentiated by exposure to penicillin; *M. catarrhalis* is a true coccus and maintains its shape but the other species will elongate. The *Moraxella* are oxidase- and catalase-positive. Many species do not utilize glucose. Susceptibility testing is not usually done.

TRUE OR FALSE

1. _____ *Moraxella lacunata* has been known to pit the agar under colonies because it can liquefy gelatin.
2. _____ All *Moraxella* spp. are oxidase-negative.
3. _____ Exposure to penicillin using a 10-unit disk can be done to differentiate true diplococci from bacillary forms.
4. _____ *M. lacunata* has been known to cause conjunctivitis.
5. _____ *M. canis* could be a pathogen in a bite wound.

ANSWERS

True or False

1. T
2. F
3. T
4. T
5. T

REFERENCES

Nagano N, et al: Presumed endocarditis caused by BRO β-lactamase-producing *Moraxella lacunata* in an infant with Fallot's tetrad, *J Clin Microbiol* 41:5310, 2003.

Wong JD, Janda JM: Association of an important *Neisseria* species, *Neisseria elongate* subsp. *nitroreducens,* with bacteremia, endocarditis, and osteomyelitis, *J Clin Microbiol* 30:719, 1992.

31 *Eikenella* and Similar Organisms

OBJECTIVES

Upon completion of this chapter, the reader should be able to:
1. Describe key morphologic and biochemical characteristics of *Eikenella corrodens*.
2. Explain the acronym HACEK and how it applies to *E. corrodens*.
3. List some pink-pigmented organisms and how to differentiate them.

SUMMARY OF KEY POINTS

Eikenella corrodens is a slow-growing gram-negative bacillus that is part of the normal human oral flora. It has been isolated from dental plaque and been implicated in increasing frequency in periodontitis, osteomyelitis, bite wound infections, bacteremias, and endocarditis. It is one of the HACEK organisms; HACEK is an acronym that represents the slow-growing gram-negative bacilli associated with endocarditis. It has also been isolated from soft tissue infections in intravenous drug abusers who lick the injection site.

    E. corrodens is a facultative anaerobe that grows slowly; small colonies will develop on blood and chocolate agars within 48 hours, but it does not grow on MacConkey agar. Two characteristics of this organism are its tendency to pit the agar and to exude a chlorine bleach odor. It is oxidase-positive and catalase-negative, reduces nitrate to nitrite, and is indole-negative. *E. corrodens* is usually susceptible to penicillin, although penicillin-resistant strains have been isolated.

    Methylobacterium species are slow-growing, gram-negative bacilli found in water and soil. They are resistant to chlorine and have been isolated from water distribution systems. They can be opportunistic pathogens but are considered to be of low virulence. Human infections reported have all involved immunosuppressed patients. These organisms may be difficult to grow on routine laboratory media. If gram-negative rods are seen in the clinical specimen but fail to grow on routine culture media, this organism should be considered. There are reports where improved growth was achieved by the use of BCYE agar. If growth is achieved, it will produce pink-pigmented colonies. *Roseomonas* is also pink-pigmented, but the two species can be differentiated by incubation at 42° C (*Roseomonas* will grow but *Methylobacterium* spp. will not) and the oxidation of methanol.

TRUE OR FALSE

1. _____ *E. corrodens* is commonly isolated from human bite wounds.

2. _____ *E. corrodens* and *Roseomonas* produce pink colonies on blood agar.
3. _____ *Methylobacterium* spp. has been isolated from tap water in hospitals.
4. _____ *Eikenella* is oxidase-negative and will not grow on MacConkey agar.
5. _____ *Eikenella* has been implicated in periodontal disease.

CASE STUDY

An emergency department nurse was working with a female patient who had been brought into the hospital by the police. The woman was apparently homeless and a known alcoholic. She was combative when the nurse tried to take her vital signs and bit the nurse on her hand. It was a deep wound. Despite cleansing and proper care, the wound became infected. Surgical drainage and excision of devitalized tissue was necessary. During surgery, culture specimens were collected. The nurse was put on broad spectrum antibiotic therapy pending culture results. The Gram stain revealed leukocytes and gram-positive cocci. After overnight incubation there were some alpha-hemolytic colonies on sheep blood agar and corresponding growth on the chocolate plate. They were alpha-hemolytic streptococci. At 48 hours of incubation, a second colony type appeared on just the blood and chocolate agars. Gram stain showed this new morphotype to be a small gram-negative coccobacillus, but there was no growth on the MacConkey plate.
1. If this second organism is gram-negative, why isn't it growing on the MacConkey agar? What are some possible organisms?
2. After 72 hours of incubation of this culture, the second colony type appeared to be surrounded by a flat, spreading growth. The technologist thought she smelled bleach. What tests can be done to arrive at an identification?
3. What is a treatment option?

ANSWERS

True or False
1. T
2. F
3. T
4. F
5. T

Case Study

1. The alpha-hemolytic streptococci seen on day 1 probably represent normal mouth flora. There are fastidious gram-negative organisms that will not grow on MacConkey. *Eikenella corrodens* is one of these that is considered normal oral flora.
2. The bleach smell is characteristic of *E. corrodens*. As the name implies, this organism corrodes or pits the agar. Look for pitting. *E. corrodens* is oxidase-positive and catalase- and indole-negative. This organism can be identified by commercial systems. Susceptibility testing should also be done.
3. Most strains are susceptible to penicillin and the beta-lactam antibiotics, although some penicillin resistance is being reported.

REFERENCES

Cercenado E, Cercenado S, Bouza E: In vitro activities of tigecycline (GAR-936) and 12 other antimicrobial agents against 90 *Eikenella corrodens* clinical isolates, *Antimicrob Agents Chemother* 47:2644, 2003.

Goldstein EJ, Tarenzi LA, Agyare EO, Berger JR: Prevalence of *Eikenella corrodens* in dental plaque, *J Clin Microbiol* 17:363, 1983.

Hornel B, et al: Systemic infection of an immunocompromised patient with *Methylobacterium zatmanii, J Clin Microbiol* 37:248, 1999.

32 *Pasteurella* and Similar Organisms

OBJECTIVES

Upon completion of this chapter, the reader should be able to:
1. Describe the growth characteristics of *P. multocida*.
2. Describe some typical biochemical reactions for *P. multocida*.
3. Explain the clinical significance of isolation of this organism in various human specimens.

SUMMARY OF KEY POINTS

The members of the genus *Pasteurella* are nonmotile, gram-negative coccobacilli that are facultative anaerobes. Most of the species are oxidase-positive and catalase-positive. The species in the genus *Pasteurella* are recovered from the respiratory tracts of dogs, cats, chickens, ducks, and other animals. The organism most frequently recovered and of clinical significance is *P. multocida*. This organism is part of the normal oral flora of dogs and cats. It is an opportunistic pathogen in humans that is transmitted through close animal contact or by bite wounds. This organism should be considered whenever there is an animal bite wound or respiratory infection in households where there are pets. *P. multocida* has been implicated in serious infections, such as meningitis and pneumonia.

The organism grows well and is nonhemolytic on blood agar, but it does not grow on MacConkey agar. Whenever a gram-negative coccobacillus is seen in the Gram stain but there is no growth on the MacConkey plate and an animal is involved, *P. multocida* should be considered. Susceptibility testing guidelines for *P. multocida* are included in the Clinical and Laboratory Standards Institute (CLSI) guidelines for fastidious organisms.

TRUE OR FALSE

1. _____ *P. multocida* appears as a coccobacillus on Gram stain and may be confused with *Haemophilus*.
2. _____ An identifying characteristic of *P. multocida* is popcorn-like odor.
3. _____ *P. multocida* can be distinguished from most of the other *Pasteurella* species by its positive indole and ornithine decarboxylase reactions.
4. _____ *P. multocida* is oxidase- and catalase-positive.
5. _____ Two gram-negative organisms that do not grow on MacConkey are *E. corrodens* and *P. multocida*.

CASE STUDY

A 75-year-old woman was brought to the emergency department by her son. The woman lives alone with her pets. He found her shaking and feverish and complaining of chest pain. At the emergency department her medical history revealed that she had chronic obstructive pulmonary disease. The woman smokes a pack of cigarettes per day and has been smoking since she was 16 years old. Blood was collected for a CBC and blood cultures, and sputum was sent for culture. Her leukocyte count was elevated, showing a predominance of neutrophils and bands. The sputum Gram stain showed many WBCs and many gram-negative coccobacilli resembling *Haemophilus* spp. The woman was admitted and treated with azithromycin.

1. The next day there was mixed growth on the blood and chocolate agars and no growth on the MacConkey plate. There were some alpha-hemolytic streptococci as well as nonhemolytic gray colonies on the blood and chocolate agars. The gray colonies were isolated but were not identified using the *Haemophilus* flowchart. The growth was identified by an automated system as *Pasteurella multocida*. The identification was verified. The woman had not been bitten by a dog or cat. How could this organism associated with animals be found in sputum?
2. The woman was initially treated for community-acquired pneumonia presumptively caused by *Haemophilus*. Is her treatment appropriate for the new organism identification?

ANSWERS

True or False
1. T
2. F
3. T
4. T
5. T

Case Study
1. There are reports in the literature that document *P. multocida* as a respiratory pathogen, particularly in patients with an underlying disease, such as bronchiectasis, COPD, or malignancy. There is even a case of *P. multocida* meningitis in a baby who had close contact with the family's pet cat. *P. multocida* is found more frequently in the oral flora of cats than in dogs.

This patient's son confirmed that the woman had two cats that she frequently held and hugged. There was probably direct inoculation with the cat oral secretions.

2. The isolate was susceptible to all tested antibiotics. The preferred drug for treating *Pasteurella* is penicillin, but amoxicillin-clavulanate may also be used. *The Sanford Guide to Antimicrobial Therapy 2006* lists azithromycin as being active in vitro.

REFERENCES

Boerlin P, et al: Molecular identification and epidemiological tracing of *Pasteurella multocida* meningitis in a baby, *J Clin Microbiol* 38:1235, 2000.

Marinella MA: Community-acquired pneumonia due to *Pasteurella multocida, Respir Care* 49:1528, 2004.

33 Actinobacillus, Kingella, Cardiobacterium, Capnocytophaga, and Similar Organisms

OBJECTIVES

Upon completion of this chapter, the reader should be able to:

1. Explain the acronym HACEK and its clinical importance.
2. Describe the clinical disease associations of *A. actinomycetemcomitans, C. hominis,* and *K. kingae.*
3. Explain the significance of *Capnocytophaga* species in cultures.
4. List some key biochemical reactions to differentiate these fastidious species.

SUMMARY OF KEY POINTS

HACEK is an acronym that represents a group of fastidious gram-negative bacilli that are similar in some respects: slow growth in culture, need for CO_2 to enhance recovery (capnophilic), and an affinity for infecting the heart valve and soft tissues. The organisms are:

- *Haemophilus aphrophilus*
- *Actinobacillus actinomycetemcomitans*
- *Cardiobacterium hominis*
- *Eikenella corrodens*
- *Kingella kingae*

All are endogenous flora of the nose, mouth, or throat. They can be recovered from routine media but may need as much as 14 days of incubation. Susceptibility testing guidelines for all of these organisms are addressed in the CLSI document M45.

The major pathogen of the genus *Actinobacillus* is *A. actinomycetemcomitans*. It causes endocarditis, severe forms of periodontal disease, and soft tissue infection. It is part of the endogenous flora of the mouth but is associated with periodontal disease. This organism is present in a large majority of young patients with localized juvenile periodontitis, a destructive form of periodontitis characterized by loss of the alveolar bone of the molars and incisors. Endocarditis can develop after dental procedures or if there is poor dentition. *A. actinomycetemcomitans* grows slowly on blood and chocolate agars and does not grow on MacConkey agar. The rods are short and stain unevenly. They are catalase-positive and oxidase-, urease-, and indole-negative.

Unlike the previous organisms, *C. hominis* rarely causes disease other than endocarditis. Many patients with endocarditis have had severe periodontitis or prior dental procedures without antibiotic prophylaxis. It is normal flora of the nose, mouth, and throat. Gram stain shows a pleomorphic appearance with bacilli whose ends are not shaped alike. The bacilli sometimes form rosettes. It grows slowly on blood and chocolate agars and not at all on MacConkey agar. It is oxidase-positive and catalase-, nitrate-, and urease-negative; these reactions distinguish it from *A. actinomycetemcomitans* and *Haemophilus aphrophilus*. Susceptibility testing is difficult to perform because of its slow growth pattern.

Kingella kingae is part of the normal flora of the mucous membranes of the respiratory tract. It is an opportunistic pathogen known to cause endocarditis, osteomyelitis, and septicemia. It is emerging as an important pathogen in children, particularly children younger than 4 years of age. Widespread immunization against *Haemophilus influenzae* and *Streptococcus pneumoniae* may have created a unique opportunity for this organism among oropharyngeal flora. Some researchers believe that because of the organism's slow growth, it may be underreported. Recovery can be enhanced by inoculation of synovial fluid or bony exudates into blood culture bottles. Isolates in blood culture broth can be detected in 1 to 3 days. It will grow aerobically on blood and chocolate agars incubated at 36° C for 2 or more days. It is the only species of the genus to be beta-hemolytic on blood agar. It is oxidase-positive and catalase-negative.

Capnocytophaga species are thin, spindle-shaped gram-negative bacilli morphologically similar to fusobacteria. They will grow aerobically in 5% CO_2 as well as anaerobically, but growth is slow and may not appear for 2 days. Capnocytophaga species are catalase- and oxidase-negative. They are part of the normal oropharyngeal flora. They may play a role in periodontitis and septicemia. *C. canimorsus* colonizes the mouths of cats and dogs. Human infections with *C. canimorsus* are associated with animal bites or close contact with dogs. Serious disease occurs if there is an underlying condition, such as splenectomy, leukemia, or renal disease. *C. canimorsus* is usually isolated from blood cultures but may be recovered from wound cultures.

KEY TERMS AND ABBREVIATIONS

Match the term in the left column with the definition on the right.

1. _____ dysgenic
2. _____ capnophilic
3. _____ HACEK
4. _____ fastidious
5. _____ microaerophilic

A. group of organisms linked to endocarditis
B. grows better with reduced oxygen
C. slow-growing
D. requires certain conditions
E. grows better with increased CO_2

TRUE OR FALSE

1. _____ An organism that is being isolated more frequently from young children is *Capnocytophaga* species.
2. _____ *K. kingae* is nonhemolytic on blood agar.
3. _____ *C. hominis* and *A. actinomycetemcomitans* can be differentiated by their catalase reactions.
4. _____ The microbiologist can enhance recovery of fastidious pathogens by inoculating bony aspirates or synovial fluid into blood culture bottles.
5. _____ If *Capnocytophaga* infection is suspected, growth can be enhanced by incubation of the plates in CO_2.

CASE STUDY

A 3-year-old child was feverish for 2 days. The mother brought the child to the emergency department (ED). The clinical history showed no recent problems. The child had surgery 6 months earlier for the insertion of ear tubes and had been healthy since that procedure. Blood was collected for CBC and blood cultures. The leukocyte count was elevated. The child was given a dose of ceftriaxone and discharged. The mother was instructed to follow up with her pediatrician. Four hours later the mother brought the child back to the ED because her condition had worsened. The child was unresponsive and died a short while later. The family was distraught and requested that a postmortem be performed to determine the cause of death. The postmortem revealed vegetations on the heart valve indicative of endocarditis. By this time the blood culture had become positive with gram-negative bacilli that were later identified as *Kingella kingae*.

1. What is the significance of *K. kingae* bacteremia and endocarditis?
2. How could this child have acquired *K. kingae?*

ANSWERS

Key Terms and Abbreviations

1. C
2. E
3. A
4. D
5. B

True or False

1. F
2. F
3. T
4. T
5. T

Case Study

1. *K. kingae* is a well-documented cause of endocarditis. It is one of the HACEK organisms.
2. *K. kingae* is part of the normal oropharyngeal flora. Children have particularly high carriage rates for this organism. The ear surgery made a breach in immune defenses and allowed the organism to be seeded into the bloodstream. It is unknown whether there were congenital heart defects, but endocarditis has been reported in people with no previous heart disease.

REFERENCES

Kiang KM, et al: Outbreak of osteomyelitis/septic arthritis caused by *Kingella kingae* among child care center attendees, *Peds* 116:206, 2005.

Yagupsky P: Use of blood culture systems for isolation of *Kingella kingae* from synovial fluid, *J Clin Microbiol* 37:3785, 1999.

Yagupsky P, Peled N, Katx O: Epidemiological features of invasive *Kingella kingae* infections and respiratory carriage of the organism, *J Clin Microbiol* 40:4180, 2002.

34 *Haemophilus*

OBJECTIVES

Upon completion of this chapter, the reader should be able to:

1. Describe the spectrum of diseases caused by *Haemophilus* spp.
2. Explain how to differentiate *H. influenzae* from the other species.
3. Explain the porphyrin test.
4. Describe the disease caused by *H. ducreyi*.

SUMMARY OF KEY POINTS

Haemophilus species are normal residents of the upper respiratory tracts of humans and other animals. Some colonize the gastrointestinal and urogenital tracts. They also cause a wide spectrum of human infections. Clinically encountered species include *H. influenzae, H. parainfluenzae, H. ducreyi, H. aphrophilus, H. para-phrophilus, H. haemolyticus, H. parahaemolyticus,* and *H. segnis. H. influenzae* was first described in 1892 by Pfeiffer who recovered it from the sputa of patients with viral influenza. The genus name was proposed in 1920 and the six capsular serotypes were described in 1931.

These pleomorphic gram-negative coccobacilli are facultative anaerobes having optimal growth at 35° to 37° C in 5% CO_2. They are differentiated by their requirements for exogenous nicotinamide adenine dinucleotide (NAD) (V factor) and/or hemin (X factor). Many species have fastidious nutritional requirements. Most species grow well on chocolate agar but may not grow on blood agar. *Haemophilus* spp. can be grown on blood agar by cross-streaking with *S. aureus*. Satellite colonies will form along the staphylococcal line of growth because X factor is released during lysis of RBCs and V factor is excreted by *S. aureus* during growth. *H. influenzae* requires both X and V factors for growth. *H. aphrophilus* is the only species that does not require X or V factors.

Haemophilus influenzae has been one of the most common causes of acute bacterial meningitis in young children. Encapsulated strains belong to one of six serotypes. *H. influenzae* type b (Hib) caused the majority of invasive *Haemophilus* infection in the United States before the widespread use of vaccines in the 1970s. Unencapsulated strains cause noninvasive respiratory

tract infection in children and community-acquired pneumonia in adults. About 16% of children with cystic fibrosis grow out nontypeable *H. influenzae* from respiratory tract specimens. In young children this is a common cause of otitis media along with *S. pneumonia*. A subgroup of *H. influenzae, H. influenzae* biogroup *aegyptius*, causes purulent conjunctivitis.

Haemophilus infections were uniformly susceptible to ampicillin until the 1970s when some strains developed resistance to ampicillin, the drug of choice for *H. influenzae* meningitis. Plasmid-mediated beta-lactamase production causes resistance to the penicillins. Another resistance mechanism involving penicillin-binding proteins has also been described. Susceptibility testing should be done on all clinical isolates.

Another pathogen of this genus is *H. ducreyi*. It causes sexually transmitted chancroid. Chancroid is a genital ulcerative disease common in Africa, Asia, and Latin America. It is an uncommon sexually transmitted disease in the United States. The lesion begins as a tender papule that becomes pustular and ulcerated. This is not the same type of lesion as chancre (syphilis). Genital ulcerations increase the risk of HIV infection during homosexual or heterosexual contact; the ulcers could also facilitate the transmission of HIV by the shedding of virus through the lesion. *H. ducreyi* has a low optimum growth temperature (33° to 35° C). This is a fastidious organism that is difficult to isolate from ulcer specimens. Culture media needs to be enriched with growth factors, but also usually contains vancomycin to inhibit growth of gram-positive bacteria. Culture media may not always be available, so transport media can maintain viability of the organism. Studies have shown good recovery rates using a thioglycolate-hemin-based media with swabs refrigerated at 4° C for up to 4 days.

H. parainfluenzae is considered part of the commensal flora of the upper respiratory tract. It is not commonly isolated as a pathogen but has been implicated in bacteremia, sinusitis, bronchitis, and cellulitis. It requires only V factor for growth.

All clinically relevant species require exogenous X and/or V factor. Most species will grow on conventional chocolate agar but not on 5% sheep blood. Body fluids, conjunctival swabs, and bronchoscopy specimens should be inoculated onto both chocolate and blood agar and incubated at 35° in 5% CO_2. Colonies tend to be small and translucent with a "mousy" odor (due to production of indole from tryptophan). Encapsulated strains form glistening colonies. To identify an isolate, its X and V factor requirements need to be determined. This may be done by placing disks containing X and V factors on unsupplemented media or by putting the supplemental factors into the media. The plates are incubated overnight and examined for growth. There may be some inconsistencies with this method. To avoid that problem the porphyrin test may be done. The porphyrin test determines an isolate's X factor requirement. Species that require X factor (heme) do not excrete porphobilinogen and porphyrins during growth because of enzymatic deficiencies. This is a direct test of the organism's ability to synthesize protoporphyrin intermediates from δ-aminolevulinic acid (ALA). Beta-lactamase testing and susceptibility testing should be done on all isolates.

TRUE OR FALSE

1. _____ H. parainfluenzae requires both X and V factors for growth.
2. _____ The Haemophilus spp. are all susceptible to ampicillin.
3. _____ H. influenzae isolated from CSF should be serotyped.
4. _____ Small colonies that only grow near S. aureus in a sinus culture should be investigated as possible Haemophilus.
5. _____ All H. influenza isolates should be tested for beta-lactamase production.

CASE STUDY

A 7-month-old baby was brought to a clinic because the child had been feverish. The child's eye was also red and producing a discharge. Blood was collected for a CBC and blood culture and the eye discharge was cultured. The Gram stain of the eye showed WBCs and gram-negative coccobacilli. After overnight incubation, the eye culture had a predominant growth of creamy colonies on the chocolate agar and a few white colonies. The only colonies growing on the blood agar were the white ones. These were coagulase-negative staphylococci.

1. What should the technologist do to identify the predominant colony type?
2. Colonies grew around both X and V disks and the ALA test was negative. What is the identification of this organism?

ANSWERS

True or False

1. F
2. F
3. T
4. T
5. T

Case Study

1. A Gram stain of the creamy colonies should be done. Gram-negative coccobacilli were seen in the clinical specimen, and the expectation is that these colonies are that same organism. The colonies should be subcultured for isolation. If there are clearly isolated colonies, these may be used to check for X and V factor growth requirements. A rapid test for porphyrin synthesis should be done. Beta-lactamase testing and susceptibility testing should also be done.
2. Haemophilus influenzae. To differentiate biotypes within this species, additional tests must be performed. The indole, urease, and acid production from xylose tests can be used to differentiate biogroup aegyptius from the other biogroups.

REFERENCES

Centers for Disease Control and Prevention: Sexually transmitted diseases treatment guidelines—2006, Morb Mortal Wkly Rep 51:RR-11, 2006.

Lyczak JB, Cannon CL, Pier GB: Lung infections associated with cystic fibrosis, Clin Microbiol Rev 15:194, 2002.

35 *Bartonella* and *Afipia*

OBJECTIVES

Upon completion of this chapter, the reader should be able to:
1. List the diseases associated with *B. henselae*.
2. List the diseases associated with *B. quintana*.
3. List some methods to detect and diagnose cat-scratch disease.

SUMMARY OF KEY POINTS

The genus *Bartonella* has been changed and rearranged several times over the last 20 years. Currently, the genus represents a group of bacteria that have a wide distribution in both wild and domestic animals. Infected animals are the reservoirs for human infection.

Several insects have been implicated in transmission; these include the human body louse, cat flea, sand flies, and ticks. Microscopically, all *Bartonella* spp. are gram-negative bacilli or coccobacilli. They are fastidious and may be able to grow on chocolate agar but incubation requires at least 12 days and as long as 45 days. Cell culture methods using shell vials have been used. Identification is difficult with commercially available methods because *Bartonella* spp. are biochemically inert in routine identification tests. Gas-liquid chromatography and molecular methods have been used.

B. quintana is found worldwide. It is the agent of trench fever. Outbreaks have been sporadic and widely separated. They are associated with poor sanitation and personal hygiene; transmission involves the body louse. Bouts of chills and fever can last as long as 5 days.

Bacillary angiomatosis is a proliferative disorder that involves the skin and lymph nodes, as well as a variety of internal organs. It is mostly seen in patients with HIV disease but may also occur in immunosuppressed transplant patients or cancer patients. The agents of this vascular proliferative disease are *B. henselae* and *B. quintana*.

Oroya fever and verruga peruana are two clinical entities caused by *B. bacilliformis*. Infections are geographically limited and seen only in the river valleys of the Andes mountains. Transmission is by the sandfly. After insect bite, fever develops. Onset of symptoms may be abrupt and include fever, headache, and anorexia. Severe anemia results due to red blood cell destruction by the organisms.

Peliosis is a disease of the internal visceral organs that develop blood-filled lesions. Before the HIV epidemic, this condition was rare. The number of cases involving the liver and spleen are increasing in association with HIV infection. *B. henselae* infection is associated with this disease.

In addition to bacillary angiomatosis and peliosis, *B. henselae* is associated with cat-scratch disease (CSD). CSD is frequently seen in children and adolescents and presents as lymphadenopathy. It occurs after exposure to cats or a cat scratch or bite. A lesion forms several days after a bite or scratch. Low-grade fever, headache, and muscle aches may be present. Lymphadenopathy in the region of the bite develops. Histologic examination of the lymph nodes stained with Warthin-Starry silver stain may show clusters of organisms. Serology tests for the detection of IgG and IgM antibodies specific for *B. henselae* are commercially available.

The genus *Afipia* is named for Armed Forces Institute of Pathology where *Afipia felis* was first described as a cause of cat scratch fever. It is now generally accepted that *B. henselae* is the etiologic agent of CSD. It now appears that *Afipia* species are widespread in nature and associated with water. They may also have a relationship with free-living amoebae.

TRUE OR FALSE

1. _____ The *Bartonella* spp. are best visualized in tissue with the Warthin-Starry silver stain.
2. _____ *Bartonella* are fastidious organisms that would be difficult to culture in a routine hospital laboratory.
3. _____ *B. quintana* is recognized as the cause of Oroya fever.
4. _____ Peliosis is a proliferative disease characterized by blood-filled lesions.
5. _____ Groups of homeless people in the United States are developing *B. quintana* infections similar to trench fever.

CASE STUDY

A 27-year-old male veterinary technician had been suffering with joint pain, malaise, and muscle aches for some time. His physician ordered a battery of tests that included a CBC, chemistry profile, and C-reactive screen. These tests were all normal and unremarkable. The physician also ordered IgG and IgM specific antibody tests to the following organisms: *Bartonella henselae, Babesia microti, Ehrlichia chaffeensis,* and *Rickettsia rickettsii.* These tests were all negative except for *B. henselae* IgG. The antibody titer was 1:64. The range 1:64 to 1:128 is considered equivocal. A positive result must be 1:256 or greater.

1. What is the significance of this test result?
2. If the physician strongly suspected this patient had cat-scratch disease, what other options exist to diagnose this disorder?

ANSWERS

True or False

1. T
2. T
3. F
4. T
5. T

Case Study

1. The presence of IgG antibody can indicate past exposure or infection, whereas the presence of IgM antibodies would indicate recent or current infection. No conclusions can be drawn from equivocal results because they are not clearly negative or positive. Repeat testing can be done in 2 weeks to determine whether there have been any changes in antibody concentration.
2. *Bartonella* species are fastidious organisms that grow slowly in culture. Most laboratories do not have the means to perform culture for this organism. If lymph node tissue or blood/tissue from lesions were recovered, the Warthin-Starry silver stain could be used to examine the specimens. Some reference laboratories offer *Bartonella* culture, but this test requires an incubation period of 21 days.

REFERENCES

Moosvi SA, et al: Isolation and properties of methane sulfonate-degrading *Afipia felis* from Antarctica and comparison with other strains of *A. felis, Environ Microbiol* 7:22, 2005.

36 Campylobacter, Arcobacter, and Helicobacter

OBJECTIVES

Upon completion of this chapter, the reader should be able to:
1. Describe the clinical syndromes associated with *Campylobacter* infection.
2. Describe culture and identification methods for the *Campylobacter* spp.
3. Describe disease associated with *H. pylori*.
4. List the methods used to detect and identify *H. pylori*.

SUMMARY OF KEY POINTS

Campylobacter species are microaerophilic, capnophilic, curved bacteria that are motile. They are nonfermentative and nonoxidative. *Campylobacter* spp. are found in the gastrointestinal tracts of a variety of animals, including poultry, dogs, and cattle. *C. jejuni* is the most common cause of bacterial gastroenteritis. It is estimated that there are more than 2.5 million cases each year in the United States. Humans become infected by ingesting raw milk, partially cooked poultry, or contaminated water, or by exposure to infected animals (including pet dogs and cats). There are also reports of sexual transmission and person-to-person transmission. Enteritis from this organism is characterized by abdominal pain, bloody diarrhea, chills, and fever, which usually last 3 to 7 days. Gastroenteritis is a self-limiting disease that does not usually require treatment with antibiotics. In severe disease with bacteremia, patients can be treated with erythromycin; fluoroquinolone resistance has been reported.

Since the eradication of polio in most of the world, the most common cause of acute flaccid paralysis is Guillain-Barré syndrome (GBS). In 1978 there was an outbreak of gastroenteritis caused by *C. jejuni* that affected more than 5000 people in Jordan. The outbreak was linked to contaminated water; 16 people developed GBS days after the onset of diarrhea. There is a connection between *Campylobacter* infection and GBS, but the exact cause is not known.

For cultivation, an enriched selective agar (e.g., Campy-BAP) should be used. *Campylobacter* spp. will grow at 35° C, but incubation at 42° C will suppress the growth of other bacteria. The media should be put in a microaerophilic atmosphere (5% oxygen). There is a filtration method for isolation of *Campylobacter* spp. that does not require selective agar. The hippurate hydrolysis test and susceptibility to nalidixic acid and cephalothin are used to differentiate species. Susceptibility testing is not routinely performed.

In 1979 it was observed that curved gram-negative organisms were often present in gastric biopsy specimens in the mucous layer. By 1984 it was clear that *Helicobacter pylori* infection was associated with chronic superficial gastritis and chronic active gastritis. Once acquired, *H. pylori* persists for life unless treated with antibiotics. *H. pylori* colonizes the mucous layer of the antrum and fundus of the stomach. It does not invade the epithelium. This organism is a major cause of peptic ulcer disease and has been linked to development of adenocarcinoma of the stomach and gastric non-Hodgkin's lymphoma. Because there is no known reservoir for this organism other than the human stomach, fecal-oral and oral-oral transmission has been proposed.

Diagnosis of infection is by two general means: (1) endoscopy to retrieve tissue for histology, culture, urease testing, and molecular testing and (2) nonendoscopic methods that include breath tests to detect urea, serology testing for IgG and IgA, and stool antigen tests. The treatment approved by the Food and Drug Administration for peptic ulcer disease is triple therapy—bismuth subsalicylate, metronidazole, and tetracycline.

Two other human pathogens within this genus are *H. cinaedi* and *H. fennelliae*. These inhabit the gastrointestinal tract of humans and may be part of the resident flora. They are sexually transmitted among homosexual men.

TRUE OR FALSE

1. _____ *Campylobacter* grows best in a reduced-oxygen environment.
2. _____ Peptic ulcer disease has been linked to infection with *C. jejuni*.
3. _____ *Campylobacter* spp. are thin gram-negative rods that have been described as "gull's wings."
4. _____ Susceptibility testing is not routinely done with *Campylobacter* isolates.
5. _____ *C. jejuni* can be differentiated from the other species by its positive hippurate hydrolysis test.

CASE STUDY

A 30-year-old woman went to her physician for treatment of diarrhea and abdominal pain that had lasted for 3 days. The woman claimed she was having bloody diarrhea. A stool specimen was obtained for culture.
1. After overnight incubation, there was normal stool flora on all the selective media except the Campy-BAP plate. How should the technologist proceed with the identification workup?
2. Should susceptibility testing be done?

ANSWERS

True or False

1. T
2. F
3. T
4. T
5. T

Case Study

1. Gram stain the colonies on the Campy-BAP to ensure that they have the characteristic morphology of *Campylobacter*. *Enterococcus* will also grow on this media. A hippurate hydrolysis test may be done as well as susceptibility to cephalothin and nalidixic acid. *C. jejuni* is hippurate hydrolysis–positive and resistant to cephalothin.

2. Susceptibility testing for *Campylobacter* spp. is not standardized. Testing is not routinely performed. Antimicrobial therapy is not usually prescribed because disease is usually self-limited.

REFERENCES

Dunn BE, Cohen H, Blaser MJ: *Helicobacter pylori*, *Clin Microbiol Rev* 10:720, 1997.

Nachamkin I, Allos BM, Ho T: *Campylobacter* species and Guillain-Barré syndrome, *Clin Microbiol Rev* 11:555, 1998.

On SL: Identification methods for campylobacters, helicobacters, and related organisms, *Clin Microbiol Rev* 9:405, 1996.

Solnick JV, Schauer DB: Emergence of diverse *Helicobacter* species in the pathogenesis of gastric and enterohepatic diseases, *Clin Microbiol Rev* 14:58, 2001.

Wassenaar TM: Toxin production by *Campylobacter* spp, *Clin Microbiol Rev* 10:466, 1997.

37 Legionella

OBJECTIVES

Upon completion of this chapter, the reader should be able to:
1. Explain the epidemiology of legionellosis.
2. List some diagnostic tools.

SUMMARY OF KEY POINTS

There is only one genus in the family *Legionellaceae*. There are many species within the genus *Legionella*, but only one that is a human pathogen, *Legionella pneumophila*. Legionellae are ubiquitous in aquatic habitats. Humans become infected from environmental sources that include man-made facilities, such as air-conditioning ducts and humidifiers, as well as from natural water sources. Legionellae are also found in hospital settings (e.g., nebulizers) and can cause nosocomial infections. These organisms can survive an extreme range of environmental conditions, probably because they are found within biofilms and free-living amoeba.

Pathogenic *Legionella* species are facultative intracellular pathogens. They survive within alveolar macrophages and persist even when antimicrobials penetrate these macrophages. There are three clinical disease manifestations: pneumonia, Pontiac fever, and other site infections. The predominant manifestation is pneumonia. Those most at risk are older persons, heavy smokers, and immunocompromised patients.

Diagnosis can be by direct detection of antigens in the specimen. A urine antigen test and a direct fluorescent test can be used on respiratory secretions and abscess material. For culture, special media must be used. Legionellae are fastidious and require cysteine for growth; buffered charcoal yeast extract (BCYE) agar is used. Plates should be incubated at 35° C in air for at least 7 days. Because legionellae are biochemically inert, identification is made by a monoclonal immunofluorescent stain. Most diagnoses are made by serology testing. Diagnosis of acute infection can only be made with a fourfold rise in titer between acute and convalescent sera. Susceptibility testing is not performed. Treatment is with the fluoroquinolones and newer macrolides.

> **INTEREST POINT**
> The Environmental Protection Agency has developed a drinking water fact sheet for the general public. It can be accessed at *www.epa.gov/waterscience/ criteria/humanhealth/microbial/legionellafs.pdf.*

TRUE OR FALSE

1. _____ There is evidence that legionellae can be spread by person-to-person contact.
2. _____ Legionellae appear as thin gram-negative bacilli.
3. _____ All specimens for *Legionella* culture should be handled in a biological safety cabinet.
4. _____ *Legionella* spp. can be spread to patients in a hospital through nebulizers.
5. _____ *Legionella* spp. can be grown on media supplemented with blood and incubated for 7 days.

CASE STUDY

A 40-year-old woman presented to the emergency department with shortness of breath, fever, chills, nausea, and vomiting. Chest x-ray showed a left upper lobe density. She had a history of rheumatoid arthritis, diabetes mellitus, and significant history of tobacco use. Her leukocyte count was elevated. She was admitted with a diagnosis of pneumonia and was empirically treated with ceftriaxone and azithromycin. The consulting physician suggested additional tests. They were mycobacterial culture, blood cultures, sputum culture, urine pneumococcal antigen test, and urine *L. pneumophila* antigen test.
1. The *L. pneumophila* antigen test was positive. What risk factors does she have for legionella?
2. What other tests could have been done to diagnose legionella?

ANSWERS

True or False
1. F
2. T
3. T
4. T
5. F

Case Study
1. This patient's risk factors include heavy smoking, underlying disease (diabetes), and immunosuppression (antiinflammatory drugs given for arthritis).
2. Other tests include sputum for DFA stain and serology tests.

OBJECTIVES

Upon completion of this chapter, the reader should be able to:
1. Describe the pathology of brucellosis.
2. Explain how to detect and diagnose brucellosis.
3. Describe safety precautions that must be followed.

SUMMARY OF KEY POINTS

Brucella are gram-negative coccobacilli that are non-motile. These are facultative intracellular parasites. They travel through the bloodstream in neutrophils and enter cells in the spleen, liver, and bone marrow. They evade killing and establish a systemic infection. Symptoms can include fever, chills, sweats, headache, fatigue with splenomegaly, and lymphadenopathy. Brucellosis is a zoonotic disease with domestic animals serving as the reservoir. The species that are pathogenic for humans are *B. abortus, B. melitensis, B. suis,* and *B. canis. B. abortus* commonly infects cattle. *B. melitensis* infects goats and sheep. Transmission of disease can result from ingestion, direct contact via skin lesions and mucous membranes, and inhalation. Risk factors for infection include the handling of infected animals, ingestion of contaminated animal products (e.g., unpasteurized milk), and the handling of cultures in the laboratory. People at greatest risk for contracting this disease are dairy farmers, slaughter-house employees, veterinarians, and laboratory personnel. There are about 100 cases/year reported in the United States. Disease may present as acute, subacute, or localized disease. Subacute brucellosis may be confused with tuberculosis.

Brucella spp. are most commonly isolated from blood and bone marrow. The organisms will only grow in aerobic blood culture bottles after 2 to 4 days. The organisms will grow on *Brucella* agar, blood agar, and chocolate agar when incubated at 35° C in 5% CO_2. Colonies may appear after 48 hours. Growth is improved by the addition of serum or blood, but X and V factors are not essential. Many strains require CO_2 for growth. Because of the fastidious nature of the organism, a serum agglutination test is widely used. *Brucella* are catalase-, oxidase-, and urea-positive, but the catalase test should not be done because of the risk of nebulizing the organisms. Identification should not be attempted with commercial identification systems. *Brucella* is a potential bioterrorist agent. Sentinel laboratory guidelines are available from the American Society for Microbiology and should be followed: *www.asm.org/policy/index.asp?bid=6342.*

Brucellosis is one of the most commonly reported laboratory-acquired infections. Aerosolization is the primary mechanism of transmission. It is essential that the microbiology laboratory be notified if brucellosis is suspected. Manipulation of specimens and culture should be done under biological safety level 3 precautions. Plates should be taped shut or enclosed in sealable plastic biohazard bags. Level A laboratories should consult with the public health laboratory director and immediately notify infection control if *Brucella* cannot be ruled out. Available vaccines are directed against *B. abortus* or *B. melitensis* in animals. Human vaccines are under development.

TRUE OR FALSE

1. _____ Brucellosis is a zoonosis.
2. _____ *Brucella* spp. are capnophilic.
3. _____ *Brucella* cultures can be worked with on the benchtop as long as countertops are disinfected after use.
4. _____ *Brucella*, like *Pasteurella*, is gram-negative but will not grow on MacConkey agar.
5. _____ Brucellosis can be acquired by eating under-cooked poultry.

CASE STUDY

A man presented to the emergency department with symptoms of headache, fever, chills, and abdominal discomfort. He said he became ill with gastroenteritis just before his return home from South America where he had visited his family's dairy farm. Examination showed the man had an enlarged spleen. The astute physician suspected a connection between the dairy farm and the illness. He questioned the man and learned he had consumed unpasteurized milk. The physician had brucellosis in his differential diagnosis. Blood cultures were ordered and the microbiology department was alerted. On day 3, the aerobic blood culture bottle became positive.
1. What should the microbiologist do to process the positive blood culture bottle?
2. Gram-negative coccobacilli are seen in the Gram stain. How should the microbiologist proceed?
3. After 4 days of incubation, a fine mist of growth appeared on the blood and chocolate agars but there was no growth on MacConkey. How should the microbiologist proceed?

ANSWERS

True or False

1. T
2. T
3. F
4. T
5. F

Case Study

1. The blood culture bottles may be processed in the automated system with other bottles, but they should be tagged to alert anyone working of the potential biohazard. There should be communication within the microbiology laboratory.

2. All manipulations must be performed in the biological safety cabinet. Care must be taken not to generate aerosols. The blood broth should be inoculated to *Brucella* agar, if available, and blood, MacConkey, and chocolate agars. Plates should be taped shut or sealed in plastic biohazard bags. Incubation should be in CO_2.

3. All work should be done in the biological safety cabinet. The growth should be checked by Gram stain for morphology. Oxidase and urease tests should be done. A catalase test should not be done. If the tests are positive, *Brucella* has not been ruled out. Consult with the public health laboratory director.

Bordetella pertussis and *Bordetella parapertussis*

OBJECTIVES

Upon completion of this chapter, the reader should be able to:
1. Describe the pathology of pertussis.
2. Explain how to detect and diagnose pertussis.
3. Describe safety precautions that must be followed.

SUMMARY OF KEY POINTS

There are three human pathogens in the genus *Bordetella:* *B. bronchiseptica, B. pertussis,* and *B. parapertussis.* *B. pertussis* causes whooping cough. Classic disease has three stages: catarrhal, paroxysmal, and convalescent. The disease begins like an upper respiratory tract viral infection with mild cough (catarrhal stage lasts 1 to 2 weeks). The cough changes to episodes of severe coughing (whooping) and vomiting (paroxysmal stage). This stage can last 2 to 6 weeks. The cough subsides during the convalescent stage. Disease occurs primarily in unimmunized children and, with increasing frequency, in adolescents. Pertussis is highly communicable, with more than 90% of susceptible household contacts also contracting the disease. Although there is widespread childhood immunization, immunity wanes 5 to 10 years after the last vaccine dose. The Advisory Committee on Immunization Practices has recommended a single-dose vaccination for adolescents 11 to 18 years of age and for adults 19 to 64 years of age. Recommended treatment and prophylaxis are the macrolide antibiotics.

Pathogenesis involves attachment to epithelial cells and damage to the respiratory epithelium. *B. pertussis* is a uniquely human pathogen, whereas *B. parapertussis* is found both in humans and lambs. *B. bronchiseptica* causes kennel cough in dogs. Nasopharyngeal swabs or aspirates are the most common specimens. For culture, direct plating at the bedside or in the office should occur. Regan-Lowe transport media may be used. Smears for direct fluorescent antibody (DFA) stain do not require viable organisms and are rapid tests, hence their popularity. The sensitivity of the test is low and DFA testing should only be done with simultaneous culture. These are small gram-negative coccobacilli. All are catalase-positive and strict aerobes with simple nutritional requirements. *B. pertussis* grows slowly and is susceptible to cold and drying.

TRUE OR FALSE

1. _____ The recommended transport medium for pertussis specimens is Cary-Blair.

2. _____ The current recommendation is for childhood and booster pertussis vaccination.
3. _____ Pertussis in humans is similar to kennel cough in dogs.
4. _____ Sputum is an acceptable specimen for *Bordetella* culture.
5. _____ The DFA stain should always be performed in conjunction with culture.

CASE STUDY

A laboratory assistant working in an outpatient clinic had orders to collect specimens from an 11-year-old child for *Bordetella pertussis* DFA and culture, rapid influenza testing, and RSV testing. The child had a nonproductive cough for 2 weeks. The laboratory assistant collected two nasopharyngeal swabs for the *Bordetella* tests and did a nasopharyngeal wash for the other tests. Two days later the laboratory assistant was contacted by the infection control practitioner. The *Bordetella* tests were positive; the employee needed to have a postexposure evaluation.

1. The infection control practitioner explained the nature of the disease and the risk of transmission. When questioned about the use of personal protective equipment, the laboratory assistant had worn gloves when collecting the specimens but no mask. What is the significance of this information?
2. The infection control practitioner required that the employee be evaluated by a physician. The laboratory assistant was given two options. She could either take 10 days of leave or take postexposure prophylaxis and continue to work. Why are these measures important?
3. The child had received all the required childhood vaccinations. How could she have contracted pertussis?

ANSWERS

True or False

1. F
2. T
3. T
4. F
5. T

Case Study

1. The child has been coughing and generating aerosols. Pertussis is a highly communicable respiratory disease. The laboratory assistant had had close contact with the infected child. The laboratory assistant is now at risk for development of disease.

2. The incubation period of pertussis averages 7 to 10 days. If a health care worker becomes infected, the potential to spread the disease to her patients is an important risk. She could be infectious but asymptomatic. Health care facilities must have infection control protocols in place to protect both the patients and workers.
3. The incidence of pertussis dramatically decreased after the advent of vaccines and their widespread use. In recent years there has been an increase in the number of reported pertussis cases, particularly among school-age children and adolescents. Immunity to pertussis begins to wane 5 to 10 years after the last pertussis vaccine dose. The current recommendation is for booster vaccine in the 11- to 18-year-old age group.

REFERENCES

Centers for Disease Control and Prevention: Recommended antimicrobial agents for the treatment and postexposure prophylaxis of pertussis. 2005 CDC guidelines, *Morb Mortal Wkly* 54(RR14):1, 2005.

40 *Francisella*

OBJECTIVES

Upon completion of this chapter, the reader should be able to:
1. Describe the pathology of tularemia.
2. Explain how to detect and diagnose tularemia.
3. Describe the safety precautions that must be followed when handling specimens and cultures.

SUMMARY OF KEY POINTS

Francisella species are widely distributed in nature and have been isolated from a variety of animals. *F. tularensis* is the agent of animal and human tularemia. In North America the most frequent source of infection is wild rabbits, beaver, and muskrats. The domestic rabbit has not been documented as a source. Other sources of human infection are blood-sucking arthropods, such as ticks, deerflies, and mosquitoes. Annual incidence of tularemia in the United States has declined from thousands of cases in the 1930s to about 100 cases annually, with several deaths each year. Humans become infected by four methods: handling infected animal carcasses, insect vectors, bite by infected animals, and inhalation. *Francisella* is a hardy organism that can persist for weeks in mud and decaying animal carcasses. Many cases of tularemia occur in people who hunt and skin animals.

F. tularensis is an intracellular parasite that resides in the cells of the reticuloendothelial system. These are highly infectious bacteria that require as few as 10 colony-forming units as the infectious dose. The most common form of the disease in the United States is the ulceroglandular form, caused by tick bites and contact with infected animals. A red papule develops and undergoes necrosis to form an ulcer. Lymphadenopathy and bacteremia occur. Once in the bloodstream, the patient experiences fever, chills, headache, and generalized aches. The drug of choice is streptomycin.

Francisella has been classified as a potential bioterrorist agent. Biosafety level 2 precautions need to be followed when handling specimens. For cultures, safety practices must be raised to biosafety level 3. Please refer to the guidelines posted on the American Society for Microbiology website at *www.asm.org/policy/index.asp?bid=6342*.

Francisella is a fastidious organism that is difficult to culture because of its requirement for cysteine and cystine. It is a gram-negative, pleomorphic coccobacillus that is a strict aerobe. *Francisella* will grow in blood culture systems within 2 to 5 days. It stains poorly by Gram stain; acridine orange stain will show the organisms in a positive blood culture bottle. *Francisella* may be confused with *Haemophilus* and *Actinobacillus actinomycetemcomitans*. It is recommended that infectious material from suspected patients be sent to a reference or public health laboratory that is equipped to handle an organism of this nature.

TRUE OR FALSE

1. _____ A hunter can become infected with *F. tularensis* by tick bite while hunting.
2. _____ *Francisella* is fastidious and requires cystine for growth.
3. _____ *Francisella* is clearly visible and easily identifiable on Gram stain as thin gram-negative rods.
4. _____ *Francisella* can be isolated from ulcers and lymph nodes.
5. _____ *Francisella* can be misidentified as *Haemophilus*.

ANSWERS

True or False
1. T
2. T
3. F
4. T
5. T

41 Streptobacillus moniliformis and Spirillum minus

OBJECTIVES

Upon completion of this chapter, the reader should be able to:
1. Explain how to detect and diagnose rat-bite fever and Haverhill fever.
2. Describe prevention methods.

SUMMARY OF KEY POINTS

There is only one species in the genus *Streptobacillus*. *Streptobacillus moniliformis* is a facultatively anaerobic, gram-variable bacillus whose natural habitat is the oropharynx of wild and laboratory rats. Human infection results either from rodent bite (rat-bite fever) or from ingestion of contaminated foods (Haverhill fever). Rat-bite fever is a rare systemic illness characterized by fever, joint pains, vomiting, and headache. Its incidence and pathogenic mechanisms are not known.

Organisms may be recovered from blood and aspirates from infected joints or lesions. The SPS anticoagulant used in blood culture bottles inhibits the growth of *S. moniliformis;* alternate blood culture methods should be used. *S. moniliformis* is fastidious but will grow on blood agar in a moist environment. Colonies are non-hemolytic and embed in the agar. This organism will grow in broth culture; growth has a characteristic "fluff ball" or "bread crumb" appearance. *S. moniliformis* is negative for indole, catalase, oxidase, and nitrate. It is motile. Serologic testing is useful but is only performed at a few reference laboratories. Penicillin is the drug of choice.

There are no vaccines. Disease prevention should focus on reducing exposure to rats. Gloves should be worn and regular hand washing should be done. Avoid hand-to-mouth contact and seek medical attention if bitten by a rat.

TRUE OR FALSE

1. _____ *Streptobacillus* can be recovered with commercial blood culture systems.
2. _____ Rat-bite fever can be acquired by eating food contaminated with rat excreta.
3. _____ *Streptobacillus* produces a characteristic "fluff ball" of growth in broth culture.
4. _____ Haverhill fever presents will acute onset of fever and chills with joint pain.
5. _____ *Streptobacillus* is fastidious and requires the presence of blood for growth.

ANSWERS

True or False
1. F
2. F
3. T
4. T
5. T

REFERENCES

Balakrishnan N, et al: *Streptobacillus moniliformis* endocarditis, *Emerg Infect Dis* 12:1037, 2006.

Centers for Disease Control and Prevention: Fatal rate-bite fever—Florida and Washington, 2003, *Morb Mortal Wkly* 53(51,52):1198, 2005.

42 | *Neisseria* and *Moraxella catarrhalis*

OBJECTIVES

Upon completion of this chapter, the reader should be able to:
1. Differentiate between *N. gonorrhoeae* and *N. meningitidis*.
2. Describe the disease states associated with each pathogen.
3. Describe types of media used for the isolation of the pathogenic species.
4. Explain how to differentiate *Moraxella* from *Neisseria*.

SUMMARY OF KEY POINTS

Neisseria species and *Moraxella catarrhalis* are kidney-bean shaped Gram-negative diplococci that do not elongate when exposed to penicillin. They are aerobic and nonmotile. These organisms are oxidase positive and catalase positive. They represent normal flora of the respiratory, alimentary, and genitourinary mucosa of humans.

Although any of these commensals can cause disease in a debilitated host, most disease is associated with *N. gonorrhoeae* (gonococcus) and *N. meningitidis* (meningococcus). *N. gonorrhoeae* is always considered a pathogen, regardless of the site of isolation. These organisms are often seen within neutrophils, an observation that helps identify a true infection.

Gonorrhea is the second most reported sexually transmitted disease to the Centers for Disease Control and Prevention after *Chlamydia trachomatis*. *N. gonorrhoeae* does not survive outside its host; it is susceptible to temperature extremes and drying conditions. *N. gonorrhoeae* is transmitted by direct, close contact between individuals. Transmission to neonates usually occurs during birth and causes ophthalmia neonatorum. Most states require prophylactic treatment with antibiotic ointments, such as erythromycin, tetracycline, or silver nitrate drops. The majority of uncomplicated gonococcal infections are lower genital tract infections caused by direct infection. Men develop acute urethritis and women usually present with endocervical infection. It is important for clinicians to communicate with the laboratory in suspected cases of gonococcal infection in nongenital sites. Special media will need to be inoculated.

Neisseria species grow best on enriched media in humid 5% CO_2 at 35° to 37° C. *N. meningitidis* will grow on blood agar but *N. gonorrhoeae* needs chocolate agar. Modified Thayer-Martin, Martin-Lewis, and New York City media contain added growth factors to enhance recovery of gonococci. Beta-lactamase testing should be performed on all isolates. Susceptibility testing can be done using the disk diffusion method following CLSI guidelines.

Identification can be based on carbohydrate utilization and conventional biochemical tests. There are also chromogenic tests and particle agglutination methods. Molecular methods have been developed for direct detection of gonococci in clinical specimens. These assays are useful for screening populations. Amplified assays are not acceptable as evidence in medicolegal cases.

N. meningitidis is an exclusively human pathogen with no known reservoir outside of humans. Asymptomatic carriers are usually the source of transmission; the organism colonizes the nose and throat. Transmission is by direct contact or via droplets. Meningococci are engulfed by epithelial cells and can survive and multiply in the bloodstream. There may be chills, acute fever, low back pain, thigh pain, or generalized muscle aches. Endotoxin release is a virulence factor that can lead to septic shock. These bacteria can invade the meninges. Skin hemorrhages are the hallmark of invasive meningococcal disease. Acute meningococcal disease can be fatal within a few hours. Once the bacteria cross the meninges and reach the subarachnoid space, their proliferation is uncontrolled. Survivors can suffer from neurologic sequelae that may include deafness and mental retardation.

Using the capsule or outer membrane, the species can be divided into serogroups. Serogrouping is necessary for epidemiologic purposes and is done by public health laboratories. Isolates of *N. meningitidis* should be sent to these laboratories for serogrouping. There is a quadrivalent vaccine for serogroups A, C, W-135, and Y. This vaccine is only protective in children older than 2 years of age. Primary contacts of patients with meningitis may be treated prophylactically with rifampin or ciprofloxacin.

For penicillin-resistant strains, broad-spectrum cephalosporins (e.g., ceftriaxone) is recommended.

Other species are occasionally reported to cause endocarditis, meningitis, empyema, pneumonia, and ocular infections. *N. cinerea* has been reported to cause ocular infections in newborns. This organism is often mistaken for *N. gonorrhoeae*. *N. lactamica* and *N. flavescens* do not grow on gonococcal selective media and often have a yellow pigment. These are residents of the throat and respiratory tract and not associated with infection.

Moraxella catarrhalis is a normal commensal of the upper respiratory tract and has been implicated in sinusitis, pneumonia, otitis media, septicemia, and meningitis.

M. catarrhalis had been susceptible to penicillin, but currently it is estimated that 85% of strains produce beta-lactamase. This would make them resistant to amoxicillin, which is frequently prescribed for ear infections. *M. catarrhalis* grows well on blood and chocolate agars. Colonies are white and dry-looking. Colonies typically can be "nudged" across the plate like a "hockey puck." An acceptable abbreviated identification scheme for gram-negative diplococci that grow on chocolate and blood agars is to do the oxidase and rapid butyrate esterase test. *M. catarrhalis* is positive for both.

TRUE OR FALSE

1. _____ *Neisseria* species are true cocci that do not elongate when exposed to penicillin.
2. _____ The beta-lactamase test should be performed on all isolates of *M. catarrhalis*.
3. _____ *N. meningitidis* isolates should be serogrouped.
4. _____ *Neisseria* species are facultative anaerobes.
5. _____ Yellow colonies on chocolate agar in a throat culture are potential pathogens and should be identified.

MULTIPLE CHOICE

1. _____ The most common form of gonococcal infection in neonates is
   A. impetigo.
   B. conjunctivitis.
   C. urethritis.
   D. pharyngitis.
2. _____ Martin Lewis media is used to isolate
   A. *N. meningitidis*.
   B. *N. gonorrhoeae*.
   C. *M. catarrhalis*.
   D. *H. influenzae*.
3. _____ The recommended treatment for close family contacts of a patient with meningococcal meningitis is
   A. rifampin.
   B. penicillin.
   C. ampicillin.
   D. erythromycin.
4. _____ Dry white colonies that can be nudged along the chocolate agar in a sinus culture could be
   A. *Haemophilus*.
   B. *E. coli*.
   C. *Moraxella*.
   D. staphylococci.

5. _____ A characteristic of all *Neisseria* species is that they
   A. are oxidase-negative.
   B. are oxidase-positive.
   C. ferment maltose.
   D. are not inhibited by SPS.

CASE STUDY

A 30-year-old man presented to a clinic complaining of pain on urination. He also thought there was some blood in his urine. A urinalysis and culture were done. There were many WBCs in his urine as well as some blood. Few bacteria were noted. The physician also ordered an amplification test for *C. trachomatis* and *N. gonorrhoeae*. The next day about 15 colonies were observed on the blood agar from the urine culture. The technologist did a Gram stain of these colonies; they were bean-shaped gram-negative diplococci. He subcultured them to chocolate agar.

1. What organism could this isolate possibly be?
2. What additional tests could be performed to identify this isolate?

ANSWERS

True or False

1. T
2. T
3. T
4. F
5. F

Multiple Choice

1. B
2. B
3. A
4. C
5. B

Case Study

1. There are only two pathogenic species that are true diplococci: *Neisseria* and *Moraxella*. The most likely organism based on the specimen type is *N. gonorrhoeae*.
2. The first test that should be done is oxidase. There are coagglutination test kits for the identification of *N. gonorrhoeae* that will give rapid results. A beta-lactamase test should be done for all *N. gonorrhoeae* isolates. This organism was *N. gonorrhoeae*. These culture results were confirmed by the positive amplified DNA test for *N. gonorrhoeae*.

REFERENCES

Centers for Disease Control and Prevention: Sexually transmitted diseases treatment guidelines—2006, *Morb Mortal Wkly Rep* 51:RR-11, 2006.

National Committee for Clinical Laboratory Standards: Abbreviated identification of bacteria and yeast; M35-A, Wayne, Pa, 2002, NCCLS.

43 Overview and General Considerations

OBJECTIVES

Upon completion of this chapter, the reader should be able to:
1. Differentiate between acceptable and unacceptable specimens for anaerobic culture.
2. List some anaerobic media and the organisms they select for.
3. Explain optimum specimen recovery and transport.
4. Describe some equipment used in a microbiology laboratory to achieve anaerobic conditions.

SUMMARY OF KEY POINTS

Anaerobic bacteriology deals with a group of organisms that grow better with little or no oxygen. A strict obligate anaerobe cannot grow on agar surfaces exposed to oxygen. Oxygen is toxic to these organisms. Many *Clostridium* species are in this category. A large number of organisms are facultative anaerobes; they grow under either aerobic or anaerobic conditions. The *Enterobacteriaceae* are facultative anaerobes. Microaerophiles, such as *Campylobacter*, grow better in higher concentrations of CO_2. The obligate aerobes require normal concentrations of oxygen. These include the mycobacteria. Most anaerobic infections are polymicrobic; they involve a mixture of aerobic and anaerobic organisms.

Pathogenic anaerobes are in the environment (exogenous source). But many anaerobes are commensals in the human body (endogenous source); they cause infection when their microenvironment changes. There are five ways to acquire an anaerobic infection or disease:
- Endogenous flora take advantage of a break in a barrier to gain access to normally sterile sites (bite wound).
- Existing wounds become contaminated with anaerobes (tetanus).
- Preformed toxin is ingested. This is actually an intoxication that causes disease (botulism).
- Toxigenic organisms colonize the gastrointestinal tract (infant botulism).
- Person-to-person spread (nosocomial spread of *C. difficile*).

It is important that appropriate specimens be collected for anaerobic culture. Specimens from certain anatomic sites should not be cultured anaerobically. In the colon, anaerobes far outnumber aerobes. Feces, colostomy drainage, and urine are unsuitable specimens. Swabs should be avoided, if possible. Aspirates and tissue biopsies are optimal. If swabs must be used, they should be put immediately into an oxygen-free transport system. There are times when these rules will need to be modified. To test for infant botulism, fresh stool is required to test for both the presence of botulinum toxin and the causative organism, *C. botulinum*. Specimen transport is important as well. Specimens should not be exposed to air or anaerobes will die. There are anaerobic transport systems that can be purchased. Temperature is another consideration. Specimens should be held at room temperature if there will be delays in processing. Refrigeration oxygenates the specimen.

Specimen processing involves making slides for stains, inoculating appropriate media, and incubating that media under suitable conditions to recover anaerobes. Media should not have been stored for long periods of time because peroxides accumulate and inhibit growth. Media can be prereduced to eliminate oxygen. PRAS (prereduced anaerobically sterilized) media are prepared and packaged under anaerobic conditions. There are several different types of anaerobic media that target different groups of organisms. No single medium will support the growth of all anaerobes while inhibiting aerobes. *Brucella* blood agar is an enriched nonselective medium, whereas LKV agar is selective for *Bacteroides* and *Prevotella*. There are a number of ways to produce anaerobic conditions that include anaerobe jars, anaerobe chambers, and holding jars.

The toxins that anaerobes produce can be extremely potent. Penetrating wounds that could be contaminated with *C. tetani* should have administration of the tetanus vaccine included in the wound management protocol. For a major wound contaminated with soil or feces, human tetanus immune globulin (TIG) should be given.

KEY TERMS AND ABBREVIATIONS

Match the term in the left column with the definition on the right.

1. _____ anaerobic
2. _____ microaerophilic
3. _____ facultative anaerobe
4. _____ myonecrosis
5. _____ PRAS
6. _____ botulism

A. prereduced media
B. poisoning
C. grows best in higher CO_2
D. muscle tissue death
E. can grow aerobically or anaerobically
F. cannot grow in presence of oxygen

TRUE OR FALSE

1. _____ *C. tetani* produces a potent toxin that is considered a potential bioweapon.
2. _____ The best material for anaerobic culture is aspirated fluid or tissue biopsy.
3. _____ All anaerobic specimens should be refrigerated if they cannot be cultured within 1 hour of collection.
4. _____ Anaerobe jars have an indicator that shows whether anaerobic conditions have been achieved.
5. _____ Culture plates stored for more than 2 weeks accumulate peroxides that inhibit growth.
6. _____ A rectal swab is not suitable for anaerobic culture but aspirate from an abscess is.
7. _____ LKV agar is selective for clostridia.
8. _____ It is not possible to acquire an anaerobic infection by person-to-person spread.
9. _____ Most anaerobic infections are polymicrobic.
10. _____ Sputum should be screened for epithelial cells before culturing it anaerobically.

ANSWERS

Key Terms and Abbreviations

1. F
2. C
3. E
4. D
5. A
6. B

True or False

1. F
2. T
3. F
4. T
5. T
6. T
7. F
8. F
9. T
10. F

44 Laboratory Considerations

OBJECTIVES

Upon completion of this chapter, the reader should be able to:
1. Explain an aerotolerance test.
2. Explain how K, V, C, nitrate, bile, and SPS disks can be used to presumptively identify anaerobes.
3. Be able to list key reactions for frequently isolated anaerobes.
4. Explain how definitive identification can be done.

SUMMARY OF KEY POINTS

Processing of specimens for culture involves evaluating the specimen for suitability for culture, performing a Gram stain, choosing appropriate culture media, and incubating the media under the appropriate conditions (temperature, atmosphere, humidity). Inoculated plates should be incubated at 35° to 37° C for 48 hours. Cultures should not be exposed to air before then because oxygen-sensitive organisms would be inhibited during their growth phase.

Most laboratories do a presumptive identification of anaerobes using a few key rapid tests. The common approach to anaerobic identification involves examining the media for growth and morphotypes. If the culture has mixed growth, colonies may be subcultured to purity plates. Gram stains should be done to determine Gram reaction and cell morphology and spore production.

Presumptive identification includes several strategies: aerotolerance testing, fluorescence (many strains fluoresce brick red under UV light), special potency disks (SPS, bile, kanamycin, vancomycin, colistin, nitrate disk), catalase test, and indole test. An aerotolerance test is done to determine whether there are true anaerobes or facultative anaerobes. The isolate is subcultured to two plates: a chocolate agar plate for incubation in the CO_2 incubator and a blood agar plate for anaerobic incubation. The special potency disks to add to the pure culture include kanamycin (K), colistin (C), and vancomycin (V). These disks are not intended for susceptibility testing; their purpose is for identification. If the isolate is a gram-negative bacillus, then K, V, C, nitrate disk, and bile disk should be placed on the subculture plate. If the organism is a gram-positive coccus, the SPS and nitrate disks should be placed in the first quadrant of the purity plate. Indole and catalase tests will provide additional useful information. Refer to the tables in the text for additional tests and interpretation of results. It is important not to expose the plates to air for more than a few minutes; some species of obligate anaerobes may be killed by exposure to atmospheric oxygen for as little as 10 minutes.

Definitive identification is only done by larger laboratories and by reference and research facilities because of the expense of the instrumentation. These laboratories may use an anaerobic glove box and identify organisms using gas-liquid chromatography (GLC) to analyze metabolic end products or cellular fatty acid. The many smaller clinical laboratories use disposable anaerobic plastic bags or anaerobic jars to achieve anaerobic conditions. In some commercial systems, biochemical assays provide a minisystem in which identification can be arrived at in 4 to 6 hours of incubation once there is a pure culture of the isolate.

Standard susceptibility testing methods have been established for testing anaerobic bacteria, but many clinical laboratories do not perform susceptibility testing. Those isolates requiring testing are referred to reference laboratories.

The following is a list of frequently encountered anaerobes and information useful in presumptive identification.

Anaerobic Gram-Positive, Spore-Forming Bacilli
- These are the *Clostridium* species. *C. perfringens* is the most frequent isolate and produces a characteristic double-zone hemolysis on blood agar plate. The Gram stain shows gram-positive boxcars with no spores. Not all bacilli may have spores and some species appear gram-negative. The *Clostridium* species are involved in gas gangrene and myonecrosis

Anaerobic Gram-Positive, Non–Spore-Forming Bacilli
- Included in this group are the genera *Propionibacterium, Eubacterium, Bifidobacterium, Lactobacillus, Actinomyces,* and *Mobiluncus. Actinomyces* spp. produce branching bacilli.
- *Propionibacterium acnes* is normal skin flora that appears as diphtheroids. It can often be seen in blood cultures, but is considered a contaminant.
- *Mobiluncus* organisms are curved rods that are susceptible to vancomycin and resistant to colistin. These organisms play a role in bacterial vaginosis.
- *Actinomyces* spp. may be involved in pelvic inflammatory disease associated with intrauterine devices.

Anaerobic Gram-Negative Bacilli
- This group includes *Bacteroides* spp., *Porphyromonas, Prevotella,* and *Fusobacterium.* Within the *B. fragilis* group, growth is enhanced by bile. There is resistance to colistin, vancomycin, and kanamycin. These organisms turn BBE agar brown.

- *Porphyromonas* produces tan colonies that fluoresce brick red. These bacteria are inhibited by vancomycin and bile, but are resistant to kanamycin and colistin.
- *Prevotella* can be pigmented or not. The pigmented species fluoresce red.
- *F. nucleatum* is a thin rod with tapered ends. It is resistant to vancomycin but sensitive to kanamycin.

Anaerobic Cocci

- *Peptostreptococcus* is the most clinically significant of the gram-positive cocci, which also includes *Streptococcus, Finegoldia, Micromonas, Peptococcus, Anaerococcus,* and *Schleiferella. Peptostreptococcus anaerobius* is sensitive to SPS, while most other gram-positive cocci are resistant. *P. magnus* is commonly isolated and has been implicated in osteomyelitis and septic arthritis.
- The gram-negative cocci include *Veillonella, Megasphaera,* and *Acidaminococcus. Veillonella* is resistant to vancomycin but sensitive to colistin and kanamycin.

INTEREST POINT

In July 2005, the Food and Drug Administration (FDA) issued a public health advisory following the deaths of four women associated with *Clostridium sordellii* infection. In each case there was a link to a pharmaceutical. The MedWatch program is an FDA safety program that provides a means for the reporting of adverse events. More information can be accessed at *www.fda.gov/medwatch/SAFETY.htm.*

TRUE OR FALSE

1. _____ Definitive identification is usually done in large reference laboratories that perform gas-liquid chromatography.
2. _____ Special potency disks containing colistin and vancomycin are used in presumptive identification.
3. _____ A key characteristic of the *B. fragilis* group is the ability to grow in 20% bile.
4. _____ Beta-lactamase testing should be done for all *Bacteroides* isolates.
5. _____ An aerotolerance test is done to see if the bacteria can grow in the presence of air.

ANSWERS

True or False

1. T
2. T
3. T
4. T
5. T

REFERENCES

Midura TF: Update: infant botulism, *Clin Microbiol Rev* 9:119, 1996.

Murdoch DA: Gram-positive anaerobic cocci, *Clin Microbiol Rev* 11:81, 1998.

45 Mycobacteria

OBJECTIVES

Upon completion of this chapter, the reader should be able to:

1. Describe the characteristics that are unique to mycobacteria.
2. Describe the processes of digestion and decontamination of clinical specimens for the isolation of mycobacteria.
3. List three acid-fast stains and the merits of each stain.
4. Describe the Runyon classification scheme.
5. Define the terms: *photochromogen, scotochromogen, nonphotochromogen.*
6. List media (both solid and liquid) commonly used for isolation of mycobacteria.
7. Describe the following biochemical tests and their use in distinguishing species: arylsulfatase, catalase, iron uptake, niacin accumulation, nitrate reduction, Tween 80 hydrolysis, tellurite reduction, and inhibition by thiophene-2-carboxylic acid hydrazide (TCH).
8. List the various molecular methods for organism identification.
9. Describe the different methods available for antimicrobial susceptibility testing.
10. Use electronic resources to find the most current treatment guidelines published by CDC.

SUMMARY OF KEY POINTS

Mycobacteria are nonmotile, non–spore-forming bacilli that are ubiquitous in nature. The genus *Mycobacterium* is the only genus in the family *Mycobacteriaceae*. These organisms are strict aerobes and are characterized by their "acid-fastness." They have a very high lipid content in their cell walls and do not stain with the common stains, such as the Gram stain. They can be induced to stain by prolonged application of dyes or application of heat. A distinguishing characteristic of these organisms is their resistance to decolorization by acidified alcohol, hence the description of acid-fastness. These organisms are also slow growers compared to other bacteria; generation times vary from 8 to 24 hours.

The mycobacteria are divided into two broad groups based on disease association: *Mycobacterium tuberculosis* complex *(M. tuberculosis, M. bovis, M. africanum)* and the nontuberculous mycobacteria. Mycobacteria other than *M. tuberculosis* (MOTT) have historically been divided into four working groups, the classic Runyon grouping system, based on growth rate and colony pigmentation. With the advent of liquid media and the need to decrease turnaround times plus newly discovered strain variability, this grouping system is no longer used. MOTT are ubiquitous in soil and water and not usually associated with person-to-person transmission.

M. avium complex (MAC) is ubiquitous in nature and had been considered to have low pathogenicity for man. With the advent of the AIDS epidemic, it has become an important pathogen that can cause disseminated disease in the immunocompromised and lymphadenitis in children.

Specimens for culture must be decontaminated to reduce overgrowth of normal flora. NaOH is a common decontamination agent, but the method used must be compatible with the automated liquid media system in use. The mucolytic agent NALC is used to digest mucus and free trapped mycobacteria. To increase the recovery rate, specimens are concentrated by centrifugation at a relative centrifugal force of at least 3000 *g*. Smears are then prepared and stained. Most laboratories currently use the fluorochrome stain auramine O because it is more sensitive than the Kinyoun stain. The Kinyoun and Ziehl-Neelsen stains can be used to confirm a positive fluorochrome stain or to look for contamination. Studies have shown that microscopy requires 5000 to 10,000 bacilli/mL of sputum for direct observation, whereas culture can detect as few as 10 to 100 viable organisms.

The current culture recommendations are to use a liquid medium as the primary method for *M. tuberculosis* (MTB) isolation. Optimal recovery is achieved by inoculating both liquid and solid media. Nonselective solid media include the egg-based Löwenstein-Jensen agar and the agar-based Middlebrook 7H10 or Middlebrook 7H11. Selective media or isolate-specific media may also be used (e.g., *M. haemophilum* grows on chocolate agar). The automated systems have been validated for a 6-week incubation period, whereas conventional media requires a minimum incubation of 8 weeks.

The traditional identification protocol was to perform biochemical testing. This requires a pure culture and more than 100 colonies. Tests used to differentiate the mycobacteria include arylsulfatase, catalase, growth rate and pigment production, iron uptake, niacin accumulation, nitrate reduction, Tween 80 hydrolysis, and others. Difficulties associated with biochemical testing include poor reproducibility of results and the fact that the organism must be at the correct phase in the growth curve for accurate results. The current trend is to use DNA sequencing for identification. New species are continually being identified with that identification based solely on DNA sequencing.

With the emergence of multidrug resistance in MTB, susceptibility testing is vital. The Centers for Disease Control and Prevention (CDC) and American Thoracic Society recommend the first isolate of MTB from a patient have susceptibility testing performed. Testing can be by direct or indirect methods. If more than 1% of the bacilli in the test population are resistant, a poor clinical outcome is predicted. Molecular approaches have been developed for detection of rifampin and isoniazid resistance. Other novel approaches using luciferase and chemiluminescence have been developed. The impetus is to detect drug resistance as quickly as possible to ensure appropriate antimicrobial therapy.

INTEREST POINT

Included in the genus *Mycobacterium* are the organisms that cause tuberculosis and leprosy. Evidence of the presence of tuberculosis has been found in Neolithic sites that are 4000 years old. Tuberculosis and leprosy were well recognized in the oldest civilizations from China, Egypt, and India. Leprosy appears to have originated in the Near East or Africa and spread with human immigrants to the Americas in the last 500 years. Although these are ancient organisms and disease conditions, we are still wrestling with their unique problems of diagnosis and control.

Mycobacterium leprae is noncultivatable. It has a cell doubling time of 12 to 14 days only in a select group of animals. It has been laboratory grown in armadillos and in the footpads of mice. Diagnosis is still based on clinical symptoms; modern diagnostic tools include demonstration of acid-fast bacilli in smears made from skin lesions and detection of IgM specific antibodies to the glycolipid PGL-1. In 1991, the World Health Assembly passed a resolution to eliminate leprosy as a public health problem by the year 2000. Although about 4 million leprosy cases have been cured since 2000, there were still 410,000 new cases detected in 2004. In nine countries in Africa,

Asia, and Latin America, leprosy is still considered a public health problem; these countries account for about 75% of the global disease burden. Several recent studies have reported relapse rates of 16% to 39% among patients with multibacillary leprosy (positive skin smears) 4 to 10 years after completion of drug therapy. Molecular methods are being explored for both diagnosis and drug susceptibility testing.

About one third of the world's population is infected with *Mycobacterium tuberculosis*. There was a rise in tuberculosis (TB) cases in the United States in the 1980s and early 1990s. CDC recommendations were published in 1993 that supported the use of rapid detection methods, species identification, and drug susceptibility testing. Fluorescence microscopy, liquid media, and rapid identification methods have allowed reporting of smear results within 1 day of specimen collection. The goal was also to report identification of *M. tuberculosis* complex within 21 days and susceptibility results within 30 days. With the goal of accomplishing the *Healthy People 2010* initiative objectives, the CDC issued its *National Plan for Reliable Tuberculosis Laboratory Services Using a Systems Approach* in the April 15, 2005, *MMWR*. Using nucleic acid amplification testing, fluorescence in situ hybridization, and fluorescence high-performance liquid chromatography of mycolic acids, the new goal is to confirm and report 75% of TB cases within 2 days of culture confirmation (i.e., to have an organism identification within 2 days of growth). The way to accomplish this rapid turnaround time and comply with competency and quality assurance issues is to regionalize services. We will be seeing much change in laboratory operations and organization as laboratories struggle to meet these turnaround time goals. The full report can be accessed at *www.cdc.gov/MMWR/preview/MMWRhtml/rr5406a1.htm*.

In December 2005, the CDC issued guidelines for a newly FDA-approved test, the QuantiFERON-TB Gold (QFT-G) test for detecting MTB infection. This test differs from the tuberculin skin test in that the QFT-G test measures the in vitro release of interferon-gamma in fresh heparinized whole blood specimens. This test may be used in all situations where the tuberculin skin test is used, including contact investigations, evaluation of recent immigrants who have had BCG vaccination, and MTB screening of health care workers. Limitations to widespread use of this test include high test cost and the need to process/test specimens within 12 hours of specimen collection. Complete guidelines may be accessed at *www.cdc.gov/mmwr/preview/mmwrhtml/rr5415a4.htm*.

The nail care business is a multibillion dollar industry in this country. But is it safe to get a pedicure? The first known outbreak of *M. fortuitum* cutaneous infections acquired from whirlpool footbaths was reported in October 2000 in California. Since then, similar outbreaks have been reported in 2002 in California and 2003 in Georgia. Various rapid-growing mycobacteria species can be found in municipal water supplies. It is believed that these bacteria colonize parts of the foot spas, particularly the drain areas and inlet screens. People at greatest risk for furunculosis (large boils on the skin) are those who have shaved their legs within 24 hours of the pedicure or who have open wounds on their legs. Customers can protect themselves by observing how the foot spas are cleaned between customers, not shaving before a pedicure, knowing the local health department regulations for nail salons, and using their personal bottles of nail polish. If the customer is not satisfied with the foot spa cleaning process or the disinfection of nail care tools, the customer should leave that salon and go to one that follows health department regulations. Helpful information for customers can be found in the following fact sheets: *www.barbercosmo.ca.gov/formspubs/manicure_factsheet.pdf* and *www.license.state.tx.us/cosmet/forms/footsparegulations.pdf*.

KEY TERMS AND ABBREVIATIONS

Match the term in the left column with the definition on the right.

1. _____ acid-fastness
2. _____ BCG
3. _____ PPD
4. _____ Runyon groups
5. _____ photochromogen
6. _____ scotochromogen
7. _____ nonphotochromogen
8. _____ rapidly growing NTM
9. _____ ubiquitous
10. _____ Hansen's disease
11. _____ Ziehl-Neelsen
12. _____ mucolytic agent
13. _____ decontaminant and digestant

A. colonies become pigmented when exposed to light
B. tuberculin skin test
C. staining method for acid-fast bacilli
D. NaOH
E. resists decolorization by acidified alcohol
F. colonies produce no pigment regardless of how they are grown
G. attenuated strain of *M. bovis*
H. existing everywhere
I. colonies are pigmented whether grown in dark or light
J. classification system based on pigmentation and growth rate
K. NALC
L. leprosy
M. nontuberculous mycobacteria that appear on solid media in 7 days or less

TRUE OR FALSE

1. _____ *M. gordonae* is a nonpathogen found in tap water.
2. _____ Although the QuantiFERON-TB Gold test is a promising new test for tuberculosis, it is not widely used because specimens must be tested within 12 hours of collection.
3. _____ The Ziehl-Neelsen carbolfuchsin stain is more sensitive than the fluorochrome stain.
4. _____ Good laboratory practice to prevent cross contamination of stained smears is to wipe the oil immersion objective after each positive smear.
5. _____ Because *M. leprae* cannot be cultivated on artificial media, diagnosis is based on the clinical picture and AFB-positive skin smears.
6. _____ Swabs in Stuart's media are acceptable wound specimens for mycobacterial culture.
7. _____ A chocolate agar plate is required for the recovery of *M. haemophilum*.
8. _____ An attenuated strain of *M. tuberculosis* has been used extensively to immunize against tuberculosis.
9. _____ The PPD test is highly sensitive and a positive reaction signals the presence of disease.
10. _____ A commonly isolated nontuberculous species seen in respiratory infections of AIDS patients is *M. fortuitum*.

MULTIPLE CHOICE

1. _____ Rough, buff-colored slow-growing colonies on a Löwenstein-Jensen slant should be tested for ___ as a preliminary identification of *M. tuberculosis*?
   A. Tween 80 hydrolysis
   B. iron uptake
   C. niacin production
   D. arylsulfatase
2. _____ Members of the *M. tuberculosis* complex include
   A. *M. bovis*.
   B. *M. leprae*.
   C. *M. kansasii*.
   D. *M. avium*.
3. _____ Specimens requiring digestion and decontamination prior to culture include
   A. sputum.
   B. CSF.
   C. pleural fluid.
   D. bone marrow aspirate.
4. _____ A fisherman from Louisiana developed a papular nodule on his finger 2 weeks after a boating accident. Culture yielded an acid-fast bacillus that grew best at 30° C and was identified as
   A. *M. avium*.
   B. *M. simiae*.
   C. *M. scrofulaceum*.
   D. *M. marinum*.
5. _____ Which charateristic best distinguishes *M. tuberculosis* from *M. avium* complex?
   A. Niacin production
   B. Tween 80 hydrolysis
   C. Iron uptake
   D. Pyrazinamidase

CASE STUDY

A 2-year-old female child presented to the emergency department with symptoms of fever and seizures. The following laboratory tests were ordered: CBC, basic metabolic panel, ASO, mononucleosis screen, urinalysis, blood culture. The child had a high WBC count ($16.2 \times 10^3/\mu L$) with a differential showing 75% neutrophils, 15% lymphocytes, and 10% monocytes. The ASO and mono screens were negative. A lumbar puncture was performed. The CSF was colorless but cloudy. The CSF cell count showed 460 WBC/mm^3 with a distribution showing 10% neutrophils, 78% lymphocytes, and 12% mononuclear cells. The WBC and RBC normal reference counts on CSF were 0 to 5 cells/mm^3. The CSF RBC was 12 RBC/mm^3, glucose was 79 mg/dL (reference range 40 to 70 mg/dL), and protein was 260 mg/dL (reference range 15 to 60 mg/dL). A cryptococcal antigen test on CSF was negative. Additional tests were ordered on the CSF; they were bacterial culture, fungus culture, AFB culture, enterovirus by PCR, and herpes simplex virus by PCR.

1. What is the significance of a cloudy CSF?
2. In bacterial meningitis, what kind of values (high or low) would you expect to see for CSF glucose and protein? Why would the results be distributed in this manner?
3. The CSF Gram stain showed many WBCs but no organisms. With the limited information the physician had on the initial visit, what pathogens should he suspect?
4. Over the next 5 days, the following results became available:
   - CSF had no growth at 72 hours.
   - Blood culture had no growth at 5 days.
   - AFB smear had no acid-fast bacilli seen.
   - Fungus smear had no fungal elements seen.
   - Enterovirus by PCR was negative.
   - Herpes simplex virus by PCR was negative.
   At 4 weeks, the fungus culture was finalized as negative. The reference laboratory performing the AFB culture called with a critical value—the liquid culture media had growth in it.
   Why didn't the AFB smear and culture results match?
5. To expedite the process, the pediatrician ordered a direct DNA probe for *M. tuberculosis* complex on the broth sediment. *M. tuberculosis* was identified by direct probe. Susceptibilities were performed but those results were not available for an additional 3 weeks. What are the current CDC recommendations for antimicrobial therapy for this organism?
6. What are the laboratory's responsibilities regarding reporting of this AFB culture both to the ordering physician and health department?

ANSWERS

Key Terms and Abbreviations
1. E
2. G
3. B
4. J
5. A
6. I
7. F
8. M
9. H
10. L
11. C
12. K
13. D

True or False
1. T
2. T
3. F
4. T
5. T
6. F
7. T
8. F
9. F
10. F

Multiple Choice
1. C
2. A
3. A
4. D
5. A

Case Study
1. A cloudy or turbid CSF is indicative of the presence of many leukocytes.
2. In bacterial meningitis the CSF is usually cloudy due to the presence of many neutrophils. The glucose concentration is decreased due to the utilization of glucose during bacterial metabolism. The protein concentration is usually elevated. Protein in CSF increases due to meningeal inflammation and changes in capillary permeability.
3. In viral meningitis the CSF is usually clear with a slight increase in protein and a preponderance of mononuclear cells. No organisms would be seen on the Gram stain but lymphocytes and monocytes would make up the majority of the cells seen. In tuberculous meningitis, the glucose would be decreased, protein would be increased, and there would be many mononuclear cells.
4. The sensitivity of the AFB culture is much greater than that for the AFB smear. Microscopy requires 100 times more cells for direct observation than for recovery in culture. AFB smear results are commonly negative while cultures will yield growth.
5. In June 2003, the CDC in conjunction with the American Thoracic Society and the Infectious Diseases Society of America published guidelines for the treatment of tuberculosis. Tuberculous meningitis is a disease associated with high morbidity and mortality despite prompt initiation of therapy. Tuberculosis in infants and children younger than 4 years of age is more likely to disseminate; prompt treatment is critical

in this patient population. Patients presenting with more severe neurologic symptoms have a greater risk of neurologic sequelae and a higher mortality. Chemotherapy should begin with a regimen of four drugs: isoniazid (INH), rifampin (RIF), pyrazinamide (PZA), and ethambutol (EMB). After 2 months if the organism is a susceptible strain, the PZA and EMB may be discontinued. The INH and RIF should be continued for 7 to 10 months.

6. Positive AFB smear or culture results should be regarded as critical values and reported to the physician via phone call. The local health department should be notified both by phone and in writing. The occurrence of TB among children indicates the recent transmission of the bacillus from an infected adult in the community or family. The most important step to detect and prevent tuberculosis among children is prompt identification and adequate treatment of infected adults.

REFERENCES

American Thoracic Society, CDC, and Infectious Diseases Society of America: Controlling tuberculosis in the United States, *Morb Mortal Wkly Rep* 54:RR-12, 2005.

American Thoracic Society, CDC, and Infectious Diseases Society of America: Treatment of tuberculosis, *Morb Mortal Wkly Rep* 52:RR-11, 2003.

Centers for Disease Control and Prevention. Guidelines for using QuantiFERON-TB Gold Test for detecting *Mycobacterium tuberculosis* infection, United States, *Morb Mortal Wkly Rep* 54:RR-15, 2005.

Centers for Disease Control and Prevention: National plan for reliable tuberculosis laboratory services using a systems approach, *Morb Mortal Wkly Rep* 54:RR-06, 2005.

Scollard DM, Adams LB, Gillis TP, et al: The continuing challenges of leprosy, *Clin Microbiol Rev* 19:338, 2006.

Vugia DJ, Jang Y, Zizek C, et al: Mycobacteria in nail salon whirlpool footbaths, California. *Emerg Infect Dis* [serial on the Internet]. 2005 Apr [date cited]. Available from *www.cdc.gov/ncidod/EID/vol11no04/04-0936.htm.*

46 Obligate Intracellular and Nonculturable Bacterial Agents

OBJECTIVES

Upon completion of this chapter, the reader should be able to:

1. Describe how *Chlamydia trachomatis* is transmitted and describe the diseases it causes.
2. List the diagnostic tools for detection of chlamydial infection.
3. Describe the epidemiology of psittacosis.
4. Explain the clinical significance of *Chlamydophila pneumoniae*.
5. List the disease syndromes associated with rickettsiae and their vectors.
6. Differentiate between human granulocytic ehrlichiosis and human monocytic ehrlichiosis.
7. Describe the clinical picture, cause, and transmission of Q fever.
8. List the disease conditions associated with *Tropheryma whippleii* and *Calymmatobacterium granulomatis*.

SUMMARY OF KEY POINTS

All of the organisms addressed in this chapter are very small obligate intracellular parasites or are extremely difficult to culture.

Chlamydia are common pathogens throughout the animal kingdom. They replicate within the cytoplasm of the host cell and form characteristic inclusions (reticulate bodies). They have often been called energy parasites because they cannot manufacture adenosine triphosphate (ATP) and they use the ATP produced by the host cell. *C. trachomatis* causes trachoma, inclusion conjunctivitis of the newborn, lymphogranuloma venereum, and genital tract diseases. It is the most common bacterial sexually transmitted disease (STD) in the United States and infects hundreds of millions of people worldwide. Genital *Chlamydia* infections have been associated with increased rate of HIV transmission; chlamydia-induced inflammation causes the recruitment of CD4 lymphocytes. *C. psittaci* infects birds; humans become infected by aerosol inhalation upon contact with infected birds. *C. pneumoniae*, however, is strictly a human pathogen that causes pneumonia, sinusitis, and pharyngitis. It has also been implicated in atherosclerotic cardiovascular disease.

The *Rickettsia* species infect vascular endothelial cells, particularly the skin, brain, and lung. They gain entrance to the human body via bite by an infected arthropod. The common vectors are fleas, ticks, and the human body louse. Rickettsial disease can be divided into three groups: typhus, spotted fever, and scrub typhus. Typhus epidemics have sporadically killed thousands of people throughout history. In 430 BC, Thucydides wrote that half the population of Athens had been killed during an epidemic that was probably attributable to returning soldiers. In the United States, however, the most important rickettsial infection is Rocky Mountain spotted fever. Although the organisms can be cultured, diagnosis is based on serology testing.

Ehrlichiosis is a zoonotic disease that is transmitted to humans via tick bite. The most common vector is the Lonestar tick; these ticks have a white spot on their bodies and actively seek a host. The natural reservoirs for the *Ehrlichiae* are deer, domestic dogs, sheep, cattle, and goats. Both *E. chaffeensis* (causes human monocytic infection) and *Anaplasma phagocytophilum* (causes human granulocytic disease) produce a febrile illness with leukopenia, thrombocytopenia, and increased aspartate aminotransferase (AST) in serum. Diagnosis during the acute phase can be made by polymerase chain reaction (PCR) amplification, detection of *E. chaffeensis* morulae in the cytoplasm of infected WBCs, and culture of peripheral blood. Tetracyclines are the drugs of choice.

Coxiella burnetii causes Q fever and is an obligate intracellular pathogen, although it can survive extracellularly by forming spores. This is a successful pathogen because it can survive for long periods in its spore form (up to 1 month on meat in cold storage) and is highly infectious when aerosolized. It is an occupational hazard among people having contact with cattle, sheep, and goats. The organisms reach high numbers in the placenta and can be dispersed during live births when aerosols are generated. Diagnosis is made serologically by antibody detection. Tetracyclines are the drugs of choice.

KEY TERMS AND ABBREVIATIONS

Match the term in the left column with the definition on the right.

1. _____ reticulate body	A. major cause of pelvic inflammatory disease
2. _____ elementary body	B. major cause of blindness worldwide
3. _____ *C. trachomatis*	C. intracellular replicative form
4. _____ apoptosis	D. endemic pathogen of all bird species
5. _____ trachoma	E. human monocytic ehrlichiosis
6. _____ lymphogranuloma venereum	F. metabolically inert infective form
7. _____ *C. psittaci*	G. programmed cell death
8. _____ *Chlamydophila pneumoniae*	H. Whipple's disease
9. _____ *Rickettsia*	I. STD characterized by acute lymphadenitis
10. _____ *E. chaffeensis*	

11. ____ *Anaplasma phagocytophilum*
12. ____ *Coxiella burnetii*
13. ____ *Tropheryma whippleii*
14. ____ *Calymmatobacterium granulomatis*

J. Strictly human pathogen causing pneumonia
K. Rocky Mountain spotted fever
L. Q fever
M. human granulocytic ehrlichiosis
N. granuloma inguinale

TRUE OR FALSE

1. ____ The best way to prevent infection with *C. burnetii* is to avoid contact with infected animals.
2. ____ *Ehrlichia ewingii* has been identified as the causative agent of Whipple's disease.
3. ____ Immunity provides little protection from reinfection with *C. trachomatis*.
4. ____ Because chlamydiae are labile, the organisms can best be maintained for culture by keeping specimens cold.
5. ____ Psittacosis is caused by infection with *Rickettsia prowazekii*.
6. ____ The triad of symptoms—headache, rash, fever—is the primary clinical manifestation in patients who have been bitten by insect vectors.
7. ____ Culture is recommended for *C. trachomatis* detection in cases of suspected sexual abuse or suspected failure of therapy.
8. ____ *C. pneumoniae* is transmitted to humans via bird or animal reservoirs.
9. ____ In the United States, the most important rickettsial infection is Rocky Mountain spotted fever.
10. ____ Most *C. pneumoniae* infections are diagnosed serologically, but respiratory specimens may also be cultured.

MULTIPLE CHOICE

1. ____ The causative agent of human granulocytic ehrlichiosis is
   A. *Ehrlichia chaffeensis.*
   B. *Ehrlichia ewingii.*
   C. *Ehrlichia sennetsu.*
   D. *Anaplasma phagocytophium.*
2. ____ The test method recommended for detection of *C. trachomatis* in endocervical specimens is
   A. culture using HeLa cells.
   B. Gram stain for inclusions.
   C. amplified DNA testing.
   D. direct immunofluorescence.
3. ____ Rocky Mountain spotted fever is caused by
   A. *Rickettsia rickettsii.*
   B. *Rickettsia prowazekii.*
   C. *Coxiella burnetii.*
   D. *Ehrlichia chaffeensis.*

4. ____ A 19-year-old male student went to the college clinic complaining of painful urination and a urethral discharge. Gonorrhea was diagnosed and he was given an intramuscular injection of ceftriaxone. Four days later the student was back at the clinic; his symptoms had not improved with treatment. The student was given a 7-day supply of doxycycline. His symptoms improved. The student was most likely infected with
   A. *Treponema pallidum.*
   B. Herpes simplex virus.
   C. *Chlamydia trachomatis.*
   D. human papillomavirus.
5. ____ A baby was born to a mother infected with *C. trachomatis.* A week after birth the baby began to have a slight discharge from one eye. The best test method for *Chlamydia* infection in the newborn is
   A. IgM antibody.
   B. IgG antibody.
   C. amplified DNA testing.
   D. culture.

CASE STUDY

A 6-year-old boy was complaining of fever for several days. The pediatrician ordered the following tests: CBC, ASO, Epstein-Barr virus antibody panel, Rocky Mountain spotted fever (RMSF) antibody panel—IgG and IgM, Lyme antibody screen. The CBC was normal, the EBV panel was negative, and the Lyme screen was negative. The ASO was positive to a titer of 400 IU/mL. The rickettsia antibody results were as follows: IgG, 0.2; IgM, 3.4. (Reference values: ≤ 0.8, negative; ≥ 1.2, positive.)

1. This is a diverse group of tests. What do you think the rationale is for ordering an ASO? RMSF antibody panel? Lyme antibody screen?
2. Can any disease syndrome be ruled out from these results?
3. How would you interpret the RMSF antibody panel results?

ANSWERS

Key Terms and Abbreviations

1. C
2. F
3. A
4. G
5. B
6. I
7. D
8. J
9. K
10. E
11. M
12. L
13. H
14. N

True or False

1. T
2. F
3. T
4. T
5. F
6. T
7. T
8. F
9. T
10. T

Multiple Choice

1. D
2. C
3. A
4. C
5. D

Case Study

1. ASO stands for antistreptolysin O titer. It detects antibodies to antistreptolysin O, a hemolysin produced by *Streptococcus pyogenes*. It can be used as an indicator of recent infection. Fever is a symptom of strep pharyngitis and rheumatic fever. The triad of symptoms—headache, rash, fever—is the primary clinical manifestation in patients who have been bitten by insect vectors. Severe headache and fever would be symptoms of RMSF. Fever would also be a symptom of Lyme disease.

2. The Epstein-Barr virus antibody panel and the Lyme disease screen were both negative. The child does not appear to have an EBV infection or Lyme disease, although fever is one of the symptoms of mononucleosis.

3. IgG antibody titer is negative while IgM is a high positive value. A low positive IgM result would be suggestive of past infection; IgM antibodies may persist for as long as 12 months after infection. This high value would be more indicative of recent or current infection. These results, however, are inconclusive for diagnosis. The best evidence for infection is a significant change on two timed (acute and convalescent) specimens wherein both tests are performed by the same laboratory at the same time.

47 Cell Wall–Deficient Bacteria: *Mycoplasma* and *Ureaplasma*

OBJECTIVES

Upon completion of this chapter, the reader should be able to:

1. Explain how mycoplasmas and ureaplasmas are different from other bacteria.
2. Explain the clinical significance of *M. pneumoniae*, *M. hominis,* and *U. urealyticum.*
3. List the tests used to diagnose the illnesses caused by these organisms.
4. List the drugs of choice for pneumonia caused by *M. pneumoniae.*
5. List the disease conditions associated with *M. fermentans* and *M. genitalium.*
6. List the media used to isolate these pathogens.

SUMMARY OF KEY POINTS

The mycoplasmas and ureaplasmas belong to the class of bacteria known as Mollicutes. They differ from other bacteria because they lack a cell wall, have a very small genome, and have limited ability to synthesize biochemicals. Consequently, they require enriched media for growth. Because they lack a cell wall, the beta-lactam antibiotics are ineffective and they do not stain with the Gram stain.

Three significant pathogens from this class include *M. pneumoniae, M. hominis,* and *U. urealyticum. M. pneumoniae* is the most common cause of bacterial pneumonia in school-age children and adults younger than 30 years of age. Mollicutes have been implicated as a cause of nongonococcal urethritis; these organisms include *M. hominis, M. genitalium,* and *U. urealyticum.* Although Mollicutes do not cause vaginitis, they do proliferate in patients with bacterial vaginosis (BV). BV is a polymicrobic phenomenon in which there is a shift in the relative percentages of organism types. Although *M. hominis* and *U. urealyticum* have been isolated from the genital tracts of sexually active asymptomatic men and women, their presence in the lower genital tract of pregnant women has been associated with prematurity and low–birth-weight infants. *U. urealyticum* can initiate an intense inflammatory reaction and has been implicated as a cause of endometritis, chorioamnionitis (infection of the placental membranes and amniotic fluid), and premature rupture of membranes.

Although *M. fermentans* has been regarded as a tissue culture contaminant for many years, in the 1980s it was isolated from Kaposi sarcoma lesions of HIV patients. This organism is being studied for its role in HIV pathogenesis, sexually transmitted diseases, chronic fatigue syndrome, and other conditions.

M. pneumoniae can be retrieved by culturing sputum, lung tissue, and other specimen types, but polymerase chain reaction (PCR) is a more sensitive test for the detection of this organism in clinical specimens. Diagnosis, however, is usually made serologically. Acute and convalescent blood specimens for IgG and IgM antibodies are usually tested. Genital mycoplasmas are detected by culture. The specimens should be protected from drying and should be transported in a special medium such as M4.

KEY TERMS AND ABBREVIATIONS

Match the term in the left column with the definition on the right.

1. _____ Mollicute
2. _____ commensal
3. _____ *M. hominis*
4. _____ *M. pneumoniae*
5. _____ *U. urealyticum*
6. _____ *M. genitalium*
7. _____ chorioamnionitis
8. _____ community-acquired pneumonia
9. _____ bacterial vaginosis
10. _____ *M. fermentans*

A. associated with non-gonococcal urethritis
B. rapid grower that produces urease
C. polymicrobic condition
D. cause of community-acquired pneumonia
E. infectious agent living in balance with its host
F. membranes contain sterol
G. associated with HIV infection
H. has "fried egg" appearance on culture
I. lung infection not acquired in a hospital setting
J. infection of placental membranes

TRUE OR FALSE

1. _____ Swabs with wooden shafts should not be used because the wood itself may be toxic to ureaplasmas.
2. _____ Mycoplasmas are inherently sensitive to the penicillins.
3. _____ *U. urealyticum* colonies can be identified by their utilization of arginine.
4. _____ Mycoplasmas are part of the normal flora of the human oropharynx.
5. _____ Susceptibility testing is recommended on all isolates of *U. urealyticum.*

MULTIPLE CHOICE

1. _____ A nonspecific serologic test that used to be popular in diagnosing *M. pneumonia* infection is
   A. cold agglutinin assay.
   B. PCR.
   C. immunoblotting.
   D. indirect immunofluorescence.

2. _____ The drugs of choice for the genital ureaplasmas are the
   A. penicillins.
   B. cephalosporins.
   C. tetracyclines.
   D. carbapenems.

3. _____ The most common cause of pneumonia in school-age children is
   A. *Streptococcus pneumoniae.*
   B. *Mycoplasma pneumoniae.*
   C. *Staphylococcus aureus.*
   D. *Mycoplasma fermentans.*

4. _____ The required culture medium for *M. pneumoniae* is
   A. Thayer Martin agar.
   B. trypticase soy agar.
   C. Middlebrook 7H11 agar.
   D. biphasic SP-4 media.

5. _____ One should suspect *M. hominis* in an anaerobic culture of prostate secretions if
   A. pinpoint colonies show no bacteria on Gram stain.
   B. colonies are urease-positive.
   C. colonies are positive with the flagella stain.
   D. suspicious colonies hemadsorb when overlaid with red blood cells.

CASE STUDY

A 27-year-old woman presented to the obstetrics triage area with complaints of a stabbing pain from the lower rib cage to the knees for the previous 14 hours. The patient was 29 weeks' pregnant. The patient stated she rested much of the day and the pain had subsided to a dull ache. She denied regular contractions or vaginal bleeding. The patient was admitted for observation with a diagnosis of threatened labor—antepartum complications. The patient was put on a fetal monitor and the following laboratory tests were ordered: fetal fibronectin, genital culture, urinalysis, urine culture, *C. trachomatis/N. gonorrhoeae* by amplified probe, genital viral culture, and *M. hominis/U. urealyticum* culture.

The urinalysis and fetal fibronectin were performed as STAT tests. The urinalysis was normal and fetal fibronectin was negative. The obstetrics nurse noted from the fetal monitor that the baby was very active. The patient was discharged with instructions to rest the following day and was given an information sheet on preterm labor.

The remaining test results were as follows:

Genital culture	No group B strep isolated
	Normal vaginal flora isolated
Urine culture	No growth after 48 hours
C. trachomatis/N. gonorrhoeae amplified probe	Negative for both organisms
Viral culture	Negative
M. hominis/U. urealyticum culture	Positive for *U. urealyticum* Negative for *M. hominis*

NOTE: The significance of the fetal fibronectin (fFN) test is that it is used to help predict preterm delivery. fFN is a protein produced during pregnancy that functions as a kind of glue to keep the fetal sac attached to the uterine lining. If fFN is found in cervicovaginal secretions during 22 to 34 weeks of gestation, it could indicate an increased risk for preterm delivery.

1. Why is the genital culture result in two parts with a specific mention of group B strep?
2. Why was a molecular probe done to test for gonococci and chlamydia?
3. Why was a culture for mycoplasmas and ureaplasmas done?

ANSWERS

Key Terms and Abbreviations

1. F
2. E
3. H
4. D
5. B
6. A
7. J
8. I
9. C
10. G

True or False

1. T
2. F
3. F
4. T
5. F

Multiple Choice

1. A
2. C
3. B
4. D
5. A

Case Study

1. Of great significance during pregnancy is the fact that infection can be transmitted from mother to infant while still in utero or during delivery. Organisms that

can cross the placenta and have adverse effects on the developing fetus include *Listeria monocytogenes, Toxoplasma gondii,* cytomegalovirus, parvovirus B19, and enteroviruses. Organisms that can ascend from the vagina and infect fetal membranes include the group B streptococci, genital mycoplasmas, and herpes simplex virus. Approximately one third of American females are colonized with group B strep. Although this may be considered normal vaginal flora, the consequences for the neonate can include meningitis. Clinical practice guidelines for the management of pregnant women with group B strep colonization have been published by the Centers for Disease Control and Prevention.

2. *Chlamydia trachomatis* is the leading bacterial cause of sexually transmitted disease. It can ascend the genital tract and cause endometritis, salpingitis, and pelvic inflammatory disease. Neonates can be infected as they pass through the birth canal. Chlamydial infection in these infants takes the form of conjunctivitis, pneumonia, and nasopharyngeal infections. For detection of chlamydia, amplification assays are considered to be more sensitive than hybridization assays or culture.

3. The presence of *M. hominis* or *U. urealyticum* in the lower genital tract of pregnant women has been associated with prematurity and low–birth-weight infants. *U. urealyticum* can initiate an intense inflammatory reaction and has been implicated as a cause of endometritis, chorioamnionitis (infection of the placental membranes and amniotic fluid), and premature rupture of membranes.

48 The Spirochetes

OBJECTIVES

Upon completion of this chapter, the reader should be able to:
1. Describe several distinguishing characteristics of spirochetes and list the genera that are pathogenic for humans.
2. Trace the clinical picture through the stages of venereal syphilis.
3. List the diagnostic tests for syphilis.
4. Describe the clinical picture, cause, and diagnosis of Lyme disease.
5. Name the organism responsible for human relapsing fever.
6. Describe leptospirosis—its cause, transmission, and diagnosis.

SUMMARY OF KEY POINTS

Spirochetes are long, slender, helical, gram-negative rods. These organisms are differentiated using morphologic features. Three genera contain human pathogens; they are *Treponema, Borrelia,* and *Leptospira.*

Treponema pallidum causes venereal syphilis. It enters its human host by penetrating the mucous membranes or through breaks in the skin. A painless chancre appears at the inoculation site. This sexually transmitted disease (STD) progresses through several stages. Secondary syphilis takes weeks to become apparent; at this stage the patient is ill with a widespread rash, fever, and weight loss and seeks medical attention. Late or tertiary syphilis may not occur until 25 years after primary infection, when there is tissue destruction. There can be central nervous system (CNS) involvement and the formation of gummas in any organ. Patients can exhibit signs of dementia, depression, and confusion.

The most commonly performed serologic test for syphilis is the RPR. The VDRL is performed on cerebrospinal fluid (CSF). The RPR is a useful screening tool, but positive tests should be confirmed with the more specific FTA-ABS. If equivocal results are obtained, a second FTA-ABS performed 2 to 4 weeks later may prove helpful. The TP-PA may also be performed to help interpret test results.

T. pallidum can also cross the placenta to cause congenital syphilis. Symptoms may not be present at birth. Diagnosis can be made by doing microscopy of fetal lesions, cord or placenta, by the VDRL on CSF, or by serologic tests for IgM-specific antibody using the FTA-ABS.

Other species of treponemes cause nonvenereal disease that includes pinta, yaws and bejel. The organisms that cause these diseases are transmitted by direct contact among children living in unsanitary conditions. The World Health Organization (WHO) sponsored a campaign during the 1950s to 1970s that significantly reduced the prevalence of yaws. These diseases are still endemic in parts of Central and South America as well as in Africa and Western Asia.

INTEREST POINT

In 1962 the Ministry of Public Health in the People's Republic of China (PRC) declared syphilis eradicated from that country. The history of STDs in China is an interesting one. Venereal disease is recorded to have arrived in China in 1504 when Dutch and Portuguese sailors in Canton (now called Guangzhou) transmitted the "Canton sore" to prostitutes. Another form of venereal disease resembling endemic syphilis came overland from India through Tibet and Outer Mongolia. Because of political turmoil and certain social customs, syphilis and gonorrhoeae gained a foothold and flourished.

Before 1949, venereal diseases were prevalent in China with an estimated 10 million cases. But after the civil war when the PRC was established, the government closed brothels, made prostitution illegal, opened STD clinics, and provided free health care. By the 1960s, STDs in China had been virtually eliminated. With the advent of the open door policy of the 1980s and changes in China's social environment, STD cases began to increase again.

The most common vector-borne disease in the United States is Lyme disease. It is caused by *Borrelia burgdorferi* and is transmitted to humans via tick bites. The Centers for Disease Control and Prevention recommends a two-step approach to diagnosis in the absence of the typical erythema migrans rash. Serology testing by IFA or ELISA is recommended as a screening tool. If the ELISA is positive, it should be confirmed by Western blot. The Infectious Disease Society of America (IDSA) has published treatment guidelines at *www.cdc.gov/ncidod/dvbid/lyme/IDSA_2000.pdf.*

Although the prevalence of leptospirosis in the United States is very low, it is considered to be the most widespread zoonotic disease in the world. Transmission is usually indirect by contact with contaminated water or soil. Veterinarians, animal workers, workers in rice fields, travelers, and people involved with water sports such as kayaking are at risk for infection. The microscopic agglutination test is not widely available but serologic tests for IgM-specific antibody are useful.

KEY TERMS AND ABBREVIATIONS

Match the term in the left column with the definition on the right.

1. _____ spirochetes
2. _____ Vincent's disease
3. _____ venereal syphilis
4. _____ chancre
5. _____ VDRL
6. _____ FTA-ABS
7. _____ RPR
8. _____ TP-PA
9. _____ relapsing fever
10. _____ Lyme disease
11. _____ zoonosis
12. _____ leptospirosis
13. _____ gumma
14. _____ erythema migrans

A. painless ulcer
B. disease is characterized by cyclic fever patterns
C. human disease caused by contact with infected blood or urine of animals
D. nontreponemal screening test
E. bull's eye skin lesion
F. destructive lesion of the gums
G. granuloma-like lesion
H. nontreponemal test done on CSF
I. caused by *T. pallidum*
J. disease transmitted to humans via animals
K. helically curved gram-negative rods
L. caused by *B. burgdorferi*
M. treponemal indirect hemagglutination test
N. fluorescent treponemal test

TRUE OR FALSE

1. _____ Ticks transmit the spirochetes that cause Lyme disease within the first hour after attaching to their human host.
2. _____ Spirochetes are differentiated by the number of insertion disks present.
3. _____ Several treponeme species are considered to be normal oral and genital flora.
4. _____ A positive ELISA test for Lyme disease should be confirmed by Western blot.
5. _____ Diagnosis of leptospirosis is usually made by detection of IgM antibodies in acute and convalescent sera.
6. _____ Treponemes can infect the umbilical cord and cross the placenta.
7. _____ Reaginic antibodies are produced against antigens of *T. pallidum*.
8. _____ Extreme water sports are a risk factor for leptospirosis.
9. _____ Human relapsing fever is caused by the bite of the human body louse.
10. _____ Susceptibility testing of *Borrelia* spp. to doxycycline should always be done because of the incidence of treatment failure.

MULTIPLE CHOICE

1. _____ Relapsing fever is caused by
   A. *L. interrogans.*
   B. *T. pallidum.*
   C. *B. burgdorferi.*
   D. *B. recurrentis.*
2. _____ Primary syphilis is characterized by the appearance of
   A. erythema migrans rash.
   B. gumma.
   C. chancre.
   D. gingivitis.
3. _____ The test for syphilis that should be performed on CSF is
   A. VDRL.
   B. RPR.
   C. ELISA.
   D. Western blot.
4. _____ For all treponemal infections, the drug of choice is
   A. penicillin G.
   B. doxycycline.
   C. tetracycline.
   D. ceftriaxone.
5. _____ can cause false positive results in the RPR test?
   A. Rheumatoid disease
   B. Old age
   C. Tuberculosis
   D. All of the above

CASE STUDY

An 81-year-old woman presented to the emergency department (ED) with symptoms of confusion, paranoia, and delusions. The ED physician ordered the following tests: CBC, chemistry panel, urinalysis, urine toxicology screen, TSH, and RPR. The CBC results were unremarkable. The toxicology screen was negative. The urinalysis was normal. Elevated chemistry values included BUN, creatinine, glucose, alkaline phosphatase, and TSH.

1. Why order a test for venereal syphilis on an 81-year-old patient?
2. The RPR result was reported as "reactive." What additional testing should be done at this point?
3. Syphilis is a reportable disease to state health departments. At what point in the testing process should the health department be notified of the positive test results?

ANSWERS

Key Terms and Abbreviations

1. K
2. F
3. I
4. A
5. H
6. N
7. D
8. M
9. B
10. L
11. J

12. C
13. G
14. E

True or False

1. F
2. T
3. T
4. T
5. T
6. T
7. F
8. T
9. T
10. F

Multiple Choice

1. D
2. C
3. A
4. A
5. D

Case Study

1. The disease progression for syphilis can be divided into three stages. The late or tertiary stage can occur 25 years after an initial untreated infection. Although very rare now, general paresis can result from damage to the nerves of the brain. This produces neuropsychiatric disturbances such as hallucinations and delusions. Hypothyroidism can also impair cerebral function and cause depression.

2. The RPR is a nontreponemal serologic test that is useful as a screening tool. The reaginic antibodies can be produced in response to syphilis, but also to tuberculosis, measles, hepatitis, rheumatoid disease, and old age. The test must be confirmed with a more specific test, such as the FTA-ABS and/or TP-PA.

3. Because so many disease conditions and factors can cause a false-positive RPR, health departments should not be notified until the results have been confirmed.

REFERENCES

Brown I: Exploring STDs in China, *Adv Med Lab Prof* 5:14, 1993.

Cohen MS, Henderson GE, Aiello P, Zheng H: Successful eradication of sexually transmitted diseases in the People's Republic of China: implications for the 21st century, *J Infect Dis* 174(Suppl 2):S223, 1996.

LaFond RE, Lukehart SA: Biological basis for syphilis, *Clin Microbiol Rev* 19:29, 2006.

49 Laboratory Methods for Diagnosis of Parasitic Infections

OBJECTIVES

Upon completion of this chapter, the reader should be able to:

1. Explain the ova and parasite (O&P) test for stool parasites including typical stains used.
2. Explain the preparation of thick and thin blood smears for blood parasites.
3. Explain other direct detection methods for parasites, including the pinworm test.
4. Describe the life cycle of *Plasmodium* spp. and the clinical presentation.
5. List the pathogenic intestinal amoeba, flagellates, and ciliates.
6. State a characteristic identifier for *E. histolytica, Giardia lamblia, Trichomonas vaginalis,* and *Balantidium coli.*
7. List the blood parasites and how to differentiate them.
8. List the roundworms that infect humans and how to identify them.
9. List the tapeworms that infect humans and how to identify them.
10. Describe the life cycle of trematodes, the species infective to man, and how to identify them.

SUMMARY OF KEY POINTS

Human understanding of parasites was very limited up until the 1600s. External parasites such as lice and fleas were obvious as were some internal parasites, such as tapeworms and pinworms. It was the belief that humans acquired these parasites by ingesting whole free-living organisms. It is thought that the name *fluke* came from the Anglo-Saxon *floc,* which means flounder. The intestinal flukes were thought to be fish *(floc)* that had gotten trapped in the wrong environment. But it was not until 1668 that the true nature of these worms and flukes was discovered by experimentation. Francesco Redi is considered to be the grandfather of parasitology. He performed his classic experiment of putting meat into three jars; one was sealed, one was left open, and one had a gauze covering. Maggots appeared on the meat in the open jar and on the gauze of the second jar, but not on the meat in the sealed jar. He also observed maggots and flies and discovered their life cycle.

Blood and tissue parasitic infections in the United States are rare and usually involve foreign-born individuals or recent returnees from endemic areas. But to peoples in other parts of the world, parasitic infections have devastating consequences. It is estimated that globally there are 500 million cases of malaria affecting the populations in more than 90 countries. About 2 million of these people die each year, most of them are children younger

than 5 years of age and pregnant women. For parasitic infections to flourish, vectors (transmitters) are needed, as are conditions that enhance the life cycles of the parasite. Good sanitation and nutrition, and a temperate climate do not promote parasitism.

Parasites are organisms that live on or in another organism at the expense of that organism. Most parasites are obligate and must spend part or all of their lives within a particular host. Others are free-living and accidentally form an association with a host, such as *Naegleria fowleri,* a free-swimming amoeba that accidentally enters human hosts who are in contaminated waters. However, it is not beneficial to the parasite to kill its host.

There are six major divisions of parasites. These are Protozoa, Nematodes (roundworms), Platyhelminthes (flatworms), Pentastomids (tongue worms), Acanthocephala, and Arthropoda (insects, ticks). Identification of parasites is based on their morphology and direct detection in a clinical specimen. There are also some cultivation methods and serologic tests that may be done.

Specimen collection and transport is important so that the organism can be preserved. The most common specimen submitted for parasite examination is stool. The O&P examination includes a direct wet mount of fresh stool to find motile protozoans, the concentrated specimen using a formalin-ether method to observe eggs, larvae, and cysts, and the permanent stained smear that facilitates identification of intestinal protozoa. Several staining methods are available. Microscopic examination requires a skilled technologist. Another common test is the pinworm preparation that looks for *Enterobius vermicularis* eggs in the perianal area. Sometimes specimens are recovered surgically, such as in duodenal drainage or washings that should be examined for *Giardia lamblia* and *Strongyloides* larvae. Another duodenal test involves the swallowing of a gelatin capsule and string; one end of the string protrudes from the mouth. When the string is removed, mucus and parasites can be recovered.

Other specimens include vaginal and prostatic secretions, urethral discharges, and urine sediment. These can be examined for *Trichomonas vaginalis.* Sputum can contain a variety of organisms including *A. lumbricoides, S. stercoralis, P. westermani, E. granulosus, E. histolytica,* and *Cryptosporidium* spp. Aspirated material from cysts and abscesses should be examined for amoeba and hydatid sand (scolices). A muscle biopsy may be helpful in the diagnosis of trichinosis.

Blood is an important specimen that can be used to diagnose several disease syndromes. Both thick and thin blood films should be made from fresh whole blood.

117

The recommended stain is Giemsa. The edges of the thin film should be examined for malaria parasites and trypanosomes. *Babesia* spp. may also be observed. Buffy coat preparations may also be useful.

Molecular methods are available but not in widespread use. Commercially available antigen tests compare well with microscopy and can be used to confirm infection with *E. histolytica, G. lamblia,* and *Cryptosporidium parvum.* Culture for parasite detection is rarely performed by microbiology laboratories. Serologic procedures are available but not routinely offered; the Centers for Disease Control and Prevention may be a resource for this testing.

The medically important parasites are briefly reviewed.

The intestinal protozoa include ameba, flagellates, ciliates, coccidia, and microsporidia.

Ameba are free-living organisms characterized by pseudopods and trophozoite and cyst stages in their life cycles. The only human pathogen is *Entamoeba histolytica.* Trophozoites penetrate intestinal tissue and ingest red blood cells (RBCs). *E. histolytica* causes amebic colitis and can cause extraintestinal abscesses. The symptoms of amebic colitis are similar to enteric disease caused by *Salmonella* and *Shigella.* Two other ameba that affect humans are *Acanthamoeba* spp. and *Naegleria fowleri.* *N. fowleri* causes primary amebic meningoencephalitis (PAM) and *Acanthamoeba* spp. cause granulomatous amebic encephalitis (GAE). The *Acanthamoeba* spp. have also caused acanthamoeba keratitis associated with poor contact lens care.

The flagellates recovered from the intestinal tract include *Giardia lamblia, Dientamoeba fragilis, Chilomastix mesnili,* and *Pentatrichomonas hominis.* The two pathogens are *G. lamblia* and *D. fragilis.* The most common isolate is *G. lamblia,* which causes watery diarrhea that can be explosive and foul-smelling. Those most commonly affected people include children in day care centers, hikers, and immunocompromised patients. Trophozoites attach to the crypts of the duodenum but do not invade the mucosa.

The only pathogenic ciliate is *Balantidium coli,* a large organism with two nuclei, a bean-shaped macronucleus, and a smaller round micronucleus. Animal reservoirs are domestic hogs.

The coccidian genera are *Isospora, Cryptosporidium,* and *Cyclospora.* These organisms are emerging as important pathogens for patients with AIDS and have been associated with several outbreaks linked to contaminated imported basil and strawberries. A modified acid-fast stain can be done to show the oocysts in stool. *Toxoplasma gondii* includes the cat in its life cycle; humans become infected by ingesting oocysts.

The microsporidia are obligate intracellular parasites that have been recognized as tissue parasites in immunocompromised patients. Spores have thick walls and are passed in the stool. Eight genera have been recognized in humans. *Enterocytozoon* and *Encephalitozoon* species can cause disseminated disease.

Blood parasites include the *Plasmodium* spp., *Babesia* spp., and the hemoflagellates (*Leishmania* and *Trypanosoma* spp.). The genus *Plasmodium* consists of many species that infect a wide range of animals, but only four species infect humans. *P. falciparum* is the most deadly and accounts for almost all the deaths. The other three human pathogens are *P. vivax, P. malariae,* and *P. ovale.* The vector for transmission is the female *Anopheles* mosquito. This parasite has a complex life cycle that begins when humans are bitten by the mosquito and sporozoites are discharged into the puncture wound. The sporozoites migrate to the liver where they transform into merozoites. This is the preerythrocytic cycle. Merozoites are released into the bloodstream, where they invade RBCs. This is the erythrocytic cycle. Merozoites invading RBCs become trophozoites and appear as ring forms. The merozoites multiply asexually within the RBC (schizogony) and cause the RBCs to rupture and release toxic materials into the bloodstream. Patients experience the classic paroxysm of fever, shaking chills, and sweats. Some of the released merozoites become male and female gametocytes and the sexual cycle (sporogony) begins. A banana- or sausage-shaped macrogametocyte is characteristic of *P. falciparum.* The gametocytes are the infective stage for mosquitoes. *P. falciparum* can cause severe and fatal complications that include the plugging of capillaries in internal organs, cerebral malaria, and sudden intravascular hemolysis. Some genetic variations in RBCs may provide natural immunity. Hemoglobin S, glucose-6-phosphate dehydrogenase (G6PD) deficiency, and Duffy antigen-negative cells appear to interfere with parasitic growth and multiplication.

Babesia spp. are transmitted by ticks and have a life cycle similar to that of *Plasmodium.* The organisms can be confused with one another. *Babesia* trophozoites are smaller than *Plasmodium* and may have four or five rings per RBC.

The hemoflagellates include the *Leishmania* spp. and *Trypanosoma* spp. These are obligate intracellular parasites that are transmitted to humans by the bite of flies. The trypanosomes have three species pathogenic to man. *T. cruzi* causes Chagas' disease, *T. brucei gambiense* causes West African sleeping sickness, and *T. brucei rhodesiense* causes East African sleeping sickness. The trypomastigotes are found in the blood of human hosts. This form has a long body with an undulating membrane and a polar flagellum. Three *Leishmania* spp. cause disease in humans. *L. tropica* causes cutaneous leishmaniasis and *L. braziliensis* causes a mucocutaneous leishmaniasis. Kala-azar or visceral leishmaniasis is caused by *L. donovani.* Diagnosis is made by recovery of promastigotes in culture or identification of the amastigote form in clinical specimens. The amastigote is small and not flagellated. These are also known as L-D (Leishman-Donovan) bodies that are seen in macrophages, where they multiply.

The intestinal helminths that infect humans include the nematodes (roundworms) and platyhelminths (flatworms). Organisms in this group include *Enterobius, Trichuris, Ascaris, Ancylostoma, Necator, Strongyloides,* and *Trichinella.* The nematodes or roundworms are small to large parasites living primarily in the intestinal tract as adult worms. Their life cycles typically require no intermediate host. All of the nematodes of humans have separate sexes and larval stages. The infective stage of *S. stercoralis* is one of the larval stages (filariform); the rhabditiform larva is the noninfective stage that passes out of the body in feces. Diagnosis depends on finding eggs in feces. *Enterobius vermicularis* is the pinworm; it has worldwide distribution. It is primarily a parasite of young children. Adult female worms migrate out of the anal orifice at night and lay their eggs in the perianal areas. Regular tape can be used to recover the eggs, which have a characteristic flattened side. *Ancylostoma* and *Necator* are referred to as hookworms because of the way they attach themselves to the intestinal wall. The eggs of the two species look alike but diagnosis is dependent on finding eggs in stool.

The cestodes are the tapeworms. The four most common adult tapeworm parasites of the human small intestine are *Diphyllobothrium latum, Taenia saginata, Taenia solium,* and *Hymenolepis nana*. All of the adult tapeworms require an intermediate host except *H. nana,* which infects humans directly by fecal-oral transmission of eggs. *H. nana* is the smallest adult human tapeworm and the most common tapeworm infection in the United States. Humans get infected by accidentally eating infected beetles (often in dry cereals) or directly in institutional and family settings where hygiene is poor. Diagnosis depends on finding eggs in feces. Adult tapeworms have a scolex at the anterior end and a body made up of segments called proglottids. As tapeworms increase in age and size, the most posterior gravid proglottids break off or disintegrate and pass in the feces. *T. saginata* is known as the beef tapeworm. Diagnosis is made by finding gravid proglottids in feces. *T. saginata* has 15 to 30 lateral branches on each side of the central uterine stem and *T. solium* has 7 to 12 lateral uterine branches. *Diphyllobothrium latum* is known as the fish tapeworm. Diagnosis is made by finding operculated eggs in feces.

The trematodes are the flatworms or flukes. Adult trematode parasites of humans live in the intestine, liver, lung, or blood vessels. Two types of parasitic flukes infect humans. One is hermaphroditic and lives in the intestine, liver, or lungs of the host. The other type consists of unisex adult males and females within blood vessels. These are the schistosomes or blood flukes. The flukes all have a complex life cycle that involves snails as first intermediate host. Many have a second intermediate host. Freshwater molluscs, specific for each species of trematode, are infected by ciliated larvae (miracidia), which emerge from the trematode egg. Within the tissues of the snail the larva goes through several reproductive cycles and emerges as a tailed, free-swimming larva called a *cercaria*. Cercariae are released into the water and may directly infect humans (e.g., schistosomes). In most species, the cercariae invade a second intermediate host (e.g., fish, crabs) and develop into encysted, infective forms called *metacercariae*. Trematode infections are usually diagnosed by identification of eggs in feces. The eggs of most human trematodes have an operculum through which the ciliated larva (miracidium) escapes. Schistosomes do not have an operculated egg. Human lung fluke infections are caused by a number of species of *Paragonimus. P. westermani* is widespread and is the most important pathogenic species. Adult flukes usually live in pairs in the lung parenchyma. The eggs are passed up the bronchial tree and may be found in sputum or feces. Crabs and crayfish serve as the second intermediate host. Humans are usually infected when eating raw or undercooked crustaceans. Raw crab is often marinated in wine or vinegar, but this does not kill the metacercariae. Metacercariae migrate from the intestine, through the diaphragm into the thoracic cavity, then into the lungs where the worms mature and begin to lay eggs. These infections can last 10 to 20 years. Diagnosis depends on finding eggs in feces or sputum. Eggs are thick-shelled and yellow-brown, with a prominent operculum.

INTEREST POINT

A health care agency in California recently reported an unusual parasitic infection that had affected two people who developed fluke infection after consuming live, imported, freshwater crabs in a restaurant. More information can be accessed at *www.ochealthinfo. com/press/2006/08-11.htm* and *www.ochealthinfo. com/epi/paragonimus.htm.*

Filarial worms are arthropod-transmitted parasites of the lymphatic, subcutaneous, and cutaneous tissues of humans. All share the characteristic that the adult female worm produces a primitive larva called a *microfilaria*, which is found in the peripheral blood or skin. Some species circulate in the blood in a well-defined rhythm or periodicity. Diagnosis depends on finding microfilariae in blood or skin. These parasites are not endemic in the United States, but are often seen in immigrants or travelers from endemic areas. *Wuchereria bancrofti* is the most common and widespread species of filarial worm infecting humans. The adult worms live in the lymphatic system and cause lymphadenitis and obstructive fibrosis, which results in lymphedema. *Onchocerca volvulus* adult worms are embedded in fibrous nodules in the subcutaneous tissues.

There are drugs to treat these parasitic infections, but many of them have serious side effects, require long treatment regimens, and may not completely eradicate the organism from its human host. Resistance to some drugs in use has been reported. More than six antimalarial drugs are in use and, unfortunately, there have been reports of resistance to all of them. Newer therapies are in development, but some researchers believe that the way to combat malaria and other prevalent parasitic diseases, such as amebiasis, is with vaccination. Developing a malaria vaccine is a challenge because exposure does not seem to stimulate a protective immune response. An effective vaccine also needs to target the stage in the life cycle that produces the symptoms. Another approach to the control of vector-borne diseases involves the interruption of the life cycle with vector controls; malaria was successfully eradicated from the United States by controlling the mosquito population. Improvements in hygiene, water treatment to eradicate fecal contamination, and adequate cooking of meats and seafood are additional methods of control.

KEY TERMS AND ABBREVIATIONS

Match the term in the left column with the definition on the right.

1. _____ oocyst
2. _____ trophozoite
3. _____ sporozoite
4. _____ gametocyte
5. _____ merozoite
6. _____ ova and parasite examination
7. _____ scolex
8. _____ proglottid
9. _____ microfilariae
10. _____ amastigote
11. _____ babesia
12. _____ kala-azar
13. _____ Chagas' disease
14. _____ rhabditiform larvae
15. _____ metacercariae
16. _____ vector
17. _____ string test
18. _____ pinworm test
19. _____ cercariae
20. _____ operculum

A. leishmanial form in humans
B. anterior end of tapeworm
C. motile, feeding form
D. released from RBCs
E. test for *Giardia*
F. leishmaniasis
G. three-part test to sediment and stain stool
H. cellophane tape test for *Enterobius*
I. living carrier for parasites
J. cell that produces gametes
K. *T. cruzi*
L. embryo stage of filarial in blood
M. form in the mosquito
N. infective stage for humans in fluke life cycle
O. encysted reproductive form
P. noninfective larval stage
Q. tapeworm segment
R. larvae released from snails into water
S. caplike cover on eggs
T. intracellular parasite transmitted by ticks

TRUE OR FALSE

1. _____ Although the eggs of *Necator americanus* and *Ancylostoma duodenale* are almost identical, diagnosis is based on the location of eggs in feces.
2. _____ Parasites that can be observed in sputum specimens include *Paragonimus westermani* and *Strongyloides stercoralis*.
3. _____ A characteristic of *E. vermicularis* eggs is their spherical shape with an operculated end.
4. _____ A proven method of controlling parasitic disease is to eradicate the vector.
5. _____ A commonly seen parasite associated with sexual transmission is *Trichomonas vaginalis*.

MULTIPLE CHOICE

1. _____ An ameba associated with keratitis is
   A. *Entamoeba histolytica*.
   B. *Acanthamoeba* spp.
   C. *Entamoeba coli*.
   D. *Entamoeba gingivalis*.
2. _____ Which observation is helpful in differentiating the trophozoite of *E. histolytica* from *Entamoeba coli*?
   A. Glycogen mass
   B. Shape of the nucleus
   C. Ingested bacteria
   D. Ingested RBCs
3. _____ Thick and thin blood smears are useful in detection and identification of
   A. *Babesia* spp.
   B. *Plasmodium* spp.
   C. *Leishmania donovani*.
   D. all of the above.
4. _____ *Enterobius vermicularis* infection can be diagnosed by finding
   A. eggs in feces.
   B. adult worms in feces.
   C. eggs in perianal specimens.
   D. proglottids in feces.
5. _____ The formalin-ether sedimentation concentration method is recommended for routine use with stool specimens because it
   A. preserves most parasites.
   B. recovers eggs.
   C. recovers cysts.
   D. all of the above.

CASE STUDY

A 14-year-old male presented to the emergency department (ED) with a history of fever with temperature as high as 105° F for the last 4 days and progressively worsening vomiting over the last 3 days. He had been seen by his primary care physician 3 days earlier. Sinusitis was diagnosed and he was started on amoxicillin-clavulanic acid. He also had nose bleeds several times a day for the last several days and passed urine that was brown in color. The physical examination in the ED showed an enlarged spleen but normal liver. Blood was collected for CBC, chemistry panel, and cultures. The history of the patient revealed that he lived with his parents and siblings. He had not been out of state for the last 2 years. His immunizations were up-to-date. His only illnesses were occasional sinusitis in the past with no febrile episode in several years. The CBC had low WBC, hemoglobin, and hematocrit counts and there were only 50 platelets/µL. His total serum bilirubin was increased but not the liver enzymes. The astute technologist scanning the CBC smear noted abnormalities with RBC morphology that were identified as ring forms.

1. Although this patient had some abnormal test results, the numbers were not critically abnormal. But the RBC morphology prompted the technologist to call the physician. Thick and thin smears for pathologist

review were ordered. What are some diseases in the differential diagnosis?
2. What additional tests could be done to help rule out diseases?
3. The infectious diseases specialist and health department were consulted. Blood films were sent to the state health department to confirm the original diagnosis of *P. vivax*. Another teenager from the area was also diagnosed with *P. vivax* during that same time period. The county is near a large airport for international flights. What is a possible explanation for this small cluster of disease?

ANSWERS

Key Terms and Abbreviations
1. O
2. C
3. M
4. J
5. D
6. G
7. B
8. Q
9. L
10. A
11. T
12. F
13. K
14. P
15. N
16. I
17. E
18. H
19. R
20. S

True or False
1. T
2. T
3. F
4. T
5. T

Multiple Choice
1. B
2. D
3. D
4. C
5. D

Case Study
1. Significant findings are the low hemoglobin and hematocrit and platelet count, high serum bilirubin but normal liver enzymes, enlarged spleen, fever, vomiting, and the presence of ring forms in RBCs. Malaria and babesiosis are in the differential diagnoses. The issue is that the boy had not traveled out of the area.
2. A malaria smear was ordered as was *Babesia* serology. The patient was admitted and consults were ordered with an infectious disease specialist and a hematologist. A diagnosis of malaria, nonfalciparum, was made.
3. This is an example of an autochthonous malaria outbreak. The two teenagers had not been out of the country or the state, had not had blood transfusions or organ transplants, and had not shared needles. The belief is that a traveler arriving on an international flight at the nearby airport had malaria. The parasite was transferred to the local mosquito population. This was a locally acquired mosquito-transmitted malaria that occasionally occurs in the United States. In 2003, eight cases were reported in Florida with large outbreaks being reported in California in 1952, 1986, and 1988. Fever, chills, headache, and vomiting are common symptoms. The common hematologic findings are thrombocytopenia and lymphopenia with or without anemia. The patients were treated with chloroquine, an antimalarial drug.

REFERENCES

Chandler AC, Read CP: *Introduction to parasitology*, New York, John Wiley & Sons, 1967.
Haque R, et al: Amebiasis, *N Engl J Med* 348:1565, 2003.
Perez MT, et al: Hematological laboratory findings in patients of an autochthonous *Plasmodium vivax* malaria outbreak, *Lab Med* 35:420, 2004.
Phillips RS: Current status of malaria and potential for control, *Clin Microbiol Rev* 14:208, 2001.

OBJECTIVES

Upon completion of this chapter, the reader should be able to:

1. Explain the difference between yeasts and molds.
2. Explain the difference between an ectothrix and endothrix infection.
3. Define the following terms: blastoconidia, conidiophore, mycelium, pseudohypha, rhizoid, saprophyte, septa, sporangiophore, spore, thallus.
4. Differentiate between dematiaceous and hyaline forms.
5. Explain dimorphism in fungi, its clinical significance, and give examples of organisms that exhibit this trait.
6. Differentiate between mycoses and mycotoxicoses.
7. Explain the clinical conditions mycetoma, tinea, chromoblastomycosis, and phaeohyphomycosis.
8. List the dermatophyte fungi.
9. List the etiologic agent and describe the disease state for each of the following mycoses: black piedra, tinea versicolor, sporotrichosis, paracoccidioidomycosis, coccidioidomycosis, blastomycosis, histoplasmosis, aspergillosis, white piedra
10. Explain the clinical significance of *Pneumocystis* infection.
11. Explain how to test for *Cryptococcus neoformans*.
12. List the zygomycetes and how to differentiate them in culture.
13. Explain the following tests: germ tube, KOH, wet prep, tease mount, in vitro hair penetration, calcofluor white stain.
14. Explain the purpose of cycloheximide in fungal media.
15. Explain safety practices in a medical mycology laboratory.

SUMMARY OF KEY POINTS

The word *mycology* is derived from the Greek word for mushroom, *mykes*. Fungi were among the first organisms recognized because they can be seen without a microscope and they have fruiting structures. They were originally classified with the plants, but now fungi are in their own kingdom, Myceteae. Fungi are ubiquitous in nature and function in the energy cycle as decomposers. All fungi are heterotrophs and saprophytes; they lack chlorophyll and get the required preformed carbon compounds from dead and decaying organic matter. Fungi secrete digestive enzymes (cellulases, proteases, nucleases) into their environmental substrate and then transport soluble nutrients across their cell membranes. Because fungi secrete a variety of metabolic products that can be highly toxic, fungi can cause poisonings (mycotoxicoses) as well as infections (mycoses).

Fungi are eukaryotic. Their cell membrane contains ergosterol instead of cholesterol and their rigid cell wall contains chitin. Fungi can be thought of as consisting of two groups: molds and yeasts. Molds are multicellular and filamentous, whereas yeasts are generally unicellular. Fungi can reproduce sexually or asexually. Yeasts generally reproduce asexually by budding; the buds or daughter cells are called *blastoconidia*. If the blastoconidia stay attached to form chains of cells, these are called *pseudohyphae*. Germ tubes are elongated buds and are the beginnings of true hyphae; true germ tubes lack a constriction at their bases. True hyphae are tubelike structures that are septated (have cross walls); there is no constriction at these cross walls as there is in pseudohyphae.

Molds are multicelled organisms. The filamentous mat of growth is called the *mycelium*; the mycelium is composed of the threadlike hyphae. The mycelium can extend down into the substrate; this vegetative mycelium absorbs water and nutrients. Hyphae can extend up away from the substrate; this aerial mycelium is the reproductive portion of the organism. Fungi reproduce by forming spores either sexually or asexually. Spores that arise directly from the vegetative mycelium include arthrospores, chlamydospores, and blastospores. Spores that arise from aerial fruiting bodies are known as *conidia*.

Hyphae can be lightly pigmented or darkly pigmented due to melanin in the cell wall. Hyaline hyphae are light in color while dematiaceous hyphae produce dark-colored molds. Coloring, type of septation in hyphae, type of conidia, dimorphism, and other characteristics are used by clinical microbiologists to identify those fungi that have clinical importance in fungal cultures.

Some fungi are dimorphic and can exist as either a yeast form or mold form. The mold form is the environmental and infective form. When the organisms gain entrance to the body and a 35° to 37° C environment, they can change to yeast forms. The yeast form is the invasive form; yeast forms can be seen in clinical specimens. Dimorphic fungi can be virulent and cause systemic infection, especially in an immunocompromised host. Species in this group include *Blastomyces dermatitidis*, *Coccidioides immitis*, *Histoplasma capsulatum*, *Paracoccidioides braziliensis*, and *Penicillium marneffei*.

Fungi exhibit a variety of virulence factors. Mycoses are frequently acquired by the inhalation of spores; small size and the ability to invade mucosal surfaces are advantages to the establishment of an infection. *Cryptococcus neoformans* has a polysaccharide capsule that allows it to go unrecognized by phagocytes. Pathogenic fungi must be able to grow at body temperature and some show dimorphism and conversion to a yeast form at 35° C.

125

The dermatophytes secrete extracellular enzymes that allow them to colonize and invade keratinous tissues. Mycotoxicoses usually result from eating contaminated foods; mycotoxicoses are poisonings due to toxins produced by filamentous fungi. Mycotoxin exposure is almost always accidental and is more likely to occur among populations where there are poor food handling, poor storage of food, and malnutrition. Preventive measures include good agricultural practice and sufficient drying of crops after harvest. An example of a relatively recent veterinary crisis linked to fungal toxins occurred in England in 1962 when 100,000 turkey poults died. The ground meal these animals had been fed was contaminated with an aflatoxin produced by *Aspergillus flavus.* Another interesting mycotoxin is the group of fungal metabolites known as ergot alkaloids. Lysergic acid comes from these ergot alkaloids. Ingestion of these alkaloids causes ergotism or St. Anthony's fire, a condition common throughout Europe during the Middle Ages.

INTEREST POINT

"Mould" or "mold," which is it?

A search in Webster's English Dictionary produces three nouns with the spelling *mold.* The first noun means soil rich in humus and comes from the Old English *molde*; Latin *molere* (to grind). The second noun comes from the Old French *modle* and from Latin *modulus* and refers to the frame on or around which an object is constructed. The third noun comes from the Middle English *mowlde* and means the superficial wooly growth on decaying matter; a fungus. There are several well known mycologists who feel that the etymology of the word "mould" is from the Old Norse *mygla,* which means to grow moldy, dating from the fourteenth century. They maintain that "mold" is derived from the Old French *modle* and means shape or pattern. Using this etymology, the correct spelling for fungal growth would be "mould." The American Society for Microbiology has adopted this spelling with the "u." There is, however, no consensus and both spellings appear in the various published texts. An excellent web-based mycology site that addresses this question with humor is *www. doctorfungus.org.*

The classic approach to medical mycology has been to classify organisms into categories based on infection site, for example, systemic, subcutaneous, cutaneous, and superficial. Systemic infections have typically been caused by the dimorphic fungi. With the increase in the number of immunocompromised patients, fungi that had been considered as contaminants are now causing devastating disease. *Sporothrix schenckii* had been known to cause a subcutaneous infection, but it may also cause an invasive systemic disease. *Malassezia furfur* had been thought to cause only the superficial dermatomycosis known as tinea versicolor. We now know that it can cause disseminated infections in patients receiving parenteral nutrition

through indwelling catheters. And intravenous drug abusers have been reported to have developed endocarditis caused by a variety of fungi.

Fungal cultures typically require incubation periods of 4 weeks at 30° C. Inoculated media should include plates or slants with and without cycloheximide; cycloheximide inhibits the growth of contaminating molds and bacteria. All fungal cultures and clinical specimens should be processed and handled in a class II biological safety cabinet. As a further precaution against laboratory-acquired infection, cultures of pathogens should be sealed with tape and autoclaved. Swab specimens are generally inadequate for the recovery of fungi; aspirated material and tissue are the preferred specimen types. Skin, nail scrapings, and hair can be examined microscopically after treatment with KOH or calcofluor white stain. With hairs, a mosaic arrangement of spores may be seen on the hair shaft (ectothrix infection) or hyphal elements and arthroconidia may be seen internally after invasion of the hair shaft (endothrix infection).

The Zygomycetes are a class of fungi that have wide hyphae and occasional septa. They are widely distributed in nature and are found on decaying matter and soil. Human infection is usually through the inhalation of spores but could also occur by ingestion of contaminated food (common bread mold) and traumatic breaks in the skin. Severe disease (zygomycosis) primarily occurs in immunocompromised patients and those with underlying disease, such as diabetes or malnutrition. These organisms have a propensity to invade and block blood vessels that results in thrombosis and tissue necrosis. The two most frequently encountered genera are *Rhizopus* and *Mucor.* The zygomycetes are easily recognized in culture because they produce fluffy, grayish-white colonies that grow quickly.

Superficial mycoses involve the skin, hair, and nails. These types of infections are caused by the dermatophyte fungi of the genera *Trichophyton, Epidermophyton,* and *Microsporum.* These organisms are capable of invading keratinous tissue because they utilize keratin as a source of nitrogen. These infections are widespread globally and are increasing in prevalence. In North America the species most frequently associated with nail infections are *T. rubrum* and *T. mentagrophytes.* Nail infections are difficult to cure and recur in as many as 40% of cases. *Microsporum* spp. infect the hair and skin. *Trichophyton* spp. infect nails, hair, and skin. *Epidermophyton floccosum* infects nails and skin, but not hair.

Cutaneous mycoses are common and are referred to as *tinea* (from Medieval Latin meaning "worm" or "moth"). These fungi produce ring-like lesions that are named for their locations on the body (e.g., *tinea capitis* is a lesion on the scalp and *tinea cruris* refers to lesions in the groin area). *Trichophyton tonsurans* is the predominant species that causes *tinea capitis* in the United States. *Microsporum audouinii* used to be the classic cause of epidemic prepubertal scalp ringworm. Hairs infected with *M. audouinii* fluoresce green using a Wood's lamp while hairs infected with *T. tonsurans* do not.

Laboratory diagnosis can involve direct microscopic observation of a hair shaft. *T. mentagrophytes* invades hair shafts (endothrix), whereas *T. rubrum* does not. The hair penetration test is used to differentiate these two species. *T. rubrum* produces tear-shaped microconidia distributed on either side of the hyphae; this has been described as a "bird on the fence" pattern. As the name implies, *T. rubrum* produces red colonies. *T. mentagrophytes* frequently produces helically coiled hyphal appendages and is urease-positive. *Epidermophyton floccosum* is a common cause of athlete's foot *(tinea pedis)*. It produces club-shaped macroconidia with thin walls. This genus lacks microconidia, a characteristic that can be used to differentiate it from *Trichophyton* species.

The fungi that are hyaline and septate and cause invasive opportunistic infections include the genera *Aspergillus, Fusarium, Geotrichum, Acremonium, Penicillium, Paecilomyces,* and *Scopulariopsis.* Aspergillosis is one of the most common fungal infections requiring hospitalization in the United States. Risk factors for infection include neutropenia, transplantation, granulocytopenia in leukemia patients, and cytotoxic drug therapy. Aspergilli are ubiquitous with conidia dispersed into the environment. Mode of infection is inhalation of the conidia. More than 22,000 solid organ transplants are performed annually in the United States; as many as 15% of these patients develop an *Aspergillus* infection. It has been estimated that 9% to 16% of all deaths in transplant recipients in the first year are due to invasive aspergillosis. Rapid diagnosis is essential. Culture of respiratory secretions lack sensitivity, and detection of antifungal antibodies is unreliable. There is a double-sandwich ELISA assay that can detect very small amounts of galactomannan; this is a promising tool for early diagnosis. Galactomannan is a component of the cell wall that is released into the circulation during fungal growth in the tissues. Another cell wall component found in pathogenic yeasts and filamentous fungi is 1,3-β-D-glucan. Studies are underway to determine how measurement of this substance can be used to diagnose infection. Molecular assays for fungal detection are not standardized or commercially available.

Fusarium is a common environmental fungus that causes disease in major crop plants and humans. *Fusarium* has long been regarded as an important ophthalmic pathogen. *Paecilomyces* and *Acremonium* are found worldwide in soil and decaying vegetation. *Paecilomyces* is resistant to most sterilizing procedures and has been known to contaminate sterile solutions and culture media. Documented infections have followed surgical procedures. *Paecilomyces* along with *Penicillium* and *Scopulariopsis* spp. produce conidia in chains.

Systemic mycoses have become increasingly important as the number of immunocompromised individuals increases. Human systemic mycoses are caused by the hyaline dimorphic fungi that are inhaled when their conidia become aerosolized. The yeast forms are also infectious if aerosolized (e.g., during specimen processing). More than 95% of these infections are self-limiting and produce few symptoms. The small percentage of infections that advance to disseminated disease are associated with predisposing factors, such as pregnancy, immunosuppression, and defects in T-cell mediated immunity.

Blastomyces dermatitidis is endemic to the Ohio and Mississippi River valleys. The organism has been found in riverbank soil and in beaver dams. There may be a self-limited illness or localized pulmonary lesion. But in disseminated disease, one or more organs will become involved. *Coccidioides immitis* is found in the arid soil of the southwest and Mexico. Outbreaks occur when drought is followed by heavy rains. Dissemination can result in bone lesions and arthritis. Definitive diagnosis of this group of pathogens had been made by observing both the mold and yeast forms. *C. immitis* does not produce yeast-like colonies at 35° C on routine mycology media.

Paracoccidioides brasiliensis is found in Central and South America with the highest incidence in Brazil. Infection is thought to occur by inhalation of the conidia or by direct inoculation through trauma. *P. braziliensis* is a slow grower and is best diagnosed by demonstrating the characteristic multiply-budding yeast cells ("mariner's wheel") in clinical specimens.

Outbreaks of histoplasmosis have been associated with exposure to certain animal reservoirs, such as starlings, chickens, and bats. The mycelial form is present in soil, especially where there is an accumulation of bat guano and bird droppings. It is endemic in the United States in the Ohio, Mississippi, and Missouri River valleys.

Histoplasma capsulatum is a parasite of the reticuloendothelial system; it is seldom seen extracellularly and yeast forms may be seen in blood or bone marrow specimens. Disseminated histoplasmosis is often seen as an AIDS-defining illness. *H. capsulatum* is a slow grower that produces white to brown colonies with a fine cottony texture. DNA probes can be done on the immature colonies. Diagnosis can be made serologically by antibody detection or antigen detection in urine specimens.

Sporotrichosis is a cutaneous to subcutaneous chronic infection that may include systemic spread, often with lymphatic involvement. It is caused by *Sporothrix schenckii,* which is found worldwide in soil and decaying vegetation. It is often introduced into the skin by trauma (rose thorn prick or splinter) and has become known as the *rose handler's disease.* It is a dimorphic fungus that grows rapidly in culture and produces delicate, hyaline, septate hyphae with flower-like clusters of oval conidia.

Penicillium marneffei has emerged as a pathogen in Southeast Asia. It is the only known *Penicillium* species that exhibits dimorphic growth, which appears to be the organism's principal virulence factor. It produces a cutaneous or mucocutaneous infection that can disseminate and become fatal, especially in HIV patients. Its spread is associated with the bamboo rat. Yeastlike cells can be seen in clinical specimens, but there is no budding. Laboratory diagnosis of infection requires demonstration of intracellular yeast cells and culture of the fungus from clinical specimens, although serologic and molecular methods have been developed.

The septate, dematiaceous molds produce a variety of superficial and subcutaneous mycoses. The fungi are usually present in soil and get introduced into tissues by trauma. These fungi produce darkly pigmented colonies. They can be grouped by clinical presentation. This group

127

of disorders can produce a wide range of opportunistic mycoses ranging from cosmetic cutaneous infections to fatal cerebral infections. The superficial infections affect the outermost layer of skin or hair. Tinea nigra *(Exophiala werneckii)* causes dark patches on the skin of the hands and feet. Black piedra *(Piedraia hortae)* causes hard black encrustations on the hair shafts. These diseases are endemic in tropical areas. Treatment involves removal of infected hairs and topical fungicides.

A mycetoma is a chronic granulomatous infection in subcutaneous tissue. The infection is characterized by swollen tumor-like lesions that produce a granular pus through draining sinuses. Bacterial mycetomas are caused by the actinomycetes *Nocardia, Actinomadura*, and *Streptomyces.* Fungal mycetomas (eumycotic) are caused by *Pseudallescheria boydii, Acremonium* spp., *Exophiala jeanselmei, Curvularia,* and *Madurella* spp. These are typically tropical diseases, but *P. boydii* causes a white grain mycetoma common in the United States. These organisms gain entry through penetrating wounds. Pigmented hyphae may be seen in tissues. *P. boydii* undergoes both sexual and asexual reproduction; conidia produced asexually are golden brown and predominate in cultures from clinical specimens.

Chromoblastomycosis is another subcutaneous mycosis characterized by chronic infection that causes raised, rough, cauliflower-like lesions usually on the lower extremities. This disease is usually seen in Africa and Latin America. The most common worldwide cause of chromoblastomycosis is *Fonsecaea pedrosoi*, but other etiologic agents include the genera *Cladosporium* and *Phialophora.* Histologic examination of crusted lesions in KOH shows characteristic copper-colored yeast (sclerotic bodies) that resemble copper pennies.

Another form of subcutaneous infection is phaeohyphomycosis caused by the genera *Alternaria, Bipolaris, Curvularia,* and *Exophiala.* Disease is characterized by the presence in tissue of dematiaceous yeastlike cells, pseudohyphae, hyphae, or any combination of these forms. Identification of these organisms is best done microscopically.

Pneumocystis jiroveci is an atypical opportunistic fungus. It was originally named *Pneumocystis carinii* and classified as a protozoan. At an international workshop in 2001, a nomenclature system was adopted to recognize the genetic differences and host specificities among populations of *Pneumocystis.* The nomen legitimum is now *Pneumocystis jiroveci.* It is a unicellular eukaryotic organism with a tropism for the respiratory surfaces of mammals. It cannot be grown in culture. The natural reservoir is unknown, but it is probably widespread in the environment. Clinical conditions associated with pneumocystis pneumonia include malnutrition, corticosteroid therapy, cytotoxic therapy, advanced malignancy, HIV-1 infection, chronic lymphocytic leukemia, organ transplantation, Hodgkin's disease, old age. The prominent characteristic in the lung is a foamy exudate in the alveolar spaces. A variety of stains can be used for identification in respiratory specimens, but methenamine silver (GMS) is the common one. GMS stain shows the cyst form of

the organism. Intravenous trimethoprim-sulfamethoxazole is usually the first treatment selected. Widespread use of prophylaxis in the HIV-1–infected population has decreased but not eradicated apparent infections.

Yeasts are ubiquitous in the environment. They are found on fruits, vegetables, and other plants. Some live in our bodies and may be found in specimens but have no clinical significance; they are considered normal flora in the oropharynx and gastrointestinal tract. Yeasts are opportunistic pathogens, particularly in the immunocompromised host. They are unicellular, eukaryotic, budding cells that reproduce by forming blastoconidia (buds). When blastoconidia are formed one from the other in a linear fashion without separation, a pseudohypha is formed. Cultures of yeasts are moist and creamy, and may be hyaline or darkly pigmented. Most yeasts grow well on common mycologic and bacteriologic media. The ability to grow at 37° C is an important characteristic; most pathogenic species grow readily at body temperature whereas saprophytes fail to grow at the higher temperature. The most commonly isolated species from humans are *Candida albicans, C. tropicalis, C. parapsilosis*, and *C. glabrata.* They are responsible for bloodstream infections, oral candidiasis (a defining feature for AIDS), vaginitis and intestinal infections *(C. tropicalis),* and otitis externa and peritonitis *(C. parapsilosis).*

There are several commercial identification systems available. All fungi stain gram-positive and appear blue-purple with Giemsa stain. *Candida albicans,* the most frequently isolated species, can be identified by the production of a germ tube. Care should be taken in interpreting this test; a true germ tube has no constriction at the point of origin. A constricted germ tube is a pseudogerm tube; *Candida tropicalis* produces pseudogerm tubes. *C. dubliniensis* is also germ tube–positive, but this species is not encountered frequently.

Current recommendations when yeasts are isolated from clinical specimens include the following: (1) identify all yeasts recovered from sterile body fluids (e.g., CSF, blood, urine, paracentesis); (2) identify yeasts isolated from immunocompromised patients or patients in whom mycotic infection is suspected; (3) do not identify yeasts from routine respiratory cultures; (4) screen respiratory cultures for *Cryptococcus neoformans.*

Cryptococcus neoformans is a widely distributed saprobe that is associated with pigeon, chicken, and turkey droppings. Cells are characterized by the presence of a capsule. *C. neoformans* was first detected in the environment in the late 1800s when it was recovered from peach juice. Cryptococcal infection begins with inhalation of the fungus with spread to the central nervous system. Infection with *Cryptococcus* is one of the AIDS-defining diseases and is a risk for transplant patients and those with diabetes or lymphoreticular malignancies.

The capsule is a virulence factor. An India ink preparation had traditionally been done to visualize the yeast cells and capsule. This test, however, is less sensitive than the cryptococcal latex agglutination test that can be done on serum or CSF.

Trichosporon species are yeastlike fungi that cause disease in immunocompromised patients. They can cause disseminated disease as well as endocarditis and endophthalmitis. This genus can also cause an infection around hair shafts known as *white piedra*. The nodules around the hair can be removed and observed after treatment with KOH.

Malassezia furfur is a yeast that requires fatty acids for growth. It is a common commensal on skin and can cause tinea versicolor, a superficial infection characterized by dark lesions on light skin or light areas on dark skin. It can also cause septicemia and systemic infection, particularly in those receiving total parenteral nutrition. Detection can be made by observing skin scrapings for bottle-shaped cells.

In 1997, NCCLS (now known as Clinical and Laboratory Standards Institute, or CLSI) approved document M27-A. This document took 15 years to develop and defined a microdilution method for antifungal testing for *Candida* spp. CLSI has since published standards for broth macrodilution and disk diffusion methods for in vitro susceptibility testing of *Candida* species. Some common antifungal drugs include the azoles (fluconazole, itraconazole, ketoconazole, and voriconazole), antimetabolites (flucytosine), glucan synthesis inhibitor (capsofungin), polyenes (amphotericin B, topical nystatin), and the systemic drug griseofulvin. Yeasts have developed resistance to these agents. Mechanisms of resistance to the azoles are well understood. Resistance can arise in one of several ways: a modification in the quality or quantity of the target enzyme, reduced access of the drug to the target, or a combination of these mechanisms. Adequate dosing of the patient is important because it has been documented that subtherapeutic doses of fluconazole when treating infection with *C. glabrata* can lead to resistance to fluconazole and other azoles, such as itraconazole.

KEY TERMS AND ABBREVIATIONS

Match the term in the left column with the definition on the right.

1. _____ saprophytic
2. _____ dermatophytes
3. _____ dimorphic
4. _____ yeasts
5. _____ molds
6. _____ blastoconidia
7. _____ germ tube
8. _____ pseudohyphae
9. _____ hyphae
10. _____ mycelium
11. _____ dematiaceous
12. _____ hyaline
13. _____ mycoses
14. _____ microconidia
15. _____ macroconidia

A. can exist in two different forms
B. darkly pigmented
C. elongated buds that remain joined but lack true septations
D. toxin produced by filamentous fungi
E. large, usually multicelled conidia
F. moist, creamy colonies on solid media
G. fungal infections
H. elongated bud with no constriction at the base
I. asexual spores on the end of hyphae

16. _____ mycotoxin
17. _____ endothrix
18. _____ ectothrix
19. _____ conidia
20. _____ fungus ball

J. within the hair shaft
K. living on dead or decaying matter
L. small, usually single-celled conidia
M. multicellular filamentous fungi
N. loose network of hyphae
O. tangled mat of hyphae in tissue
P. infects skin; grows in keratin layer
Q. clear, colorless
R. outside the hair shaft
S. budding yeast forms
T. tubelike projections.

TRUE OR FALSE

1. _____ The optimal culture method for recovery of dimorphic fungi in blood is one that lyses WBCs before incubation at 30° C.
2. _____ Colistin, an antifungal agent that prevents overgrowth of rapidly growing molds, should be included in the battery of culture media for fungal culture.
3. _____ A KOH preparation or calcofluor white stain may be used for direct microscopic examination of specimens.
4. _____ *Pneumocystis jiroveci* has a tropism for respiratory surfaces in mammals.
5. _____ The India ink preparation has greater sensitivity to detect *C. neoformans* than the cryptococcal antigen test.
6. _____ A true germ tube has a constriction at the point of origin.
7. _____ *Epidermophyton floccosum* causes tinea pedis.
8. _____ Yeasts do not need to be identified in routine sputum cultures.
9. _____ Fluconazole has excellent activity against most *Candida* species, except *C. glabrata*.
10. _____ Patients with diabetes are at high risk of developing rhinocerebral zygomycosis.

MULTIPLE CHOICE

1. _____ The fungus that is positive for the hair penetration test is
   A. *Trichophyton mentagrophytes.*
   B. *Trichophyton rubrum.*
   C. *E. floccosum.*
   D. *Aspergillus flavus.*
2. _____ Neonatal intensive care unit babies on total parenteral nutrition are considered to be at high risk for infection with
   A. *H. capsulatum.*
   B. *Fusarium* spp.
   C. *Malassezia furfur.*
   D. *Microsporum audounii.*

3. _____ The clinical hallmark of zygomycosis is
   A. formation of a fungus ball in a lung cavity.
   B. vascular invasion resulting in tissue necrosis.
   C. foamy exudates in the lungs.
   D. crusty, cauliflower-like lesion.
4. _____ An occupational hazard of florists and gardeners is
   A. mucormycosis.
   B. sporotrichosis.
   C. candidiasis.
   D. endophthalmitis.
5. _____ A middle-aged farm worker from South America developed a chronic respiratory illness that appeared to be tuberculosis. The AFB culture of sputum was negative. A lung biopsy was done and sent for both AFB and fungus culture. Yeastlike cells were seen on the Gram stain. Some yeast had multiple buds radiating out like the spokes of a wheel. The likely infective agent is
   A. *Trichosporon* spp.
   B. *Fusarium spp.*
   C. *Fonsecaea pedrosoi.*
   D. *Paracoccidioides braziliensis.*

CASE STUDY

A 24-year-old woman residing in a rural area on the East Coast presented to the emergency department (ED) complaining of lethargy, abdominal pain, and tachycardia (rapid heart rate). She had been ill for 2 weeks with generalized weakness, headache, and body aches and had been admitted to another hospital for several days where she was treated with antibiotics. Although her discharge instructions were to follow up with a specialist, the patient did not do that. The patient chose to treat herself with herbal remedies. Shortly after presentation to the ED, the patient became hypoxic and had to be intubated and placed on a ventilator. Admission tests included a CBC, chemistry panel, blood culture, urinalysis, urine culture, PT, and PTT. Some abnormal test results are listed below. The urinalysis was positive for protein and leukocyte esterase, blood, and bacteria. Abdominal examination showed hepatosplenomegaly.

Test	Patient Result	Reference Range
WBC	2.1	4.8-10.8 $10^3/\mu L$
RBC	3.21	3.80-5.40 $10^3/\mu L$
Hemoglobin	8.8	11.7-15.5 g/dL
Hematocrit	24.9	27.0%-49.5%
PT/PTT	19.9/63.8	10.6-12.8/21.6-34.0 sec
BUN	43	6-20 mg/dL
Creatinine	2.20	0.5-1.4 mg/dL
AST (SGOT)	551	5-40 U/L
Alkaline phosphatase	641	38-126 U/L
LDH	>9000	313-618 U/L

1. To complete the CBC, a manual differential had to be performed. When the medical technologist was scanning the peripheral blood smear, she noted inclusions in the WBCs. There were intracellular, stained forms that appeared to be surrounded by a nonstaining capsule. What could the inclusions be?
2. After these initial results were released, additional tests were ordered by the infectious diseases consultant. See below. How are ehrlichiosis, histoplasmosis, and the CD4 count relevant to this patient's symptoms?

Additional Tests Ordered the Following Day		
Ehrlichia chaffeensis IgG and IgM	IgM <1:16 IgG <1:64	<1:16 <1:64
Histoplasma antigen on urine	93.9 units	<1.0 negative >10 high positive
CD4 absolute count	27	381-1469 cells/µL

3. The patient was given a dose of doxycycline while in the emergency department. When the test results were all in, the patient was given amphotericin B. Why was the antimicrobial changed?

NOTE: Peripheral blood smears were stained with a periodic acid-Schiff stain (PAS) in addition to the usual Giemsa stain used in hematology. PAS and methenamine silver (GMS) stains are used to show the cell wall of fungi. Upon transfer of this patient to the tertiary care facility where she had been previously, it was learned that an HIV antibody screen had been performed during that earlier admission and this test was positive.

ANSWERS

Key Terms and Abbreviations

1. K
2. P
3. A
4. F
5. M
6. S
7. H
8. C
9. T
10. N
11. B
12. Q
13. G
14. L
15. E
16. D
17. J
18. R
19. I
20. O

True or False

1. T
2. F
3. T
4. T
5. F
6. F
7. T
8. T
9. T
10. T

Multiple Choice

1. A
2. C
3. B
4. B
5. D

Case Study

1. Leukocyte inclusions could be transient morphologic abnormalities such as cytoplasmic vacuoles, morulae of *Anaplasma phagocytophilia* that causes human granulocytic ehrlichiosis, the yeast form of *Histoplasma capsulatum*, or parasites (*Toxoplasma* or *Leishmania*).

2. The patient presented with symptoms of headache, body aches, and malaise. Ehrlichiosis is a common tick-borne illness. The targeted cells are the macrophages and granulocytes where cytoplasmic vacuoles house the infecting organism. The arthropod-borne disease is common in this geographic location. The same symptoms along with abdominal pain are characteristic of histoplasmosis. Hepatosplenomegaly is consistent with acute disseminated histoplasmosis. *Histoplasma* infection is frequently asymptomatic in immunocompetent individuals. However, it is a hallmark disease for those with AIDS. Another clue is the very high LDH.

Studies have shown that a high LDH can be used as an adjunct clinical marker to differentiate between infection with *H. capsulatum* and *Pneumocystis jiroveci*. This patient's CD4 count is very low, another hallmark of AIDS.

3. Doxycycline is the drug of choice for ehrlichiosis but amphotericin B, an antifungal agent, is used to treat histoplasmosis.

REFERENCES

Al-Agha OM, Mooty M, Salarieh A: A 43-year-old woman with acquired immunodeficiency syndrome and fever of undetermined origin, *Arch Pathol Lab Med* 130:120, 2006.

Bennett JW, Klich M: Mycotoxins, *Clin Microbiol Rev* 16:497, 2003.

Corcoran GR, Al-Abdely H, Flanders CD, et al: Markedly elevated serum lactate dehydrogenase levels are a clue to the diagnosis of disseminated histoplasmosis in patients with AIDS, *Clin Infect Dis* 24:942, 1997.

Cushion MT: *Pneumocystis*. In *Manual of clinical microbiology*, Washington, DC, ASM Press, 2003.

Pfaller MA, Diekema DJ, Sheehan DJ: Interpretive breakpoints for fluconazole and *Candida* revisited: a blueprint for the future of antifungal susceptibility testing, *Clin Microbiol Rev* 19:435, 2006.

Singh N, Paterson D: *Aspergillus* infections in transplant recipients, *Clin Mircobiol Rev* 18:44, 2005.

Thomas PA: Current perspectives on ophthalmic mycoses, *Clin Microbiol Rev* 16:730, 2003.

Vanittanakom N, Cooper CR, Fisher MC, Sirisanthana T: *Penicillium marneffei* infection and recent advances in the epidemiology and molecular biology aspects, *Clin Microbiol Rev* 19:95, 2006.

Wheat J, Sarosi G, McKinsey D, et al: Practice guidelines for the management of patients with histoplasmosis, *Clin Infect Dis* 30:688, 2000.

Woodfolk JA: Allergy and dermatophytes, *Clin Microbiol Rev* 18:30, 2005.

OBJECTIVES

Upon completion of this chapter, the reader should be able to:

1. Explain what a virus is by giving a brief description of its structural components and infectious cycle.
2. Briefly explain how viruses are classified.
3. List the common respiratory viruses infecting man.
4. List the population(s) most at risk for respiratory syncytial virus (RSV) infection and mode of transmission.
5. Differentiate between antigenic drift and antigenic shift, and relate this to the effectiveness of vaccines.
6. List the viruses associated with skin eruptions (exanthemas); include the six classic childhood rashes.
7. List the conditions associated with AIDS.
8. List the viruses associated with gastrointestinal infections.
9. List the population(s) most at risk for rotavirus and the mode of transmission.
10. List the viruses associated with central nervous system (CNS) disease.
11. List appropriate testing measures to detect the following viruses: influenza, RSV, enterovirus, HIV, hepatitis A virus (HAV), hepatitis B virus (HBV), hepatitis C virus (HCV), rubeola, rubella, human T-cell lymphoma virus (HTLV), rotavirus, West Nile virus, rabies, human papilloma virus (HPV), herpes simplex virus (HSV), cytomegalovirus (CMV), Epstein-Barr virus (EBV), and varicella-zoster virus (VZV).
12. List the two most common viral sexually transmitted diseases (STDs).
13. List the different types of HPV and their preferred tissue types for infection.
14. Explain the relationship between HPV infection and cervical carcinoma.
15. Explain the antibody responses to infection with HBV and how an acute infection can be differentiated from a chronic one.
16. Describe several viral infections and the syndromes caused by their latency and reactivation.
17. List several antiviral agents.
18. Discuss viral infection from the perspective of the transplant patient and list the common viral complications.

SUMMARY OF KEY POINTS

Viruses are obligate intracellular parasites and among the smallest of all life forms. Viral diseases have caused some of the great pandemics throughout history. In the twentieth century, we had three influenza pandemics and the AIDS pandemic. Although we have eliminated some of the more lethal viral diseases such as smallpox, viruses are still common pathogens that cause a vast array of illnesses. We have made great advances with vaccines for polio, rabies, and hepatitis and have managed to control measles, mumps, and rubella, but we still have no cures for many of these pathogens.

Viruses have a nucleic acid core surrounded by a protein coat (capsid). This DNA or RNA genome and capsid are referred to as the *nucleocapsid*. Viruses are classified on the basis of their structure: DNA or RNA, single- or double-stranded, presence or absence of a lipoprotein envelope. The International Committee on the Taxonomy of Viruses (ICTV) approves the categorization of viruses, which is different from the taxonomy of bacteria. Virus families are designated by the suffix *viridae*. Subfamilies are designated by the suffix *virinae*, and genera are designated by the suffix *virus*.

Viruses can only replicate inside an appropriate host cell. Steps in the replication or infectious cycle include attachment, penetration, uncoating, synthesis, assembly, and release. Viruses display tropisms, that is, each virus type only infects particular cell types. This may be a function of the mode of transmission. Release of the viral particles often causes the death of the host cell. Local infection with the presence of viruses in the blood (viremia) may allow a secondary target tissue to become infected.

Some viruses, such as herpes and VZV, can remain latent in their human hosts until periodically activated. The virus enters sensory ganglia; there is limited transcription of the viral genome during this latency period. Once activated, the viruses cause lesions; shingles are the result of the reactivation of VZV.

The viruses that cause respiratory ailments include influenza viruses, parainfluenza viruses, RSV, human metapneumovirus, adenoviruses, rhinoviruses, coronaviruses. The influenza and parainfluenza viruses both have an affinity for mucopolysaccharides on cell surfaces, but they belong in two separate groups. Influenza is a highly contagious acute respiratory disease that has caused epidemics and pandemics. There are three types of influenza viruses (A, B, and C), but A and B account for almost all epidemic respiratory disease. There are two glycoprotein antigens on the virion surface that are important for pathogenesis and epidemiology. These are the hemagglutinin (H) and neuraminidase (N) antigens. These antigens are constantly changing, making vaccine development a challenging problem. When there are large changes in hemagglutinin, we have antigenic shift and the potential for an epidemic. The hemagglutinin H2 was responsible for the Asian pandemic of 1957 and H3 caused the Hong Kong pandemic of 1968. Recently, an

H5 strain of avian influenza killed several people in Hong Kong and Southeast Asia. There is concern that this "bird flu" could lead to another influenza pandemic. The primary control measure is vaccination with a trivalent inactivated vaccine. Amantadine and rimantadine have been licensed for prevention and treatment. Diagnosis techniques include cell culture, antibody titer, and direct detection of viral antigens in clinical specimens.

The parainfluenza viruses (PIV) cause an upper respiratory disease in children and adults. It has been estimated that almost all children will have been infected by PIV type 3 by 2 years of age. PIV-1 is the principle cause of croup and PIV-3 is second in prevalence after RSV. These are community-acquired pathogens. Certain factors can predispose to infection; these are malnutrition, environmental smoke, and lack of breastfeeding.

The parainfluenza virus is in the family *Paramyxoviridae*, as is the mumps virus. Mumps is an acute, self-limited illness characterized by parotitis (inflamed salivary gland) along with high temperature and fatigue. Humans are the only natural host. Transmission is by droplet spread and contact with saliva. Since the licensure of the live, attenuated vaccine in 1967, there has been a drop of more than 99% in the number of reported cases. Children receive a trivalent vaccine against mumps, measles, and rubella. Even so, outbreaks in both vaccinated and unvaccinated populations do occur. After reviewing data from the recent outbreaks in 2005-2006, the Advisory Committee on Immunization Practices (ACIP) has revised its recommendations for mumps vaccination. The recommendations for school-age children as well as health care workers can be found at *www.cdc.gov/mmwr/preview/mmwrhtml/mm5522a4.htm.*

RSV is the most common viral respiratory pathogen. It is estimated that this organism causes 45% of all hospital admissions for acute respiratory disease in children younger than 2 years of age. This is a seasonal disease causing bronchiolitis and pneumonia with the highest incidence between November and March. Some clinicians have also reported RSV to be a major health concern in older adults. Transmission is through contact with infected droplets. RSV can survive on environmental surfaces for 6 hours. A hallmark of RSV infection is, as the name implies, fusion of the host cells into syncytial cells. There are rapid tests for the detection of RSV in nasopharyngeal secretions; the best specimens are nasal washes or direct aspiration of secretions. Antiviral therapy for respiratory viruses other than the influenza virus has had limited effectiveness. Use of ribavirin therapy for RSV has been tried but is controversial.

In 2001, a novel virus was isolated from children in The Netherlands who had respiratory tract illness. Using sequence data, the virus appeared to be related to an avian pneumovirus; it was given the name human metapneumovirus (hMPV). This virus has been completely sequenced and classified as a *Paramyxoviridae* in the genus *Metapneumovirus*. It is closely related to RSV, and clinical disease presentation is the same for both viruses. hMPV has a worldwide distribution, seasonal peak activity coinciding with RSV, and appears to be responsible for a considerable proportion of lower respiratory tract infections in infants and young children. Serologic epidemiology studies have shown seroprevalence of hMPV-specific antibodies in adults is nearly 100% and is greater than 90% in children younger than 5 years of age. hMPV grows poorly in cell culture; immunofluorescence and real-time polymerase chain reaction (RT-PCR) are the more common diagnostic methods.

Adenoviruses were first detected when they caused spontaneous degeneration in adenoid tissue cultures. Adenoviruses can cause a wide range of infections that includes pharyngitis, acute respiratory disease, pneumonia, gastroenteritis, and meningoencephalitis. Illnesses occur throughout the year and appear to be more common in school-age children. Laboratory diagnosis is by cell culture of the affected tissue.

The common cold is predominantly caused by two virus groups: the rhinoviruses and the coronaviruses. Together they cause as many as 55% of colds. These infections are spread by person-to-person transmission of contaminated respiratory secretions or by the aerosol route. The viruses are present in the highest concentrations in the nose, where they infect nasal epithelial cells. There are approximately 100 rhinovirus serotypes based on neutralization tests; because of this variety, it has been difficult to develop tests for viral antigen detection. Some recent treatment advances include intranasal administration of ICAM-1 (intercellular adhesion molecule 1 is the cell receptor for many rhinoviruses) and zinc gluconate lozenges.

In 2003, a novel coronavirus was identified as the cause of the worldwide syndrome that became known as SARS (severe acute respiratory syndrome). The disease is characterized by rapid onset of high temperature, radiographic evidence of pneumonia, thrombocytopenia, and leukopenia. Respiratory distress may require hospitalization and mechanical ventilation. During the initial outbreaks in China and Vietnam, a secondary attack rate of more than 50% was noted among health care workers who had cared for the SARS patients. The SARS-associated coronavirus (SARS-CoV) was added to the National Notifiable Disease Surveillance System (NNDSS) and case definitions were published by the Centers for Disease Control and Prevention (CDC). This document can be viewed at *www.cdc.gov/mmwr/preview/mmwrhtml/mm5249a2.htm.*

In a 1991 study of children with acute febrile illness and rash, 72% of the identified infectious agents were viruses and 20% were bacteria. The classic six childhood diseases that produce skin eruptions (exanthemas) are measles, scarlet fever, rubella (German measles), atypical scarlet fever, erythema infectiosum (caused by parvovirus B19), and roseola.

The measles virus is in the family *Paramyxoviridae* and is related to the virus that causes distemper in dogs. This virus causes an acute generalized infection with epidemic peaks in developed countries that coincide with the school year. The virus is spread from person to person via aerosol with infection of the mucosal cells of the respiratory tract. The virus spreads to the lymph nodes and then to circulating T and B cells and monocytes.

136

Viremia is accompanied by a rash. The hallmark of measles is the Koplik's spots on the mouth epithelium. Measles is rarely fatal in North America and Europe, but in developing countries where there is poor nutrition and hygiene, the mortality rate may be as high as 20%. Diagnosis is usually made by the clinical symptoms, but serum may also be tested for virus-specific IgM.

The rubella virus is a member of the family *Togaviridae*. It is found only in human populations and causes German measles. It is transmitted by direct contact with nasopharyngeal secretions or by congenital transmission. Before the widespread use of the trivalent vaccine for measles, mumps, and rubella, rubella was an epidemic disease. It is usually a mild disease characterized by rash and fever. Pregnant women exposed to rubella are in danger of intrauterine infection. Infants with congenital rubella acquired during the first trimester may present with low birth weight, mental retardation, deafness, congenital heart disease, and neurologic defects. Infection occurring later in pregnancy may result in splenomegaly, osteomyelitis, and a variety of clinical presentations. Diagnosis in the newborn is made by virus isolation. The presence of IgM in the neonate is evidence of congenital infection, but the absence of IgM does not rule out infection.

It has been estimated that 40% to 60% of the adult population is serologically positive for human parvovirus B19. This virus has a worldwide distribution and may cause two types of infection: erythema infectiosum (fifth disease) or transient aplastic crisis. The virus is transmitted through saliva and respiratory secretions or from mother to fetus. Congenital infection can cause fetal death. It can also be transmitted via blood products. This fifth disease is easily identified by the hot, red cheeks giving a "slapped cheek" appearance. The most practical diagnostic approach is to test serum for virus-specific IgM or paired acute and convalescent sera for IgG.

Roseola is caused by human herpesvirus 6. There is an acute fever that lasts 3 to 5 days followed by an abrupt drop in temperature and the appearance of a rash on the trunk. The rash spreads from the trunk to the neck and extremities. The virus is shed in the saliva. Most cases are benign and self-limited. Serologic testing for virus-specific IgG can be done on acute and convalescent sera; there is also a PCR test available.

Viral gastroenteritis is the second most common clinical disease in developed countries; the first is viral respiratory disease. Common viral agents of gastrointestinal infection include rotavirus, noroviruses, and enteric adenoviruses. Rotaviruses are the most common viral cause of gastroenteritis in children. Disease is more prevalent in the winter months; symptoms include vomiting, diarrhea, and dehydration. The most severe disease occurs in children 6 months of age to 3 years of age, but there have been disease outbreaks among the elderly in nursing homes. Rotavirus is spread by the fecal-oral route. It is a frequent cause of nosocomial infections. Virus is detected directly in stool samples using either an EIA or latex agglutination test.

The noroviruses are members of the *Calicivirus* family and are the primary cause of viral gastroenteritis in adults. These viruses are associated with contaminated food and water; symptoms include nausea, vomiting, diarrhea, and abdominal cramps. Outbreaks have occurred on cruise ships and in institutions.

Enteric adenoviruses are the second most common gastrointestinal viral pathogen in children younger than 2 years of age. Adenovirus types 40 and 41 are the intestinal pathogens that produce sporadic epidemics. Symptoms are prolonged diarrhea with a low-grade fever; there may be vomiting. Adenovirus infection can be detected by culture and serology testing of acute and convalescent serum specimens as well as antigen (40 and 41) detection in stool specimens.

The viruses that cause CNS disease are the enteroviruses and arboviruses. The enteroviruses are single-stranded RNA viruses in the family *Picornaviridae*. These include coxsackie virus A and B, echovirus, enterovirus, poliovirus, and HSV. The enteroviruses are responsible for a variety of diseases and conditions that include aseptic meningitis, paralytic poliomyelitis, and encephalitis as well as respiratory illness, myocarditis, and pericarditis. Enteroviruses have been isolated from more than 40% of patients with aseptic meningitis. Enterovirus 71 causes a polio-like paralysis. Enteroviral infection is common among infants and young children, whereas polio is more prevalent in young adults. Specimens to be tested include biopsy specimens, CSF, stool, or throat swab. Cultures can be done for detection of enterovirus, HSV, and VZV. Serum antibody testing and antigen testing using molecular methods is also available.

Encephalitis is an inflammation of the brain parenchyma. Acute viral encephalitis can be caused by a wide variety of organisms. Frequently these infections are transmitted by an arthropod vector. Neurotropic arboviruses include St. Louis, Western, and Japanese encephalitis viruses. In summer of 1999, the first domestically acquired cases of West Nile encephalitis (WNV) were documented in the United States. In 2003, the CDC issued a warning for physicians not to confuse the symptoms of WNV with viral meningitis; both can present with fever, sensitivity to light, and a stiff or sore neck. Viral meningitis typically affects children and young adults with a mild, self-limiting illness. WNV affects older people with severe illness and is acquired by the bites of mosquitoes that have fed on infected birds. Diagnosis is made by detection of IgM in CSF or serum. PCR has limited usefulness because of transient and low viremia. Two other endemic causes of viral encephalitis in the United States are HSV and rabies. Rabies is a fatal infection of the CNS acquired through the contaminated saliva of rabid animals. The only reliable method of diagnosis is examination of brain tissue; DFA tests are the preferred tests for rabies diagnosis. In cases of viral encephalitis of unknown origin, rabies should always be considered.

Other causes of viral encephalitis include the mumps virus, which causes a meningoencephalitis; the lymphocytic choriomeningitis virus (LCM), which is associated with rodent reservoirs and the inhalation of aerosolized virus; human immunodeficiency virus (HIV).

The human immunodeficiency viruses HIV-1 and HIV-2 are members of the family *Retroviridae.* HTLV-1 and HTLV-2 are also retroviruses. These are RNA viruses that produce reverse transcriptase, which allows them to replicate their viral RNA genome into DNA and then into RNA. HIV-1 is the more aggressive virus and is responsible for the AIDS pandemic. AIDS is the end stage of a process wherein the immune system and its ability to control infections and malignant proliferation is destroyed. The virus has an affinity for the CD4 surface marker of T lymphocytes. As the number of CD4+ T lymphocytes decreases, the risk and severity of opportunistic infections increases. The first clinical symptoms may appear a few days after infection; this manifestation could be flulike symptoms or aseptic meningitis syndrome.

Immunologic markers of AIDS include a steady decline in the number of CD4+ T cells, depression of T4:T8 cell ratio to less than 0.9 (normal is >1.5), functional impairment of monocytes and macrophages, and anergy to recall antigens in skin tests. Some conditions that were included in the 1993 AIDS surveillance case definition include disseminated coccidioidomycosis, cryptococcosis, cryptosporidiosis, histoplasmosis, recurrent pneumonia, and pneumocystis pneumonia.

Detection of HIV antibody is still the mainstay of diagnosis. Repeatedly reactive antibody tests should be confirmed by Western blot. Clinical management of infected persons includes the use of highly active antiretroviral therapy (HAART) and is dependent on the measurement of CD4+ lymphocytes and viral load. Molecular methods are used to quantify the viral load. Diagnosis of HIV infection in babies born to HIV-positive mothers is problematic because of maternal IgG in the baby's blood. PCR for viral DNA or RNA is recommended.

HTLV-1 is endemic in Japan, the Caribbean, Melanesia, Sub-Saharan Africa, and South and Central America. Only a small percentage (<4%) of infected people develop symptoms and disease; the mean time following infection to the development of adult T-cell leukemia (ATL) is 40 years. Volunteer blood donors in the United States, Canada, and several other countries are screened. In the United States, blood donors whose serum is reactive by EIA for antibody and confirmed by Western blot are counseled and permanently deferred from donating blood.

HPVs are members of the family *Papovaviridae.* These viruses show a tissue tropism with preference for either cutaneous or mucosal tissues. Most attention has focused on the more than 30 sexually transmitted genotypes and their role in the pathogenesis of cancer. HPVs induce epithelial cell proliferation. The viruses cannot be propagated in cell culture. Diagnosis is dependent on clinical presentation or the detection of HPV DNA; in situ hybridization can be performed on tissue. HPV is the most prevalent viral STD and causes genital warts (condyloma acuminata). More than 65 million Americans are living with an incurable viral STD such as HPV or HSV. Cutaneous infection occurs in childhood with HPV types 1-4; HPV-1 causes plantar wart on the soles of the feet whereas HPV types 2-4 cause the common wart on hands.

Many viruses can damage the liver. EBV and CMV occasionally cause symptomatic hepatitis. But the primary hepatitis viruses are a diverse group. HAV produces sporadic and infectious hepatitis that is transmitted via contaminated food and water. The most common source of infection is household contact with an infected person. Other means of transmission include illicit drug use, travel to endemic countries, and men having sex with men. HAV is the only primary virus to be cultured in vitro,

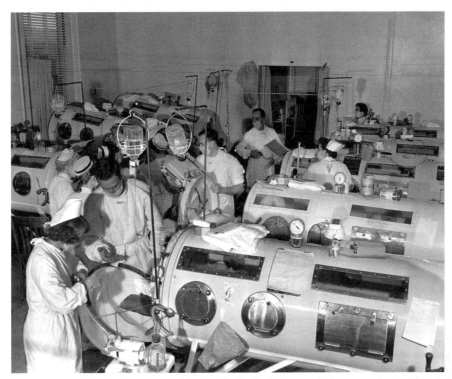

Figure 51-1 During the polio epidemics that occurred in the first half of the twentieth century in the United States, thousands of people, especially children, developed paralysis that affected their ability to breathe. Tank respirators, also known as iron lungs, were put into use. The patient was encased in an air-tight chamber; the chamber created negative air pressure around the patient's thoracic cavity, causing air to rush into the lungs. During the epidemics of the 1930s through 1950s, polio wards were established in hospitals; the iron lung machines filled the rooms and maintained respiration for the most severely affected patients. (Courtesy March of Dimes.)

but diagnosis is by serology testing for IgM antibody. There is no chronic infection. A vaccine became available in the 1990s for children older than 2 years of age and for adults.

HBV is a DNA hepadnavirus. It produces acute and chronic disease and is associated with hepatocellular carcinoma. Transmission is by parenteral means. Blood donors are all screened for HBV. Other routes of transmission include tattooing and acupuncture, sexual contact, and perinatal infection. Although this virus has not been cultured, there are a variety of diagnostic tools. Antibody to the surface, core, and e antigens can be measured. Hepatitis B surface antigen (HBsAg) is the first marker to appear in acute infection; as the infection resolves, HBsAg disappears and HBsAb appears. HBsAg is detectable either during acute or chronic infection. Viral load testing is done to confirm diagnosis and differentiate between chronic infection and an inactive carrier state. HBV genotyping is done to predict response to therapy; more than 60% of the people undergoing therapy with lamivudine develop resistance over time. Other therapeutic agents include adefovir and alpha-interferon. If the viral genome becomes incorporated into the genome of liver cells, hepatocellular carcinoma may develop. There is an effective vaccine; its use for occupational exposure and health care workers has been incorporated into OSHA's blood-borne pathogens standard (29 CFR Part 1910.1030).

After HAV and HBV were elucidated, other causes of hepatitis were recognized. HCV is an RNA virus transmitted by blood transfusion, intravenous drug abuse, hemodialysis, and contaminated instruments such as manicure devices, body piercing devices, and tattooing devices. HCV infection becomes chronic in more than 80% of patients. It is an independent risk factor for cancer after the development of cirrhosis. Diagnosis is made by antibody detection. HCV RNA is measured to assess response to treatment; alpha-interferon and ribavirin have been used in treatment regimens.

Other hepatitis viruses include the delta agent (HDV) that causes hepatitis D, hepatitis E virus (HEV), and hepatitis G virus (HGV). HDV is a defective RNA virus that is incapable of multiplication without the surface antigen of HBV. In the United States, most cases are seen in people exposed to contaminated needles and blood products. HDV can convert asymptomatic or mild chronic HBV into fulminant disease. HEV causes a self-limited illness that is transmitted enterically. Diagnosis of HEV is by serology testing for IgG and IgM. HGV infection is common worldwide and is associated with blood transfusion. The liver, however, is not a significant site of replication. Many people with HGV are co-infected with HBV, HCV, or HIV.

Transplant patients on immunosuppressive drug therapy are at great risk of infection. Viruses that have affected

139

posttransplant patients include herpes viruses, CMV, hepatitis viruses, adenoviruses, and the JC and BK viruses (polyomaviruses).

KEY TERMS AND ABBREVIATIONS

Match the term in the left column with the definition on the right.

1. _____ virion
2. _____ capsid
3. _____ syncytia
4. _____ viral tropism
5. _____ hemadsorption
6. _____ latent
7. _____ oncogenic
8. _____ viremia
9. _____ rabies
10. _____ norovirus
11. _____ SARS
12. _____ varicella-zoster virus
13. _____ EBV
14. _____ HSV-1
15. _____ rhinoviruses
16. _____ JC virus
17. _____ antigenic drift
18. _____ pandemic
19. _____ antigenic shift
20. _____ arbovirus
21. _____ parvovirus B19

A. viruses in the blood
B. gastrointestinal disease outbreak on cruise ships
C. common cold
D. multinucleated mass not separated into cells
E. capable of tumor production
F. worldwide outbreak
G. recognition of particular cell types
H. causes mononucleosis and Burkitt's lymphoma
I. dormant or hidden
J. fifth of the childhood exanthems
K. viral protein coat
L. subtle changes in H or N antigen
M. adherence to the surface of a RBC
N. infection diagnosed by FA staining of brain tissue
O. entire viral particle
P. coronavirus acute respiratory syndrome
Q. major genetic change causes pandemics
R. causes a multifocal leukoencephalopathy in organ transplant patients
S. arthropod-borne virus
T. reactivation causes a lip ulcer
U. recurrence causes shingles

TRUE OR FALSE

1. _____ Specimens for viral culture should be transported in viral transport media and stored at room temperature.
2. _____ Viral cultures are examined for cytopathic effect, which would indicate the presence of a virus.
3. _____ Adenoviruses are the most common viral respiratory pathogen and cause bronchiolitis in children younger than 2 years of age.
4. _____ Although we have influenza vaccines, the disease cannot be eradicated because of the constant changes in the neuraminidase and hemagglutinin antigens.
5. _____ The best way to detect a rotavirus infection is to do a viral culture on stool.

6. _____ Tests for CMV antigenemia and BK virus by PCR are often done to monitor transplant patients.
7. _____ HTLV-1 infection is associated with Kaposi's sarcoma.
8. _____ There is no chronic hepatitis A syndrome.
9. _____ The current recommendations for diagnosis of West Nile virus infection include testing CSF for IgM-specific antibodies.
10. _____ Two viruses associated with congenital infection are human parvovirus B19 and human herpesvirus 6.

MULTIPLE CHOICE

1. _____ Which statement about HIV detection is FALSE?
   A. Repeatedly reactive EIA procedures should be confirmed by Western blot.
   B. Diagnosis of HIV infection in babies born to HIV-positive mothers can be done by detection of antibody to HIV-1,2.
   C. HIV viral load is a good predictor of disease progression.
   D. Postexposure use of zidovudine has been shown to decrease transmission by as much as 80%.

2. _____ A hepatitis B virus panel of tests includes HBV surface antibody (HBsAb), HBV surface antigen (HBsAg), hepatitis Be antibody (HBeAb), and hepatitis Be antigen (HBeAg). A patient's results were:
   HBsAg—negative
   HBeAg—negative
   HBsAb—positive
   HBeAb—positive
   The most likely interpretation would be
   A. acute early infection.
   B. HBV vaccination.
   C. recovery of infection with immunity.
   D. chronic carrier state.

3. _____ Which statement about the human papillomavirus is FALSE?
   A. HPV types 2-4 cause the common wart often seen on children's hands.
   B. The most common types associated with a high risk of cervical cancer are HPV types 16 and 18.
   C. HPV causes genital warts.
   D. HPV is the second most prevalent viral STD in the United States.

4. _____ Viruses that cause central nervous system disease include
   A. enteroviruses.
   B. human herpesvirus 6.
   C. coxsackie viruses.
   D. both A and C.

5. _____ The two most prevalent viral respiratory pathogens in children are
   A. RSV and parainfluenza virus.
   B. coronavirus and rhinovirus.
   C. varicella-zoster virus and herpes virus.
   D. norovirus and adenovirus.

CASE STUDY

A middle-age white man had a CBC and chemistry profile done as part of his yearly physical examination. His hemoglobin and hematocrit were slightly decreased and the liver enzymes AST (SGOT) and ALT (SGPT) were slightly elevated, but all other results were in the acceptable reference range. His AST was 101 (reference range 5-40 U/L) and ALT was 122 (reference range 7-56 U/L). The physician followed up by ordering additional blood tests. Tests and results are listed below.

Test	Patient Result	Reference Range
Iron	62	49-181 µg/dL
Ferritin	260.0	17.9-464.0 ng/mL
Hepatitis C antibody (HCAb)	Positive	Negative
Reflex test: HCAb (RIBA)	Positive	Negative

After seeing the above results, the patient was referred to a hepatologist who ordered the additional testing listed below.

Alpha-fetoprotein (AFP) (tumor marker)	8	0-15 ng/mL
HC RNA quantitative by RT-PCR	7.1	<1.9 log IU
HCV genotyping	1a	

1. Why were two HCV antibody tests done?
2. Why were ferritin and iron tests performed?
3. What is the significance of performing HCV quantitative RNA testing and viral genotyping?
4. Why did the hepatologist order the AFP?
5. This patient never had a blood transfusion nor did he work in health care. How could he have acquired this viral infection?

ANSWERS

Key Terms and Abbreviations

1. O
2. K
3. D
4. G
5. M
6. I
7. E
8. A
9. N
10. B
11. P
12. U
13. H
14. T
15. C
16. R
17. L
18. F
19. Q
20. S
21. J

True or False

1. F
2. T
3. F
4. T
5. F
6. T
7. F
8. T
9. T
10. F

Multiple Choice

1. B
2. C
3. D
4. D
5. A

Case Study

1. Positive test results for HCV IgG should be confirmed by a different methodology. The common screening test method is enzyme immunoassay (EIA). Supplemental testing with a more specific assay to prevent the reporting of false-positive results is recommended. The recombinant immunoblot assay (RIBA) is the recommended method to test specimens with a low positive anti-HCV screening result.

2. Hemochromatosis is in the differential diagnosis for a middle-aged white man with abnormal liver function tests. Hemochromatosis is a hereditary disorder characterized by the accumulation of iron in body tissues; the liver is one area where excess iron is stored. This can lead to cirrhosis and an increased risk for hepatocellular carcinoma. Ferritin is the tissue form of accumulated iron and reflects the total body iron status.

3. The HCV RNA assay is used to document viremia. The assay can also be used to monitor the individual's response to therapy. There are six major HCV genotypes. Patient prognosis and disease course appear to be dependent on the genotype. The majority of HCV-infected Americans are infected with genotype 1 subtype 1a. Unfortunately, response rates to therapy are much lower in genotype 1a.

4. AFP is a protein produced by the fetal liver but is not present in healthy individuals. AFP is increased in hepatocellular carcinoma and in benign liver conditions such as acute viral hepatitis, chronic active hepatitis, and cirrhosis.

5. HCV is a major public health concern and is the most common chronic blood-borne infection in the United States. Blood transfusion used to account for the majority of HCV infections. But since the identification of

the virus about 20 years ago and the institution of HCV screening of all donor units, the most important behavioral risk factor for HCV infection in developed Western countries is injection drug use and needle sharing. Some studies have measured that illicit drug use is accountable for 60% of infections. Other methods of transmission/acquisition include hemodialysis, tattooing, acupuncture, manicure devices, razors, and occupational and nosocomial exposures.

REFERENCES

Alexander LN, Seward JF, Santibanez TA, et al: Vaccine policy changes and epidemiology of poliomyelitis in the United States, *JAMA* 292:1696, 2004.

Burd EM: Human papillomavirus and cervical cancer, *Clin Microbiol Rev* 16:1, 2003.

Centers for Disease Control and Prevention: 1993 Revised classification system for HIV infection and expanded surveillance case definition for AIDS among adolescents and adults, *Morb Mortal Wkly Rep* 41:RR-17, 1992.

Centers for Disease Control and Prevention: Outbreak of severe acute respiratory syndrome—worldwide, 2003, *Morb Mortal Wkly Rep* 52:226, 2003.

Centers for Disease Control and Prevention: Recommendations for prevention and control of hepatitis C virus (HCV) infection and HCV-related chronic disease, *Morb Mortal Wkly Rep* 47:RR-19, 1998.

Centers for Disease Control and Prevention: Resurgence of wild poliovirus type 1 transmission and consequences of importation—21 countries, 2002-2005, *Morb Mortal Wkly Rep* 55:145, 2006.

Centers for Disease Control and Prevention: Revised U.S. Surveillance case definition for severe acute respiratory syndrome (SARS) and update on SARS cases—United States and worldwide, December 2003, *Morb Mortal Wkly Rep* 52:1202, 2003.

DeClercq E: Clinical potential of the acyclic nucleoside phosphonates cidofovir, adefovir, and tenofovir in treatment of DNA virus and retrovirus infections, *Clin Microbiol Rev* 16:569, 2003.

Dufresne AT, Gromeier M: Understanding polio: new insights from a cold virus, *Microbe* 1:13, 2006.

Henderson DK: Managing occupational risks for hepatitis C transmission in the health care setting, *Clin Microbiol Rev* 16:546, 2003.

Henrickson KJ: Parainfluenza viruses, *Clin Microbiol Rev* 16:242, 2003.

Hulisz D: Efficacy of zinc against common cold viruses: an overview, *J Am Pharm Assoc (Wash DC)* 44:594, 2004.

Kahn JS: Epidemiology of human metapneumovirus, *Clin Microbiol Rev* 19:546, 2006.

Nainan OV, Xia G, Vaughan G, Margolis HS: Diagnosis of hepatitis A virus infection: a molecular approach, *Clin Microbiol Rev* 19:63, 2006.

Strader DB, Wright T, Thomas DL, Seeff LB: Diagnosis, management, and treatment of hepatitis C, *Hepatology* 39:1147, 2004.

52 Bloodstream Infections

OBJECTIVES

Upon completion of this chapter, the reader should be able to:
1. Differentiate between bacteremia and septicemia.
2. List the most frequently isolated bacterial and fungal bloodstream pathogens.
3. Explain the significance of IV catheters to bloodstream infections.
4. Describe the proper blood collection procedure.
5. Explain the importance of blood volume in a blood culture to clinically significant test results.
6. List and describe several blood culture systems.

SUMMARY OF KEY POINTS

The suffix "emia" is derived from the Greek word meaning "blood"; it refers to the presence of a substance in blood. *Bacteremia* refers to the presence of bacteria in the blood, whereas *fungemia* refers to the presence of fungi in the bloodstream. Septicemia means there is a bloodstream infection where bacteria are not only present but are also multiplying and producing toxins. Vital statistics list the major causes of death in the United States, with heart disease ranking first causing about 725,000 deaths and septicemia causing more than 22,000 deaths (0.97%). It has been estimated that more than 200,000 nosocomial bloodstream infections occur yearly in the United States. In both adults and children, the majority of these nosocomial bloodstream infections are associated with the use of an intravascular catheter. It is difficult to measure the mortality associated with these infections, but estimated costs per infection have been reported to be between $34,000 and $56,000.

Bacteremia can be transient, intermittent, or continuous. We have all experienced transient bacteremia; teething infants and people having dental procedures have had oral flora gain entry to the bloodstream through breaks in the gums. If the bacteria are cleared from the blood by scavenging leukocytes, there is no infection. But if the bacteria multiply more rapidly than the immune system can clear it, then septicemia occurs. Symptoms of septicemia include fever, chills, and malaise due not only to the presence of the microorganisms but also specifically to the various toxins associated with those organisms. The mortality rate due to septicemia rises with the increasing age of the patient.

The majority of catheter-related bloodstream infections in both adults and children are caused by gram-positive organisms (coagulase-negative staphylococci, *S. aureus,* and enterococci). Interpretation of blood cultures yielding coagulase-negative staphylococci is difficult. Are these staphylococci true pathogens or is the blood culture contaminated with skin flora? The current recommendation from the Infectious Diseases Society of America is to draw paired blood cultures; one set (aerobic and anaerobic) should be drawn through the intravenous (IV) catheter and one set should be collected by peripheral venipuncture. A positive culture collected through the IV catheter requires careful interpretation but a negative culture is diagnostic. Current practice includes the culture of removed IV catheters. The catheter tip is cultured using a semi-quantitative (roll plate) method or quantitative (vortex or sonication) technique. A positive catheter tip culture in the absence of a positive blood culture has little clinical significance.

The single most important factor in the detection of bacteremia is adequate blood volume. The total volume of blood collected should be divided between two separate venipunctures to minimize the chance of a false-positive culture due to cutaneous contamination. Single blood cultures have limited clinical utility. Automated blood culture systems have culture bottles that are designed to hold 7 to 10 mL of blood per bottle. To optimize pathogen recovery in an adult, at least 30 mL of blood should be drawn in two venipunctures and distributed evenly between two blood culture sets.

Bloodstream infections may also occur as organisms are released from a focus of infection, such as an undrained abscess or infective endocarditis. The primary causes of infective endocarditis are the viridans streptococci from the oral cavity. There is also a group of gram-negative bacilli associated with endocarditis; they are known by the acronym *HACEK* for *Haemophilus aphrophilus, Actinobacillus actinomycetemcomitans, Cardiobacterium hominis, Eikenella corrodens,* and *Kingella kingae.*

A variety of other organisms can cause bloodstream infections; these include the fungi, viruses, mycobacteria, parasites, and fastidious bacteria. Blood cultures are a primary diagnostic tool if brucellosis is suspected. Communication between the laboratory and physician is vital, however, both for provision of proper culture medium and incubation conditions and for the safety of laboratory personnel. If anthrax is suspected, the clinician needs to communicate this to laboratory personnel. If the patient is immunocompromised and the physician suspects an unusual pathogen, this should be communicated to the laboratory. Incubation times for automated blood culture systems can be modified if the suspect pathogen has a slow growth rate. If the patient is a dialysis patient, recovery of a coagulase-negative staphylococcus could be a significant pathogen rather than a contaminant.

Because false-positive blood cultures may lead to prolonged hospital stays and unnecessary treatment with antibiotics, it is very important that proper technique be used in the collection of blood cultures. The benchmark of 3% is widely used as the acceptable limit for contaminated blood cultures. Rates higher than this represent a quality assurance issue both for the hospital and the microbiology laboratory.

INTEREST POINT

The Clinical and Laboratory Standards Institute (formerly known as NCCLS) is an educational organization that promotes the development and use of voluntary consensus standards and guidelines within the health care community. The documents published by CLSI provide health care professionals with practical operating guidelines that lead to consistent practices, precision, and efficient use of resources. Their documents deal with all aspects of laboratory science. CLSI documents are fundamental tools in microbiology; laboratories worldwide use the CLSI performance standards for antimicrobial susceptibility testing, quality control testing, and interpretive guidelines. CLSI also sets the standards for the collection of diagnostic blood specimens. Document H3-A5 published in December 2003 recommended the following process for site preparation before blood culture collection:

1. Cleanse the site with 70% alcohol as normally done for venipuncture site preparation.
2. Use a 1% to 10% povidone-iodine solution or chlorhexidine gluconate to swab concentrically in a widening circle starting at the venipuncture site. Allow the solution to air dry. Chlorhexidine gluconate is recommended for patients with iodine sensitivity. It cannot, however, be used on infants younger than 2 months.
3. Remove the iodine or chlorhexidine with a 70% alcohol prep pad. Allow the alcohol to air-dry before performing venipuncture. Do not palpate the cleaned site.
4. Wipe the blood culture bottle stopper with the antiseptic solution recommended by the manufacturer.
   The CDC and OSHA work closely together to ensure the safety of the health care worker as well as the patient. In January 2001, H.R. 5178 was passed into law; this is the Needlestick Safety and Prevention Act. This act required changes in the blood-borne pathogens standard that was in effect under the Occupational Safety and Health Act of 1970. Because of the high incidence of occupational exposure to blood-borne pathogens from accidental sharps injuries, engineering controls to make sharps (e.g., needles and scalpels) safer medical devices were required. Needles used in phlebotomy had to have a built-in safety feature. Although it is recommended that blood specimens for culture be collected by venipuncture directly into the blood culture bottles and that a needle and syringe be avoided for safety reasons, there are many times a syringe must be used. If a syringe is used, the blood must be transferred to the blood culture bottles with a safety shielded transfer device.

The content of the bill can be accessed at *http://thomas.loc.gov/*.

KEY TERMS AND ABBREVIATIONS

Match the term in the left column with the definition on the right.

1. _____ bacteremia
2. _____ occult
3. _____ fungemia
4. _____ endocarditis
5. _____ septicemia
6. _____ septic shock
7. _____ SPS
8. _____ HACEK

A. complication due to the presence of toxins in the blood
B. infection of the membrane lining the heart
C. presence of bacteria in the blood
D. group of gram-negative bacilli associated with endocarditis
E. multiplication of bacteria in the bloodstream
F. presence of fungi in the blood
G. hidden
H. anticoagulant used for blood cultures

TRUE OR FALSE

1. _____ The presence of fungi in blood indicates that there is a primary infection site elsewhere in the body.
2. _____ Parasites can be found transiently in the bloodstream as they migrate to other organs.
3. _____ *Histoplasma* is the most common genus of fungus isolated from blood cultures.
4. _____ Teeth cleaning during a routine dental checkup can cause a transient bacteremia.
5. _____ In the case of an undrained abscess, bacteria is released transiently into the bloodstream. It is best to draw blood cultures before the next spike in temperature.

MULTIPLE CHOICE

1. _____ Diagnosis of which parasitic infection is dependent on observing the organisms in peripheral blood smears?
   A. *Coccidioides* spp.
   B. *Plasmodium* spp.
   C. *Malassezia furfur*
   D. *Naegleria fowleri*
2. _____ A frequent complication in hospitalized patients who have an IV catheter is
   A. aneurysm.
   B. pneumonia.
   C. suppurative thrombophlebitis.
   D. DIC.

3. _____ Alcohol is the standard antiseptic used to cleanse venipuncture sites, but for blood culture collection
   A. soap and water should be used.
   B. chlorhexidine gluconate is recommended for all patients.
   C. 2% povidone-iodine should be used on all patients.
   D. the site should be cleansed three times using alcohol and iodine or chlorhexidine.
4. _____ To determine whether a patient's fever is due to a catheter-related bloodstream infection, the current recommendation is to
   A. collect two blood cultures from the same site using one venipuncture.
   B. collect two blood cultures 15 minutes apart both drawn through the IV catheter.
   C. collect two blood cultures: one by peripheral venipuncture and one through the IV catheter.
   D. collect one blood culture through the IV catheter.
5. _____ Factors that affect successful detection of organisms in the blood include
   A. collecting 10 to 20 mL of blood per culture.
   B. collecting two or more blood cultures.
   C. using the anticoagulant SPS in broth.
   D. all of the above.

CASE STUDY

A newborn developed a fever. Nursery protocol required a blood culture be collected. One culture was ordered and collected. Within 24 hours the blood culture was positive with a Gram stain showing gram-positive cocci in clusters and the organism identified as a coagulase-negative staphylococcus. Two days later the baby's condition had not improved and a second blood culture was collected. The second culture also grew a coagulase-negative staphylococcus. Appropriate antibiotic therapy was begun. The neonatologist ordered a culture of the mother's breast milk. This culture yielded a coagulase-negative staphylococcus. The mother had been using a breast pump that was the property of the postpartum nursing unit. This pump was cultured; a coagulase-negative staphylococcus was isolated.
1. Why wasn't antimicrobial therapy initiated after the first positive blood culture?
2. Why did the neonatologist order the culture of the breast milk?
3. What infection control measures should be in place if a central piece of equipment is to be shared by patients?

ANSWERS

Key Terms and Abbreviations

1. C
2. G
3. F
4. B
5. E
6. A
7. H
8. D

True or False

1. T
2. T
3. F
4. T
5. T

Multiple Choice

1. B
2. C
3. D
4. C
5. D

Case Study

1. Coagulase-negative staphylococci are part of the indigenous skin flora. A single positive blood culture is difficult to interpret, especially when the organism isolated could be a contaminant.
2. With two positive blood cultures both growing the same organism, the question that needs to be answered is how the baby became infected. Because we know the baby was being breast fed, it was logical to examine the breast milk for pathogens.
3. Given that the mother was using the hospital-owned breast pump, it was good investigative work to determine whether the pump was a link in the chain of infection. Apparently the pump was not being adequately cleaned between uses. The infection control nurse and postpartum departments needed to work closely to ensure proper equipment disinfection and the safety of the patients. This would be considered a nosocomial infection because it was acquired in the hospital.

REFERENCES

Centers for Disease Control and Prevention: Guidelines for the prevention of intravascular catheter-related infections, *Morb Mortal Wkly Rep* 51:RR-10, 2002.

Mermel LA, Farr BM, Sherertz RJ, et al: Guidelines for the management of intravascular catheter-related infections, *Clin Infect Dis* 32:1249, 2001.

National Committee for Clinical Laboratory Standards: Procedures for the collection of diagnostic blood specimens by venipuncture; Approved standard H3-A5, ed 5, Wayne, Pa, 2003, National Committee for Clinical Laboratory Standards.

Needlestick Safety and Prevention Act *http://thomas.loc.gov/*.

Wenzel RP, Edmond MB: The impact of hospital-acquired bloodstream infections, *Emerg Infect Dis* 7:174, 2001.

Wisplinghoff H, Bischoff T, Tallent SM, et al: Nosocomial bloodstream infections in U.S. hospitals: analysis of 24,179 cases from a prospective nationwide surveillance study, *Clin Infect Dis* 39:309, 2004.

Wisplinghoff H, Seifert, H, Tallent SM, et al: Nosocomial bloodstream infections in pediatric patients in United States Hospitals: epidemiology, clinical features and susceptibilities, *Pediatr Infect Dis J* 22:686, 2003.

53 Infections of the Lower Respiratory Tract

OBJECTIVES

Upon completion of this chapter, the reader should be able to:

1. Have an understanding of the anatomic structure of the lower respiratory tract and know what the trachea, bronchi, bronchioles, and alveoli are.
2. Differentiate between the following specimens: sputum, induced sputum, endotracheal suction, pleural fluid, bronchoalveolar lavage, bronchial washing, and bronchial brush sample.
3. List the Gram stain screening criteria for an acceptable sputum specimen.
4. Explain the significance of a mucoid *Pseudomonas aeruginosa* in a respiratory culture from a cystic fibrosis patient.
5. List the normal respiratory flora as well as potential pathogens.
6. Explain the difference between community-acquired pneumonia and hospital-acquired pneumonia.
7. List the most common causes of lower respiratory tract infection in the different age groups—children, young adults, adults, and geriatric patients—and in the immunocompromised patients.
8. List the laboratory tests useful in diagnosing the less common infections caused by *Pneumocystis jiroveci*, *Legionella* spp., *Chlamydophila pneumoniae*, *Bordetella pertussis*, *Mycoplasma pneumoniae*, and *Nocardia*.

SUMMARY OF KEY POINTS

The respiratory tract can be divided into two major areas. The upper respiratory tract consists of all structures above the larynx. The lower respiratory tract follows air flow below the larynx through the trachea into the bronchi and bronchioles and finally into the alveolar spaces where gas exchange occurs. Infections of the lower respiratory tract occur if pathogens evade the various host defense mechanisms of the upper airways.

Bronchitis can either be acute or chronic. Acute bronchitis is usually due to viral agents such as the influenza virus, respiratory syncytial virus (RSV), rhinovirus, and coronavirus. This is usually a seasonal ailment. In children, however, acute bronchitis may also be due to the bacteria *Bordetella pertussis*. Although vaccination is required by many school districts, there are sporadic outbreaks of pertussis. Acute viral bronchitis may be complicated by secondary bacterial infection. Chronic bronchitis is defined as cough and sputum production on most days for at least 3 months of the year over a 2-year period. Chronic bronchitis is usually due to cigarette smoking or exposure to noxious chemicals; there may also be acute infections

during the chronic course of the chronic condition. Potential bacterial pathogens include *S. pneumoniae*, *Haemophilus influenzae*, *Moraxella catarrhalis,* and *Chlamydophila pneumoniae.*

Acute bronchiolitis is a clinical disease that affects infants and small children usually during the winter months. It is frequently caused by RSV and is characterized by wheezing, fever, and respiratory distress.

The most serious lower respiratory tract infection is pneumonia. Symptoms include fever, cough, sputum production, difficulty breathing, and chest pain. From a management perspective, pneumonia is divided into two broad types: community-acquired and hospital-acquired. The most common cause of community-acquired pneumonia (CAP) is *Streptococcus pneumoniae* with the highest incidence of pneumonia in the very young and the very old. *Mycoplasma pneumoniae* is common in children and adults younger than 30 years of age. Organisms can reach the deep lung air spaces to cause infection by one of four routes: inhalation of pathogens via airborne droplets, aspiration of oropharyngeal or gastric secretions, upper airway colonization that reaches down into the normally sterile lung, or seeding of the lung via the bloodstream. Chronic pneumonia is caused by mycobacterial or fungal infection.

A nosocomial infection is one that is acquired while hospitalized. Hospital-acquired pneumonia (HAP) is defined as pneumonia that develops more than 48 hours after admission. Closely associated with HAP is ventilator-associated pneumonia (VAP), which is a disease that occurs more than 48 to 72 hours after endotracheal intubation. HAP has a high morbidity and mortality. HAP is usually caused by bacteria and accounts for up to 25% of all intensive care unit infections. The common pathogens are gram-negative bacilli, such as *P. aeruginosa, E. coli, Klebsiella pneumoniae,* and *Acinetobacter* spp., and the gram-positive organisms such as *S. aureus* and methicillin-resistant *S. aureus.*

Key issues in diagnosing and managing patients with HAP and VAP include the collection of a lower respiratory tract culture before antibiotic therapy and the performance of either semiquantitative or quantitative cultures. Quantitative cultures increase the specificity of the diagnosis. Guidelines for the management of adults with HAP and VAP have been proposed by the American Thoracic Society in conjunction with the Infectious Diseases Society of America. The goal of these guidelines is the management of these patients with early appropriate antibiotic therapy over a minimal effective period to decrease the selective pressures for the development of multidrug-resistant bacterial pathogens.

The easiest specimen to collect for testing is an expectorated sputum. It is important to instruct the patient on specimen production to avoid contaminating the sputum with saliva. Sputa should be screened for culture by quantitating cells from the Gram stain. Specimens with more than 10 epithelial cells/low-power field (LPF) are considered to be poor specimens; sputum from the deep lung would not contain squamous epithelial cells. The presence of columnar epithelial cells is an indicator of a deep lung specimen; these cells can frequently be seen in bronchoalveolar lavages (BAL).

KEY TERMS AND ABBREVIATIONS

Match the term in the left column with the definition on the right.

1. _____ alveoli
2. _____ thoracic cavity
3. _____ pleural fluid
4. _____ mediastinum
5. _____ colonization
6. _____ caseating necrosis
7. _____ miliary tuberculosis
8. _____ aspiration pneumonia
9. _____ empyema
10. _____ thoracentesis
11. _____ BAL
12. _____ bronchial washing

A. body space that contains the heart and lungs
B. space between the lungs
C. disseminated disease
D. needle puncture of the pleural cavity
E. microscopic structures for gas exchange
F. coexistence between host and bacteria
G. mass of dead tissue resembling soft cheese
H. accumulation of fluid between the pleura
I. disease caused by inhalation of gastric or oral secretions
J. wash of the bronchial tree with 30 mL of saline
K. pus in the pleural cavity
L. deep washing of the alveolar spaces

TRUE OR FALSE

1. _____ Miliary tuberculosis is a risk to people older than 65 years of age because of latent tubercle multiplication and decreased immune function.
2. _____ *C. diphtheriae* produces disease through the action of its exotoxin.
3. _____ The best specimen for diagnosis of pertussis is a sputum culture.
4. _____ Pneumonia can be caused by anaerobes such as *Prevotella*, particularly if the patient aspirated oral secretions.
5. _____ Tracheostomy suction specimens should be treated as sputum by the laboratory.

MULTIPLE CHOICE

1. _____ An unacceptable sputum for culture is one that contains
   A. >10 epithelial cells/LPF.
   B. <10 epithelial cells/LPF.
   C. <25 WBCs/LPF.
   D. many gram-positive organisms.
2. _____ Routine culture media for sputum specimens should include the following agar types:
   A. 5% sheep blood, colistin and nalidixic acid.
   B. 5% sheep blood, MacConkey, chocolate.
   C. 5% sheep blood, MacConkey, mannitol salts agar.
   D. 5% sheep blood, MacConkey, Sabouraud's heart infusion.
3. _____ The most prevalent cause of community-acquired pneumonia regardless of age is
   A. *S. pneumoniae*
   B. *H. influenzae*
   C. *P. aeruginosa*
   D. *Mycoplasma pneumoniae*
4. _____ A mechanism by which respiratory pathogens evade the host's immune response is
   A. production of lysozyme.
   B. production of endotoxin.
   C. secretion of IgA.
   D. multiplying within host cells.
5. _____ Isolation of a mucoid *Pseudomonas aeruginosa* from sputum should always be reported because it should alert the physician to the possibility of underlying
   A. neoplasm.
   B. cystic fibrosis.
   C. pneumonia.
   D. COPD.

CASE STUDY

A 5-year-old boy had been ill with fever and malaise for 2 weeks. His family physician had diagnosed influenza and recommended rest but prescribed no medications or laboratory tests. The child continued to be ill; his mother took him back to the general practitioner who repeated the earlier diagnosis but prescribed amoxicillin. As the week progressed, the child's condition worsened. The mother brought the child to the emergency department. Upon admission, the child was feverish and had a non-productive cough. The chest x-ray showed infiltrates. A CBC and blood culture were collected. The WBC count was elevated with a preponderance of neutrophils in the differential. The child was admitted to the pediatric unit. The child's condition continued to deteriorate and a lumbar puncture was done. Tests performed on the CSF included a Gram stain and culture, glucose, and protein. There were no organisms seen on the Gram stain and the glucose and protein results were within the normal reference range. After a 24-hour incubation period, the blood culture became positive. Gram-positive cocci in clusters were seen on the Gram stain. The child went into respiratory failure and died that day.

1. What are the possible identities for the gram-positive cocci seen in the blood culture?
2. A postmortem was performed. There were abnormalities noted in the lungs and specimens were taken for culture. These cultures yielded *Staphylococcus aureus*. Postmortem diagnoses of *S. aureus* sepsis and pneumonia were made. The administration of amoxicillin failed to improve the child's condition. Why?
3. How could the child have acquired *S. aureus*?

ANSWERS

Key Terms and Abbreviations
1. E
2. A
3. H
4. B
5. F
6. G
7. C
8. I
9. K
10. D
11. L
12. J

True or False
1. T
2. T
3. F
4. T
5. T

Multiple Choice
1. A
2. B
3. A
4. D
5. B

Case Study
1. Gram-positive cocci in clusters are indicative of the staphylococci. A single positive blood culture is difficult to interpret. Using only the Gram stain result, the culture could be contaminated with coagulase-negative staphylococci or could be harboring a true pathogen such as *S. aureus*.
2. Amoxicillin is an extended spectrum penicillin. When penicillin was first introduced in the 1940s, it was successfully used against many microbes. But within 20 years resistance to this antibiotic was being reported. The current incidence of methicillin-resistant *S. aureus* may be as high as 40%. Amoxicillin, however, has activity against streptococci and *H. influenzae*, the organisms most commonly recovered from respiratory specimens from children. The *S. aureus* recovered was resistant to oxacillin; clinical evidence shows that this isolate would not respond to other beta-lactam antibiotics or the cephalosporins.
3. *S. aureus* frequently colonizes the nares and upper respiratory tract. It is a pathogen in community-acquired pneumonia and has been associated with postviral respiratory tract infection, such as influenza.

REFERENCES

American Thoracic Society, Infectious Diseases Society of America: Guidelines for the management of adults with hospital-acquired, ventilator-associated, and healthcare-associated pneumonia, *Am J Respir Crit Care Med* 171: 388, 2005.

Centers for Disease Control and Prevention: National Nosocomial Infections Surveillance (NNIS) System Report, data summary from January 1992 through June 2004, issued October 2004, *Am J Infect Control* 32:470, 2004.

54 Upper Respiratory Tract Infections and Other Infections of the Oral Cavity and Neck

OBJECTIVES

Upon completion of this chapter, the reader should be able to:
1. Describe the structures that constitute the upper respiratory tract.
2. List the causative organisms of pharyngitis.
3. Differentiate between pharyngitis, laryngitis, epiglottis, and parotitis.
4. Differentiate between disease caused by *Corynebacterium diphtheriae* and *Bordetella pertussis*.
5. Differentiate between stomatitis and thrush.
6. Explain how to process specimens for the detection of group A *Streptococcus*.

SUMMARY OF KEY POINTS

The respiratory tract is generally divided into two regions: upper and lower. The upper respiratory tract includes all the structures down to the larynx: the sinuses, throat, nasal cavity, epiglottis, and larynx. One of the most frequent illnesses that cause patients to seek medical care is acute pharyngitis. Viruses are the most common cause of acute pharyngitis. These pathogens include rhinovirus, coronavirus, adenovirus, influenza virus, parainfluenza virus, and respiratory syncytial virus. The most common bacterial cause of pharyngitis is *Streptococcus pyogenes*. Other bacteria implicated in pharyngitis include groups C and G streptococci, *Corynebacterium diphtheriae*, and less frequently *Neisseria gonorrhoeae*, *Arcanobacterium haemolyticum*, *Yersinia enterocolitica*, and *Francisella tularensis*.

Untreated pharyngitis due to group A streptococci can lead to the serious sequelae of rheumatic fever and glomerulonephritis. Rheumatic fever is uncommon now due to the widespread practice of testing for streptococcal infection and treating with antimicrobials. Several rapid antigen detection kits have been marketed for use both in physicians' offices and in laboratories. Although the sensitivity of these kits is high, a negative rapid antigen test for group A streptococci should be confirmed by either culture or a nucleic acid method.

INTEREST POINT

The Infectious Diseases Society of America (IDSA) published practice guidelines for the diagnosis and management of group A streptococcal pharyngitis in 2002. This infection is most common in school-age children, causing up to 30% of the pharyngitis cases. In adults this organism is only responsible for about 10% of the cases of pharyngitis. Because of the decreased incidence of "strep throat" in the adult population, the IDSA developed a clinical algorithm that would obviate the need for confirmatory testing among particular patient groups. The drug of choice is penicillin; more information on antimicrobial therapy can be found at *www.journals.uchicago.edu/ CID/journal/issues/v35n2/020429/020429.html*.

Other bacterial causes of pharyngitis include *C. diphtheriae* and *B. pertussis*. Although vaccination of infants for diphtheria, pertussis, and tetanus became recommended for children in the 1940s, the number of pertussis cases in adults and adolescents has been increasing since the 1980s. It is believed this is due to waning immunity as the immunized pediatric population ages. There are sporadic outbreaks of pertussis and diphtheria. These organisms require specialized media for cultivation and should be considered when diagnosing the patient with pharyngitis. Tests for pertussis include a relatively rapid direct fluorescent antibody stain, culture using Regan-Lowe media, and polymerase chain reaction (PCR). Nasopharyngeal swabs are the preferred specimens. Although diphtheria is now extremely rare in the United States, there are sporadic outbreaks of this disease among children. A gray-white membrane may cover the tonsils and pharynx in contrast to the bright red pharynx of other infections. Diagnosis is done by culture of the membrane on Loeffler's agar or cystine-tellurite agar. When collecting nasopharyngeal swabs for these tests, the health care worker should protect himself by wearing a mask. The Centers for Disease Control and Prevention published guidelines in 2006 for the prevention of tetanus, diphtheria, and pertussis among adolescents. More information can be found at *www.cdc.gov/mmwr/PDF/rr/rr5503.pdf*.

INTEREST POINT

Mumps is a viral disease causing swelling of the salivary glands (parotitis). The word *mumps* is believed to have originated from the old English word for a "grimace," possibly because of the swelling of the face and painful swallowing. There was a recent outbreak of mumps in Iowa early in 2006. In the United States there have been about 265 cases of mumps reported each year since 2001. But by March 2006, a total of 219 cases of mumps had been reported in Iowa alone. From January to May 2006 more than 2500 cases of mumps had been reported from 11 states. This is the largest mumps epidemic in the United States since 1988. Iowa has had laws mandating vaccination against measles, mumps, and rubella for entry into school since 1977. With a highly vaccinated population, how did this epidemic happen? After reviewing data from the recent outbreak, the Advisory Committee on Immunization Practices (ACIP) has revised its recommendations for mumps vaccination. The recommendations for school-age children as well as healthcare workers can be found at *www.cdc.gov/mmwr/preview/mmwrhtml/mm5522a4.htm*.

KEY TERMS AND ABBREVIATIONS

Match the term in the left column with the definition on the right.

1. _____ pharyngitis	A. bronchitis characterized by a barking cough
2. _____ nasopharynx	B. sore throat
3. _____ croup	C. mumps
4. _____ epiglottis	D. potentially life-threatening infection of the epiglottis and soft tissue
5. _____ poststreptococcal sequela	E. pertussis
6. _____ rhinitis	F. best site for collection of RSV specimens
7. _____ whooping cough	G. common cold
8. _____ thrush	H. glomerulonephritis
9. _____ parotitis	I. trench mouth
10. _____ Vincent's angina	J. oral candidiasis

TRUE OR FALSE

1. _____ Acute laryngitis is almost always caused by bacteria.
2. _____ Because epiglottitis is usually caused by viruses, swabbing the epiglottis is not recommended.
3. _____ A bacitracin filter paper disk on a throat culture plate can be used for definitive identification of *S. pyogenes* because only group A streptococci are susceptible to bacitracin.
4. _____ As many as 30% of the patients having oral surgery may develop an anaerobic infection.
5. _____ The cause of pharyngitis can be determined without testing by noting the appearance of the pharynx.

MULTIPLE CHOICE

1. _____ Organisms that have been shown to cause pharyngitis include
   A. *Haemophilus influenza.*
   B. *Staphylococcus aureus.*
   C. *Streptococcus pneumoniae.*
   D. *Streptococcus pyogenes.*
2. _____ The best culture medium for isolation of *Bordetella pertussis* is
   A. cystine-tellurite agar.
   B. Regan-Lowe agar.
   C. Thayer Martin.
   D. chocolate agar.
3. _____ A whole family (mother, father, toddler, and a cousin recently released from prison) presented to the emergency department with complaints of sore throat. The rapid strep A antigen test was negative on all four people. The physician ordered a throat culture for *N. gonorrhoeae* on each family member. What agar plates should be inoculated?
   A. 5% sheep blood agar (SBA) and Thayer Martin
   B. SBA and Loeffler's agar slant
   C. SBA and Bordet-Gengou agar
   D. SBA incubated aerobically and SBA incubated anaerobically
4. _____ Since the widespread use of the MMR vaccine in the United States, health care providers have become less likely to suspect mumps in patients with parotitis. Laboratory diagnosis should be done by
   A. IgM antibody titer.
   B. viral culture of throat swab.
   C. PCR of CSF.
   D. antigen detection in tissue.
5. _____ Which of the following organisms is never considered to be normal oropharyngeal flora?
   A. *S. aureus.*
   B. *N. gonorrhoeae.*
   C. *H. influenzae.*
   D. *M. catarrhalis.*

CASE STUDY

An 11-year-old girl complained of a sore throat for 2 days. Her mother brought the child to an outpatient clinic run by the local hospital. The child's throat was swabbed with two swabs and a "rapid strep screen" was done. The result was negative. It is the laboratory's policy to verify negative rapid group A streptococcal antigen tests with culture. The second swab was used to inoculate a 5% sheep blood agar (SBA) plate that was incubated overnight. The next day the SBA plate showed heavy growth of normal oral flora and moderate growth of beta-hemolytic colonies. The beta-hemolytic colonies were subbed to another SBA plate for isolation that had a bacitracin disk added. After overnight incubation, this pure culture was typed using a latex agglutination test for group A streptococci. This test was negative.

1. Why was the bacitracin disk added to the subplate?
2. What other beta-hemolytic organisms are known to cause pharyngitis?
3. What additional tests can be done to arrive at the identity of the beta-hemolytic colonies?

ANSWERS

Key Terms and Abbreviations

1. B
2. F
3. A
4. D
5. H
6. G
7. E
8. J
9. C
10. I

True or False

1. F
2. F
3. F
4. T
5. F

Multiple Choice

1. D
2. B
3. A
4. A
5. B

Case Study

1. *S. pyogenes* can be presumptively identified by use of a 0.04-unit bacitracin filter paper disk. A zone of inhibition around the disk indicates susceptibility. This is, however, only a presumptive test because other group A streptococci can give similar results. Another rapid test, the PYR test, can be done to confirm the identification as *S. pyogenes*. The enterococci and *S. pyogenes* are PYR-positive.
2. Groups C and G streptococci can cause pharyngitis as well as *Streptococcus agalactiae* (group B).
3. Latex agglutination tests for the Lancefield groups of beta-hemolytic streptococci, PYR test, or nucleic acid detection tests.

REFERENCES

Bisno AL, Gerber MA, Gwaltney JM, et al: Practice guidelines for the diagnosis and management of group A streptococcal pharyngitis, *Clin Infect Dis* 35:113, 2002.

Centers for Disease Control and Prevention: Mumps epidemic—Iowa, 2006, *Morb Mortal Wkly Rep* 55:366, 2006.

Centers for Disease Control and Prevention: Mumps outbreak at a summer camp—New York, 2005, *Morb Mortal Wkly Rep* 55:175, 2006.

Centers for Disease Control and Prevention: Notice to readers: updated recommendations of the Advisory Committee on Immunization Practices (ACIP) for the control and elimination of mumps, *Morb Mortal Wkly Rep* 55:629, 2006.

55 Meningitis and Other Infections of the Central Nervous System

OBJECTIVES

Upon completion of this chapter, the reader should be able to:

1. Describe the structures that constitute the central nervous system (CNS) and the routes of CNS infection.
2. Describe the functions of cerebrospinal fluid (CSF).
3. Differentiate between meningitis and encephalitis.
4. Describe the blood-brain barrier and its functions.
5. Compare the chemical and cellular findings from CSF analysis during viral and bacterial meningitis.
6. List the etiologic agents of meningitis based on prevalence by age group.
7. Describe how to process CSF for Gram stain and bacterial culture.

SUMMARY OF KEY POINTS

The central nervous system constitutes the largest part of the nervous system and consists of the brain and spinal cord. These structures have two protective coverings; one made of bone and one consisting of membranes called the meninges. The brain and spinal cord are also enveloped by a clear, colorless fluid called cerebrospinal fluid. The functions of this CSF are to cushion the brain within the skull and act as a shock absorber, circulate nutrients, and remove chemical wastes from the brain.

An important defense mechanism of the CNS is the blood-brain barrier. This barrier is produced by the endothelial cells of the capillaries that supply blood to the brain. This barrier maintains homeostasis in the brain by restricting the flow of chemical constituents from the blood. Meningitis is inflammation of the meninges. When these membranes become inflamed, the blood-brain barrier is affected. Bacteria and other pathogens cause meningitis. There are two major categories of meningitis: purulent and aseptic. Purulent meningitis is characterized by an acute inflammation with many neutrophils in the CSF. Aseptic meningitis is usually viral and is characterized by an increase of lymphocytes and other mononuclear cells in CSF. Viral meningitis is predominantly caused by the enteroviruses but neonates can acquire the herpes simplex virus during passage through the birth canal. Other pathogens causing aseptic meningitis can include the spirochetes *T. pallidum*, *Borrelia burgdorferi*, and *Leptospira* spp.

Meningitis needs to be differentiated from encephalitis. Encephalitis is an acute inflammation of the brain usually caused by direct viral invasion. Mosquito-borne arboviruses (West Nile virus, St. Louis, eastern and western equine) commonly infect humans during the summer months. A rare but devastating meningoencephalitis is due to the free-living amebae *Naegleria fowleri* and *Acanthamoeba* spp. that invade the brain via the nasal passages.

The predominance of pathogens is age-dependent with neonates having the highest incidence of meningitis. Meningitis occurs in about 25% of newborns with neonatal sepsis. The most common bacterial pathogens are group B streptococci, *Escherichia coli*, and *Listeria monocytogenes*.

Haemophilus influenza type b (Hib) was a common cause of meningitis in young children 4 months of age to 5 years of age, but with the advent of the Hib vaccine in the United States in 1985 and its incorporation into childhood immunization programs, childhood Hib disease has dramatically declined. Among young adults *Neisseria meningitidis* is the common cause of disease. *Streptococcus pneumoniae* meningitis develops from bacteremia or from infection of the sinuses or middle ear; it is frequently the cause of disease in young children and the elderly.

Other serious CNS microbial afflictions include brain abscesses usually caused by anaerobes, brain lesions due to cysticerci of *Taenia solium* or *Toxoplasma gondii*, and cerebral malaria (blockage of cerebral capillaries by *Plasmodium falciparum*).

An invaluable diagnostic tool is the CSF Gram stain and culture. As the CSF is collected, the fluid should be placed into sequentially numbered tubes. Tubes 1 and 3 or 4 may have cell counts done to differentiate a bloody tap from a subarachnoid hemorrhage. Tube 1 would be used for chemistry (glucose and protein) and immunology studies and tube 2 for culture. The sensitivity of the Gram stain can be increased if the cellular elements of the CSF are concentrated by use of a cytocentrifuge. Patients with AIDS may be tested for *Cryptococcus neoformans*. Commercially available cryptococcal antigen tests have much higher sensitivity than an India ink stain. Bacterial antigen tests have low sensitivity and specificity and have fallen out of use. For viral pathogens, molecular methods are popular. Although more expensive than culture, PCR has a sensitivity of almost 100% for herpes simplex virus, Epstein-Barr virus, CMV, and enteroviruses.

> ### INTEREST POINT
> West Nile virus (WNV) was first recognized as a human pathogen in 1937 in the West Nile District of Uganda. There were outbreaks of severe human meningitis or encephalitis in the 1950s in Israel and Egypt. And the disease made its debut in North America in 1999. From 1999 to 2001, there were 149 human cases reported in the United States to the Centers for

Disease Control and Prevention (CDC), including 18 deaths. The incidence peaked in 2003 with 9862 total reported cases, 2860 cases of meningitis/encephalitis, and 264 deaths. These rates have dropped off since 2003 with only 3000 total cases and 119 deaths in the United States in 2005.

Most people who become infected with WNV do not develop symptoms. About 20% of those who do develop symptoms complain of headache. The few who develop neuroinvasive disease usually present with headache, fever, changes in consciousness, and altered mental status.

Examination of CSF shows an increased number of leukocytes with a predominance of lymphocytes. Glucose is normal but protein is elevated. The most efficient diagnostic testing scheme is IgM antibody to WNV in serum or CSF collected within 8 days of onset of illness. Because IgM antibody does not cross the blood-brain barrier, the presence IgM in CSF is a strong indicator of CNS infection. Although PCR testing is frequently used, results must be interpreted cautiously. WNV infections have transient and low viremias; a negative PCR test does not rule out infection. More information on the CDC's guidelines for WNV surveillance, prevention, and control can be found at *www.cdc.gov/ncidod/dvbid/westnile/resources/wnv-guidelines-aug-2003.pdf.*

KEY TERMS AND ABBREVIATIONS

Match the term in the left column with the definition on the right.

1. _____ meninges
2. _____ meningitis
3. _____ encephalitis
4. _____ blood-brain barrier
5. _____ CSF

A. inflammation of the brain parenchyma
B. nutrient bath for the brain
C. defense mechanism for the CNS
D. infection within the subarachnoid space
E. membranes covering the brain and spinal cord

TRUE OR FALSE

1. _____ The rabies virus travels along sensory nerves to the brain.
2. _____ The blood-brain barrier is a homeostatic mechanism that regulates transport into the CNS.
3. _____ CMV and the BK virus typically cause encephalitis in the HIV-positive patient.
4. _____ If a subarachnoid hemorrhage is suspected, cell counts should be done on CSF in tubes 1 and 4.
5. _____ The best way to visualize amoeba in CSF is to Gram stain a refrigerated specimen.

MULTIPLE CHOICE

1. _____ The function of the CSF is to
   A. provide a means by which the brain monitors change.
   B. carry metabolites to neural tissues.
   C. cushion and protect the brain.
   D. all of the above.
2. _____ An indigent 35-year-old woman presented to the emergency department with complaints of headache, sore neck, and fatigue. Her speech was slurred. Blood was obtained for culture and serum ethanol; CSF was obtained for culture. The ethanol was elevated. Rare gram-negative diplococci were seen in the Gram stain. The most likely diagnosis is
   A. ethanol intoxication.
   B. *N. meningitidis* meningitis.
   C. *S. pneumoniae* meningitis.
   D. *H. influenzae* type b meningitis.
3. _____ Meningoencephalitis is commonly caused by
   A. *Naegleria fowleri.*
   B. West Nile virus.
   C. both A and B.
   D. none of the above.
4. _____ The best way to test for *Cryptococcus neoformans* in the CSF of an AIDS patient is
   A. India ink stain.
   B. cryptococcal antigen test.
   C. culture.
   D. PCR.
5. _____ The most sensitive and specific method to test for herpes simplex virus in CSF is
   A. culture.
   B. PCR.
   C. latex agglutination tests.
   D. IgG antibody detection.

CASE STUDY

A premature newborn became febrile. A blood culture was collected and the baby was started on ampicillin. The next day the baby had convulsions. CSF was collected; it was cloudy with a slightly decreased glucose and increased protein. Gram negative bacilli were seen in the CSF Gram stain. The blood culture collected the previous day became positive and showed gram-negative bacilli in the Gram stain of the broth. The following day growth from both the CSF and blood cultures showed a lactose-fermenting organism that resembled *E. coli* on the culture plates. Biochemical tests showed the organism to be oxidase-negative and indole-, methyl red–, and citrate-positive.

1. Is this organism *E. coli*? Why or why not?
2. Why do neonates have the highest prevalence of meningitis?
3. What infection control measures need to be put into place in the nursery when a diagnosis of meningitis is made?

ANSWERS

Key Terms and Abbreviations
1. E
2. D
3. A
4. C
5. B

True or False
1. T
2. T
3. T
4. T
5. F

Multiple Choice
1. D
2. B
3. C
4. B
5. B

Case Study
1. *Escherichia coli* is oxidase-positive, ferments lactose, is indole-positive, methyl red–positive, and citrate-negative. *Citrobacter koseri* (formerly *diversus*) resembles *E. coli* on culture media and has similar biochemical characteristics, but *C. koseri* is citrate-positive. *C. koseri* is a relatively uncommon cause of neonatal meningitis but has a high and devastating tendency to cause brain abscess. The bacteria have been found within macrophages in the ventricles of the brain and in necrotic material taken postmortem from the abscess. It has been hypothesized that *C. koseri* evades host immune responses by living and multiplying within macrophages and thus setting up a chronic infection. One study found that more than 70% of neonates with *C. koseri* meningitis developed brain abscesses. *C. koseri* is usually isolated from the urinary tract. *Citrobacter* sepsis may arise from an endogenous source such as the urinary tract. Mother to infant transmission and health care worker to infant transmission are less likely.

2. Neonates have an immature immune system. They are exposed during birth to the variety of organisms that colonize the vaginal tract. The blood-brain barrier of infants may have a greater permeability. Neonatal meningitis usually results from sepsis but may also result from scalp lesions.

3. The neonate with meningitis needs to be isolated from the other babies. There have been published reports of *C. koseri* meningitis spreading through special care units. Mortality rates of 30% to 50% have been reported and those infants who do survive have a high incidence of sequelae such as hearing loss and mental retardation.

REFERENCES

Centers for Disease Control and Prevention: Epidemic/epizootic West Nile virus in the United States: guidelines for surveillance, prevention, and control—3rd revision, 2003, available at *www.cdc.gov/ncidod/dvbid/westnile/resources/wnvguidelines2003.pdf.*

Ribeiro CD, Davis P, Jones DM: *Citrobacter koseri* meningitis in a special care baby unit, *J Clin Path* 29:1094, 1976.

Townsend SM, Pollack HA, Gonzalez-Gomez I, et al: *Citrobacter koseri* brain abscess in the neonatal rat: survival and replication within human and rat macrophages. *Infect Immun* 71:5871, 2003.

56 Infections of the Eyes, Ears, and Sinuses

OBJECTIVES

Upon completion of this chapter, the reader should be able to:

1. Briefly describe the anatomy of the eye.
2. Differentiate between conjunctivitis, blepharitis, and keratitis.
3. List some pathogens commonly associated with each of the infectious processes listed above as well as infections that affect the interior of the eye.
4. Describe the pathogens that frequently cause external ear infections.
5. Explain otitis media and list the most frequently encountered pathogens.
6. Describe culture methods for eye and ear specimens.
7. Describe the disease processes that differentiate acute sinusitis from chronic sinusitis.
8. Describe a suitable specimen for sinus culture and list the appropriate panel of culture media.

SUMMARY OF KEY POINTS

The most common type of ocular infection is conjunctivitis. It can be caused by allergies or bacteria and viruses. In adults the etiology is usually viral. Adenoviruses are the most common viral cause. In children conjunctivitis is usually due to *H. influenzae* and *S. pneumoniae*. This inflammation is characterized by redness, itching, and a discharge. Conjunctivitis is highly contagious; it can be transferred from one eye to the other by rubbing the infected eye, or it can be transferred to other individuals.

Blepharitis is an inflammation of the eyelids that is commonly caused by *S. aureus* or *S. epidermidis*. Keratitis is an inflammation of the cornea and is more serious than conjunctivitis. It can be caused by any of the classes of pathogens, but the most common bacterial pathogen is *S. aureus*. The filamentous molds, *Aspergillus* spp. and *Fusarium* spp., as well as yeast have been isolated from corneal lesions. Herpes simplex virus and *N. gonorrhoeae* can also cause infection. A free-living protozoan, *Acanthamoeba* spp., has emerged as an infectious agent among soft and extended-wear contact lens users.

Conjunctivitis can be diagnosed by swabbing the conjunctiva and plating to appropriate media. For keratitis, an ophthalmologist takes scrapings of the lesions. The scrapings should be plated directly onto the culture media that includes an enriched medium such as chocolate agar.

> ### INTEREST POINT
>
> About 30 million people use contact lenses in the United States. However, a fungus called *Fusarium* is emerging as an infectious disease associated with contact lens use and/or contact lens solutions. Beginning in November 2005, cases of *Fusarium* keratitis were reported in Asia. As of April 2006, 109 cases have been reported from 17 states in the United States; the Centers for Disease Control and Prevention is investigating this emerging problem.
>
> Fungal keratitis is rare and is usually associated with trauma to the eye, frequently involving plant matter. *Fusarium* species are ubiquitous and can be found in soil and tap water and on many plants. This infection can be serious and can lead to loss of vision and need for a corneal transplant. More information can be found at *http://www.cdc.gov/mmwr/preview/mmwrhtml/mm55d410a1.htm*.
>
> To prevent infection of the eye, the following practices should be followed:
> - Wash hands with soap and water and dry with a lint-free cloth before handling lenses
> - Follow the schedule prescribed by the physician for lens wear and replacement
> - Follow manufacturer's guidelines for cleaning and storage of the lenses
> - Keep the lens case clean
> - If redness, pain, light sensitivity, tearing, blurry vision, swelling, or discharge occur, see your physician immediately.

External ear infections are treated as any other soft tissue infections. Swimmer's ear is common among scuba divers and swimmers and is frequently due to *Pseudomonas aeruginosa*. Middle ear infection or otitis media is usually not diagnosed by culture. This is most common in children; one study found that almost one third of the visits of preschool children to pediatricians were prompted by middle ear infections. Symptoms can include fever, ear pain, dulled hearing, and drainage from the ear canal if the tympanic membrane becomes perforated.

The pathogens associated with otitis media are the same ones associated with sinusitis. Bacterial flora from the nose and throat make their way up to the inner ear and sinuses.

The most common bacterial agents in children are *S. pneumoniae* and *H. influenzae*. The viruses involved are the respiratory ones, chiefly respiratory syncytial virus (RSV) and influenza virus. When the infection becomes chronic, anaerobes and gram-negative bacilli predominate. If surgical intervention becomes necessary, aspirated fluid or swabs may be cultured.

A rare complication of chronic otitis media is mastoiditis (inflammation of the mastoid air cells). To prevent the extension of disease to the central nervous system, mastoidectomy is performed.

Sinusitis is more prevalent in winter and spring. Maxillary sinus infection causes facial pain, especially when bending forward, headache, pain that seems to originate from the upper teeth, and a purulent nasal discharge. Acute sinusitis usually follows a viral infection or common cold. Respiratory allergies can also lead to sinus infection. *M. catarrhalis* is a pathogen more frequently seen in children than in adults.

Nasal swabs are poor specimens for diagnosis. Sinus washings or aspirates that have been surgically collected are the specimens of choice. These specimens should be inoculated onto sheep blood agar, chocolate agar, and MacConkey agar.

KEY TERMS AND ABBREVIATIONS

Match the term in the left column with the definition on the right.

1. _____ conjunctivitis	A.	infection of the internal area of the eyeball
2. _____ lacrimal	B.	inflammation of the inner eyelid
3. _____ blepharitis	C.	inflammation of the mastoid air cells
4. _____ keratitis		
5. _____ endophthalmitis	D.	pertaining to tears
6. _____ otitis media	E.	inflammation of the eyelids
7. _____ otitis externa	F.	inflammation of the middle ear
8. _____ mastoiditis	G.	infection of the cornea
	H.	swimmer's ear

TRUE OR FALSE

1. _____ In orbital cellulitis cultures should include aerobic and anaerobic media.
2. _____ An increasingly common affliction among contact lens wearers is keratitis associated with *Acanthamoeba* infection.
3. _____ *Pseudomonas aeruginosa* is the most common cause of otitis media.
4. _____ Swimmer's ear usually results from softening of the ear tissue, which allows *M. catarrhalis* to infect the outer ear.

5. _____ The specimen of choice in sinusitis cases is a swab of the nasal drainage.

MULTIPLE CHOICE

1. _____ Since the widespread use of the Hib vaccine in the 1980s, the most common cause of acute sinusitis in children has become
   A. nontypable *H. influenzae*.
   B. alpha-hemolytic streptococci.
   C. *Alloiococcus otitidis*.
   D. *Moraxella catarrhalis*.
2. _____ The minimal battery of plates for an ear culture should include
   A. BAP with bacitracin disk
   B. BAP with optochin disk
   C. BAP and MacConkey
   D. BAP, MacConkey, chocolate
   (**NOTE**: BAP is 5% sheep blood agar.)
3. _____ Antibiotic drops are routinely put into the eyes of newborns to prevent infection with
   A. Group B streptococci.
   B. *Chlamydia trachomatis*.
   C. *Haemophilus influenzae*.
   D. Herpes simplex virus.
4. _____ A major difference between acute and chronic otitis media is
   A. the location of infection.
   B. chronic infection is usually due to anaerobes.
   C. acute infection usually occurs as a consequence of a viral respiratory infection.
   D. both B and C.
5. _____ Pinkeye in children is common and highly contagious. The most common viral agent and cause of epidemic disease is
   A. herpes simplex virus.
   B. respiratory syncytial virus.
   C. adenovirus.
   D. varicella zoster virus.

CASE STUDY

A 2-year-old had been suffering from chronic otitis media and sinusitis. The pediatric specialist performed surgery to look at the left ear while the child was under anesthesia. Operative findings corroborated the clinical history. The child also suffered from adenoiditis; an adenoidectomy was performed. A bilateral maxillary sinus wash was also collected and the washings were sent for sinus culture. The sinus culture Gram stain showed few leukocytes and no organisms.
1. What battery of plates should have been inoculated?
2. There was a light growth of gray colonies that had a mousy odor. Gram stain showed these colonies to be gram-negative coccobacilli. What is the probable identification of this organism?
3. Identification and susceptibility testing take an additional day. There is a rapid test that can be performed to screen these organisms for an enzyme that would make them resistant to the penicillins. What is this test?

ANSWERS

Key Terms and Abbreviations

1. B
2. D
3. E
4. G
5. A
6. F
7. H
8. C

True or False

1. T
2. T
3. F
4. F
5. F

Multiple Choice

1. A
2. D
3. B
4. D
5. C

Case Study

1. Otitis media and sinusitis occur when bacteria that populate the nose and throat invade the ear and sinuses. The majority of the cases of acute sinusitis are caused by *S. pneumoniae* and *H. influenzae*. Media used for sinus culture are similar to those used for respiratory tract pathogens. Sheep blood agar, chocolate, and MacConkey agar should be used.

2. Grayish colonies on chocolate agar that produce a mousy odor are characteristic of *Haemophilus influenzae*. This organism is gram-negative and appears as short, rounded rods. Identification can be made using a commercial system of biochemical reactions or presumptive identification made using the organism's requirements for NAD and hemin.

3. There is a high incidence of beta-lactamase–producing strains of *H. influenzae*. Susceptibility to the penicillins cannot be assumed. All isolates of *H. influenzae* should be screened for beta-lactamase production. This can be accomplished by the Nitrocefin disk test (Cefinase; BD Diagnostics Systems, Sparks, Md). But this test does not replace conventional susceptibility testing by disk diffusion or dilution because these organisms have demonstrated resistance to ampicillin by other methods.

REFERENCES

Centers for Disease Control and Prevention: Update: *Fusarium keratitis*—United States, 2005-2006, *Morb Mortal Wkly Rep* 55:563, 2006.

Marciano-Cabral F, Cabral G: *Acanthamoeba* spp. as agents of disease in humans, *Clin Microbiol Rev* 16:273, 2003.

57 Infections of the Urinary Tract

OBJECTIVES

Upon completion of this chapter, the reader should be able to:
1. Describe the structures that constitute the urinary tract.
2. List the causative organisms of both community-acquired urinary tract infections (UTIs) and hospital-acquired UTIs.
3. Differentiate between pyelonephritis, cystitis, urethritis, acute urethral syndrome, and asymptomatic bacteriuria.
4. Explain the difference between clean-catch midstream specimen, in-out catheterized and indwelling catheterized specimens, and suprapubic aspirates.
5. Explain the various screening strategies to reduce the number of contaminated urine cultures.
6. Explain how to plate urine for quantitative culture.
7. Explain how to interpret and quantitate urine cultures.

SUMMARY OF KEY POINTS

The urinary tract consists of the kidneys, ureters, bladder, and urethra. The function of the urinary tract is to make and process urine. Urine is an ultrafiltrate of blood that consists mostly of water but also contains nitrogenous wastes, sodium, potassium, chloride, and other analytes. Urine is normally a sterile fluid. But bacteria may ascend from the lower urinary tract (bladder and urethra) or be pushed up into the bladder during a catheterization procedure. The urethra is colonized with organisms such as lactobacilli, corynebacteria, and coagulase-negative staphylococci.

UTI is primarily a disorder of women; its prevalence is age- and sex-dependent. The incidence in men rises after 60 years of age or when enlargement of the prostate interferes with removal of urine from the bladder. UTIs can lead to sepsis and are the most frequent nosocomial infection reported from hospitals and nursing homes in the United States. Millions of hospitalized patients each year have urinary catheters inserted, and as many as 25% of these patients develop a catheter-associated UTI. Common urinary pathogens include *E. coli, Klebsiella* spp., *Proteus* spp., *Staphylococcus saprophyticus, Staphylococcus aureus,* enterococci, other *Enterobacteriaceae,* and *Candida* spp. Group B streptococci are important pathogens for pregnant women. Other coagulase-negative staphylococci may be recovered, but they are generally considered to be nonpathogens.

Some individuals suffer from recurrent UTIs, despite adequate antibiotic treatment. One possible explanation is that urinary pathogens may be able to evade the host immune response and antimicrobials by invading and residing in epithelial cells of the bladder. Some of these pathogens such as *Proteus* spp. have also been implicated in kidney stone formation.

The traditional concentration cutoff of 10^5 CFU/mL has been used as the indicator of infection. However, a large portion of patients whose urine cultures yield less than this amount of bacteria seek medical help for bladder infection. Urinalysis shows pyuria, which can be defined as greater than 8 leukocytes/mm^3 of uncentrifuged urine. This phenomenon is called *acute urethral syndrome.*

Interpretation of urine cultures from specimens obtained through catheters is difficult. If urine is collected by in-and-out catheterization, it should be a good specimen. The specimen should be labeled as an "in/out cath" specimen. But if a Foley catheter has been in place for more than 5 days, it is likely that a biofilm has already begun to form on the lumen. Culture of urine collected from this Foley catheter may give misleading information.

Bacterial contamination of urine cultures is a significant issue for many microbiology laboratories. Numerous studies have been done to identify the factors that contribute to contamination and to identify screening strategies that effectively detect bacteriuria. A 1998 Q-Probes study by the College of American Pathologists determined that the median contamination rate of urine cultures collected from outpatients was 18.1%. Factors that decreased this rate included rapid transportation to the laboratory, refrigeration of specimens in cases of a testing delay, and having female patients hold the labia apart during sampling. Although a Gram stain of uncentrifuged urine seems to be a very sensitive screening method to detect bacteriuria, it is not widely used because of the volume of specimens that require screening and the time required to process these specimens. Many laboratories use a screening strategy that employs dipstick and microscopic analyses.

INTEREST POINT

Group B streptococci (GBS) were first identified as a cause of puerperal sepsis during the 1930s and have been a leading bacterial infection associated with illness in newborns. Women can be colonized with GBS and carry the organisms in the vagina and rectum. Newborns become infected during the birth process or while in utero. GBS can cause bacteremia, pneumonia, meningitis, osteomyelitis, or septic arthritis in the newborn. The sequelae of infection can include long-term neurologic problems and death. Prevention of perinatal GBS disease focuses on interrupting the vertical transmission from mother to child. Maternal intrapartum colonization is a major risk factor for early-onset disease in infants.

In May 1996, the Centers for Disease Control and Prevention (CDC) in conjunction with the American

---

160

College of Obstetricians and Gynecologists (ACOG) and the American Academy of Pediatrics (AAP) issued recommendations for prevention strategies. These recommendations for prevention, diagnosis, and treatment have recently been updated and are available at *www.cdc.gov/mmwr/preview/mmwrhtml/rr5111a1.htm*.

The presence of GBS in urine in any concentration in a pregnant woman is an indicator of colonization. The laboratory's role is to report the presence of any quantity of GBS in a urine culture from a pregnant woman as well as the corresponding susceptibility patterns. Women with either symptomatic or asymptomatic GBS bacteriuria should receive appropriate antimicrobial treatment at diagnosis as well as at delivery as intrapartum prophylaxis.

KEY TERMS AND ABBREVIATIONS

Match the term in the left column with the definition on the right.

1. _____ urethra
2. _____ ureter
3. _____ bacteriuria
4. _____ Foley catheter
5. _____ hematogenous
6. _____ pyelonephritis
7. _____ cystitis
8. _____ urethritis
9. _____ pyuria

A. presence of bacteria in urine
B. tube allowing urine to leave the bladder
C. blood-borne
D. tube connecting the bladder and kidney
E. inflammation of the bladder
F. indwelling catheter
G. inflammation of the urethra
H. infection of the kidney
I. many leukocytes in the urine

TRUE OR FALSE

1. _____ In a healthy human all areas of the urinary tract below the urethra are sterile.
2. _____ Urinary tract infection is primarily a disease of females.
3. _____ *Staphylococcus aureus* in the urine can be indicative of pyelonephritis.
4. _____ When patients have a Foley catheter, it is standard procedure to obtain urine for culture by aspirating it from the collection bag.
5. _____ Urine should ideally be plated within 2 hours of collection.

MULTIPLE CHOICE

1. _____ Resident flora of the urethra include
   A. lactobacilli.
   B. nonhemolytic streptococci.
   C. all of the above.
   D. none of the above.

2. _____ A urinary pathogen that has been associated with kidney stone formation is
   A. *Proteus* spp.
   B. *Candida albicans.*
   C. *Citrobacter freundii.*
   D. *E. coli.*

3. _____ A 1-μL loop of urine was used to inoculate a 5% sheep blood agar plate. After overnight incubation there were more than 100 white colonies counted growing on the plate. This translates into
   A. >100 CFU/mL.
   C. >10^4 CFU/mL.
   B. >10^3 CFU/mL.
   D. >10^5 CFU/mL.

4. _____ The most frequently isolated urinary nosocomial pathogen from a catheterized patient is
   A. *S. aureus.*
   B. *Candida albicans.*
   C. *E. coli.*
   D. *S. saprophyticus.*

5. _____ A urine culture from a 27-year-old woman is growing three organisms that are present in approximately equal numbers of 10^4 CFU/mL. The urine is reportedly a clean-catch midstream specimen. The organisms are a coagulase-negative staphylococcus, an alpha-hemolytic streptococcus, and long, thin gram-positive bacilli. Which of the following statements is FALSE?
   A. The staphylococci should be tested to rule out *S. saprophyticus.*
   B. The alpha-hemolytic streptococci should be PYR tested to rule out *Enterococcus* spp.
   C. No work needs to be done. Report "Multiple organisms present; probable contamination."
   D. Perform a catalase test on the gram-positive bacillus. If the catalase test is negative, the presumptive identification would be lactobacilli.

CASE STUDY

A 26-year-old woman was pregnant with her first child. During her routine monthly visit to the obstetrician, she mentioned that she was experiencing a burning sensation upon urination. The obstetrician ordered a urinalysis and culture. The urinalysis was unremarkable. The culture yielded mixed gram-positive growth. The predominant colony type was white, nonhemolytic, catalase-positive, and coagulase-negative. There were about 15 white beta-hemolytic colonies that were catalase negative.

1. What further testing (if any) should the microbiologist do on the nonhemolytic colonies?
2. What further testing (if any) should the microbiologist do on the beta-hemolytic colonies?
3. What is the laboratory's responsibility in this situation?

ANSWERS

Key Terms and Abbreviations

1. B
2. D
3. A
4. F
5. C
6. H
7. E
8. G
9. I

True or False

1. F
2. T
3. T
4. F
5. T

Multiple Choice

1. C
2. A
3. D
4. C
5. C

Case Study

1. The preliminary identification of this organism is a coagulase-negative staphylococcus. It must be speciated, however, because *S. saprophyticus* is a pathogen, especially in young, sexually active women. Susceptibility testing is not performed on *S. saprophyticus*. Other coagulase-negative staphylococci rarely cause UTI; if they are pathogens, infection is usually related to catheterization.
2. The beta-hemolytic colonies are streptococci. These colonies should be identified using a commercial product for Lancefield grouping. Any group B streptococci should be reported regardless of the amount. Susceptibility testing may be required if the patient is allergic to penicillin. There is increasing resistance being reported to erythromycin and clindamycin.
3. Laboratories are expected to report the presence of GBS in any amount recovered from the urine of pregnant women. Culture and susceptibility results should be reported to both the ordering physician and the anticipated site of delivery (when known).

REFERENCES

Centers for Disease Control and Prevention: Prevention of perinatal group B streptococcal disease—revised guidelines from CDC, *Morb Mortal Wkly Rev* 51 (RR-11):1, 2002.

Loo SY, Scottolini AG, Luangphinith S, et al: Urine screening strategy employing dipstick analysis and selective culture: an evaluation, *Am J Clin Pathol* 81:634, 1984.

Nicolle LE, Bradley S, Colgan R, et al: Infectious Diseases Society of America guidelines for the diagnosis and treatment of asymptomatic bacteriuria in adults, *Clin Infect Dis* 40:643, 2005.

Richards MJ, Edwards JR, Culver DH, Gaynes RP: Nosocomial infections in medical intensive care units in the United States. National Nosocomial Infections Surveillance System, *Crit Care Med* 27:853, 1999.

Shaw KN, McGowan KL, Gorelick MH, Schwartz JS: Screening for urinary tract infection in infants in the emergency department: which test is best? *Pediatrics* 101:1, 1998.

Tambyah PA, Maki DG: The relationship between pyuria and infection in patients with indwelling urinary catheters: a prospective study of 761 patients, *Arch Intern Med* 160:673, 2000.

Valenstein P: Urine culture contamination—a College of American Pathologists Q-Probes study of contaminated urine cultures in 906 institutions, *Arch Pathol Lab Med* 144:123, 1998.

Zorc JJ, Kiddoo DA, Shaw KN: Diagnosis and management of urinary tract infections, *Clin Microbiol Rev* 18:417, 2005.

OBJECTIVES

Upon completion of this chapter, the reader should be able to:

1. List the various normal genital flora found in both males and females.
2. Describe vaginitis and list the various pathogens that can cause this disorder.
3. Differentiate vaginitis from bacterial vaginosis.
4. List the most common causes of sexually transmitted disease (STD), both bacterial and viral, and the tests that will diagnose these infections.
5. List the various organisms that can cause genital lesions.
6. Describe how genital infections in the mother can affect the fetus.
7. Describe the relationship between the human papillomaviruses (HPV) and genital warts and cancer.
8. Describe the various upper genital tract infections.
9. Explain the role of microscopy, culture, serology, and molecular technology in the diagnosis of infection with the following pathogens: *Neisseria gonorrhoeae, Chlamydia trachomatis, Trichomonas vaginalis, Treponema pallidum,* herpes simplex virus (HSV), HPV, *Mycoplasma hominis,* and *Candida albicans.*

SUMMARY OF KEY POINTS

Genital tract infections can manifest themselves as external lesions or internal infections in both men and women. External lesions can include the anogenital warts caused by HPV, the primary chancre of syphilis, the vesicular lesions caused by HSV, and other less common conditions such as chancroid *(Haemophilus ducreyi),* lymphogranuloma venereum *(C. trachomatis),* and granuloma inguinale *(Calymmatobacterium granulomatis).* Internal infections can be caused by organisms ascending the genital tract to cause inflammation in the uterus, fallopian tubes, and ovaries. Genital tract infections can be caused by endogenous organisms; the patient's own resident flora becomes pathogenic. Of public health concern are genital tract infections that are caused by exogenous organisms that are transmitted via sexual activity. Some of these infections are reportable to state health departments and/or the Centers for Disease Control and Prevention (CDC). The list of reportable diseases as of January 2006 can be accessed at *www.cdc.gov/epo/dphsi/phs/files/NNDSSeventcodelist January2006.pdf.*

Syphilis, gonorrhea, chlamydia, and AIDS are reportable diseases in every state. HIV infection and chancroid are reportable in many states.

The two most prevalent bacterial STDs in the United States are chlamydia and gonorrhea. The two most prevalent viral sexually transmitted infections in the United States are caused by HPV and HSV. The reported rates of *C. trachomatis, N. gonorrhoeae,* and HPV infection is highest among adolescents 15 to 19 years of age, particularly young females. With only a few exceptions, all adolescents in the United States can consent to confidential diagnosis and treatment of STDs without parental consent or knowledge. In many states adolescents can also consent to HIV counseling and testing.

The most frequently reported bacterial genital infection in the United States is chlamydia; and it is most prevalent in young adults younger than 25 years of age. It is common for both men and women to be infected yet be asymptomatic. Serious sequelae from *C. trachomatis* infection in women include pelvic inflammatory disease (PID), infertility, and ectopic pregnancy. The CDC has recommended annual screening of all sexually active women younger than 25 years of age and screening of older women with risk factors (e.g., a new sex partner or multiple sex partners).

Of particular concern is the identification of a sexually transmissible agent in a young child beyond the neonatal period. This could be evidence of possible child sexual abuse. A rectal or genital *C. trachomatis* infection in young children could be the result of a perinatally acquired infection. However, sexual abuse should be suspected if there is genital herpes, syphilis, gonorrhea, or nontransfusion, nonperinatally acquired HIV infection. Every state has laws that require the reporting of child abuse. If a health care provider suspects abuse, he or she must report the incident to local child-protection services. Clinicians must also be aware of the medicolegal issues regarding testing and diagnosis in this patient age group. For the diagnosis of gonococcal and chlamydial infection, only standard culture systems should be used. All presumptive isolates of *N. gonorrhoeae* should be confirmed by a different test method (e.g., biochemical, serologic, enzyme substrate, or DNA probe methodology). Nonculture tests for *C. trachomatis* infection are not specific enough to be legally useful in a suspect child abuse/assault case. Isolates should be preserved and specimens should be saved in case additional or repeat testing is required.

Although HPV is the most prevalent viral STD in the United States, it is not on the reportable diseases list. There are 20 million people in the United States who are currently infected with HPV and 5.5 million more people will become infected this year. HPV is not only associated with nonneoplastic diseases such as condyloma acuminata and recurrent respiratory papillomatosis, but HPV has also been definitively linked to cervical cancer. HPV is widely accepted as the cause of most squamous cell cervical cancers. Anal cancer is less common but is

163

increasing in frequency in both men and women and is linked to HPV. Although there are several commercially available molecular assays for HPV, the HC2 assay from Digene is currently the only test approved by the Food and Drug Administration (FDA) for HPV testing of the cervix. This test has been coupled with fluid-based cytology methods (ThinPrep) so that abnormal cytology results would automatically trigger the HPV test. In one study, it was projected that an effective HPV vaccine could prevent 1300 deaths from cervical cancer annually if all 12-year-old girls in the United States were vaccinated. There have been promising results with vaccine studies. In one recent study a vaccine for HPV-16, one of the HPV viral types with a high association with cervical cancer, yielded a 91% efficacy in preventing HPV-16 infection and may have prevented cervical cancer precursors. In June 2006, the FDA approved the first vaccine directed against the HPV-16 strain.

Also of public health concern are the infections that a mother passes to her unborn child or transmits during delivery. Transplacental infection of the fetus can occur if the mother has syphilis or is infected with the viral agents HIV, CMV, or HSV or with *Listeria monocytogenes*. As the baby passes through the birth canal, it may be exposed to *C. trachomatis, N. gonorrhoeae, E. coli*, or another enteric or group B streptococci. Ophthalmia neonatorum is a potentially serious eye infection of newborns that can lead to blindness. It is common practice to put antiseptic agents or antibiotics in a newborn's eyes as a prophylactic measure. Prophylaxis with 1% silver nitrate drops was in widespread use; this practice caused a significant decline in the incidence of gonococcal ophthalmia but had less impact on chlamydial ophthalmia. Erythromycin or 1% tetracycline ointments are now being used because of their activity against *C. trachomatis* and because they cause less chemical irritation of the conjunctiva compared with silver nitrate. While this practice has had an impact on neonatal ophthalmia, it does not prevent the nasopharyngeal colonization of the infant or prevent pneumonia.

Skin lesions or other symptoms such as urethral or vaginal discharge, painful urination (dysuria), or swollen lymph nodes may cause patients to seek medical treatment. A person can, however, be infected and have no symptoms. A common problem among women is vaginitis; this presents as an abnormal malodorous discharge accompanied by itching. It is usually caused by *Candida* spp. or *Trichomonas vaginalis*. Bacterial vaginosis produces similar symptoms but is due to a polymicrobic condition where there is a noted absence of the normal lactobacilli species and an overgrowth of anaerobic species, *Gardnerella vaginalis,* and other mixed flora. Diagnosis of bacterial vaginosis can be made if the following characteristics are observed: vaginal pH is elevated above 4.5, the vaginal discharge has a "fishy" odor because of volatile amines produced by the anaerobic bacteria, and clue cells are present. Clue cells are vaginal epithelial cells that are covered with bacteria.

Laboratory diagnosis can be made through a variety of means. Bacterial and viral pathogens can be diagnosed by culture. Culture is the only acceptable test in suspect cases of child abuse/assault and still the "gold standard"

for detection of many infections. Molecular methods are used more and more frequently for their sensitivity, specificity, and faster turnaround time. There are molecular probes that can test for both *N. gonorrhoeae* and *C. trachomatis* from a single swab. It is imperative to follow the manufacturer's recommendations regarding swab type. Swabs can have plastic, wood, or metal shafts. The swab tips can be cotton, rayon, calcium alginate, Dacron, or polyester. Some materials are toxic to the organisms being investigated. Trichomonads and fungal elements can be seen in wet mounts. A Gram stain of a urethral discharge from a male patient can yield a presumptive diagnosis of gonorrhea if intracellular diplococci are seen. Confirmation tests need to be performed. Gram stain of cervical discharge is not recommended.

INTEREST POINT

If there is an ascending infection in a pregnant woman or spread from a hematogenous source, the membranes of the placenta (chorioamnionitis) or the umbilical cord (funisitis) may become infected. Pathogens may include *E. coli, Listeria monocytogenes, Ureaplasma urealyticum,* and *Mycoplasma hominis*. These infections are associated with preterm birth and low–birth-weight infants. If a physician orders a placenta culture, proper collection is vital. The surface of the placenta will become contaminated with vaginal flora during delivery. For the culture to be meaningful, the chorion and amnion layers should be separated aseptically near the base of the umbilical cord and the culture swab inserted between these membranes.

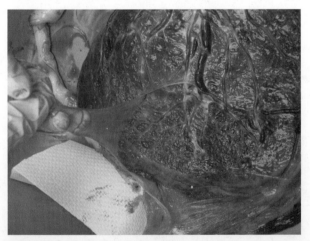

Figure 58-1 Fetal side of placenta (side with umbilical cord). The membranes are already disrupted. The thin amnion layer is grasped and gently lifted off the chorion, which is firmly attached to the placenta.

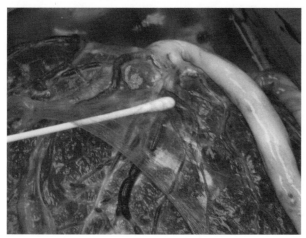

Figure 58-2 The swab is gently inserted between the amnion and chorion layers at the base of the umbilical cord.

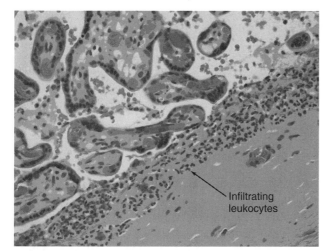

Infiltrating leukocytes

Figure 58-3 Infected placenta showing infiltration of leukocytes *(arrow)*. This is the histologic picture of chorioamnionitis. A cross-section of placenta was stained with hematoxylin and eosin. White blood cells stain purple and red blood cells stain red.

KEY TERMS AND ABBREVIATIONS

Match the term in the left column with the definition on the right.

1. _____ STDs
2. _____ chancre
3. _____ dysuria
4. _____ genital warts
5. _____ neoplasia
6. _____ urethritis
7. _____ vaginitis
8. _____ bacterial vaginosis
9. _____ proctitis
10. _____ PID

A. purulent vaginal discharge
B. abnormal, disorganized growth in a tissue than can form a mass
C. sexually transmitted diseases
D. inflammation of the fallopian tubes or ovaries
E. inflammation of the epididymis

11. _____ bartholinitis
12. _____ prenatal
13. _____ postpartum
14. _____ chorioamnionitis
15. _____ epididymitis
16. _____ orchitis

F. inflammation of the rectum
G. primary lesion of syphilis
H. after birth
I. polymicrobic condition
J. infection of the placental membranes
K. during pregnancy
L. condylomata acuminata
M. Bartholin's gland abscess
N. inflammation of the testicles
O. painful urination
P. inflammation of the urethra

TRUE OR FALSE

1. _____ *Entamoeba histolytica* has emerged as an STD, especially among homosexual groups.
2. _____ The best specimen to detect group B streptococci during prenatal testing is a culture swab of the endocervix.
3. _____ Bacterial vaginosis refers to a shift in the relative amounts of vaginal flora with a loss of lactobacilli.
4. _____ The presence of clue cells with few leukocytes is indicative of bacterial vaginosis.
5. _____ When culturing intrauterine devices, it is important to incubate the device long enough to recover *Actinomyces*.

MULTIPLE CHOICE

1. _____ The organism that outnumbers other normal flora of the vagina is
   A. coagulase-negative staphylococci.
   B. lactobacilli.
   C. corynebacteria.
   D. *Streptococcus agalactiae.*
2. _____ Vaginitis can be caused by
   A. streptococci.
   B. *Trichomonas vaginalis.*
   C. *Lactobacillus* spp.
   D. none of the above.
3. _____ The best way to diagnose congenital *T. gondii* infection is
   A. culture eye discharge.
   B. tissue biopsy.
   C. test neonatal blood for IgM.
   D. test neonatal blood for IgG.
4. _____ Infections that infants can acquire as they pass through an infected birth canal include
   A. *Listeria monocytogenes.*
   B. *Chlamydia trachomatis.*
   C. *Toxoplasma gondii.*
   D. parvovirus B19.

5. _____ The most common viral STD occurring in the United States today and the cause of most squamous cell cervical cancers is
   A. molluscum contagiosum virus.
   B. CMV.
   C. herpes simplex virus.
   D. human papillomaviruses.

CASE STUDY

A 25-year-old female presented to her local hospital in labor. It was determined she had received insufficient prenatal care and had a possible antepartum amniotic infection. The routine admission tests (CBC, urinalysis, type and screen) were done as well as an RPR, hepatitis B surface antigen, rubella antibody screen, and HIV screen. Her WBC count was $17.5 \times 10^3/\mu L$ with 73% neutrophils and 6% bands. A catheterized urine specimen was collected. The urinalysis was essentially normal but there were few bacteria seen microscopically. A urine culture was ordered. A blood culture was also ordered. The serology tests were all negative. Upon delivery it was noted that the placenta was meconium (newborn's bowel discharge) stained. The placenta was sent for culture. The placenta Gram stain showed few WBCs and gram-positive bacilli.

1. How should a placenta culture be processed with respect to culture media and incubation conditions? Given the Gram stain reading of gram-positive bacilli, what are some possible organisms?
2. The next day the blood culture bottle became positive. A Gram stain of the broth showed gram-positive bacilli. The sheep blood agar plate of the placenta culture had grayish white beta-hemolytic colonies. These bacilli were catalase-positive, bile esculin–positive, and were motile when viewed in a wet prep. What is the most likely identification of this organism? Is this a contaminant or a true pathogen?
3. The same organism grew in both the blood and placenta cultures. How could this woman have become infected? And what are the implications for the fetus?

ANSWERS

Key Terms and Abbreviations
1. C
2. G
3. O
4. L
5. B
6. P
7. A
8. I
9. F
10. D
11. M
12. K
13. H
14. J
15. E
16. N

True or False
1. T
2. F
3. T
4. T
5. T

Multiple Choice
1. B
2. B
3. C
4. B
5. D

Case Study
1. Culture media should be chosen to provide recovery of aerobes, anaerobes, and yeast. A full workup would also include culture for the genital mycoplasmas. The common placental pathogens include the enterics, beta-hemolytic streptococci, *S. aureus*, *N. gonorrhoeae*, *Haemophilus*, *Listeria monocytogenes*, and anaerobes. A standard panel of culture plates would include 5% sheep blood, chocolate, MacConkey, an anaerobe plate and could also include a Thayer-Martin plate. The gram-positive bacilli that could be present would include *Lactobacillus* spp., *Corynebacterium* spp., and *Listeria monocytogenes*.
2. *Lactobacillus* spp. are catalase-negative. Motility differentiates *Listeria* spp. from corynebacteria. *Listeria monocytogenes* has a characteristic tumbling motility in a hanging drop preparation, is able to grow in the presence of bile, and hydrolyzes esculin. *L. monocytogenes* is a pathogen. It can be recovered from the mother's lochia, cervix, blood, and diseased parts of the placenta. It can also be recovered from the umbilical cord, fetal CSF, gastric aspirate, and meconium.
3. *L. monocytogenes* is a common food contaminant that is associated with unpasteurized dairy products, raw vegetables, and processed meats. There have been a number of outbreaks recorded that have involved from a handful of people up to as many as 180 people. Infection during pregnancy can lead to intrauterine infection of the fetus. This can trigger premature labor and cause stillbirth. Infected placental tissues usually show chorioamnionitis. *L. monocytogenes* can be fatal if left untreated. The drugs of choice are ampicillin plus an aminoglycoside. It is also usually susceptible to erythromycin, trimethoprim-sulfamethoxazole, and imipenem.

REFERENCES

Bracci R, Buonocore G: Chorioamnionitis: a risk factor for fetal and neonatal morbidity, *Biol Neonate* 83:85, 2003.

Centers for Disease Control and Prevention: Increases in fluoroquinolone-resistant *Neisseria gonorrhoeae* among men who have sex with men—United States, 2003, and revised recommendations for gonorrhea treatment, 2004, *Morb Mortal Wkly Rep* 53:335, 2004.

Centers for Disease Control and Prevention: Prevention of perinatal group B streptococcal disease—revised guidelines from CDC, *Morb Mortal Wkly Rep* 51:RR-11, 2002.

Centers for Disease Control and Prevention: Sexually transmitted diseases treatment guidelines—2006, *Morb Mortal Wkly Rep* 51:RR-11, 2006.

Centers for Disease Control and Prevention and Department of Health and Human Services: Report to Congress—prevention of genital human papillomavirus infection, Jan. 2004 *www.cdc.gov/std/HPV/2004HPV%20Report.pdf.*

Gibbs RS: The relationship between infections and adverse pregnancy outcomes: an overview, *Ann Periodontol* 6:153, 2001.

Zar H: Neonatal chlamydial infections: prevention and treatment, *Pediatr Drugs* 7:103, 2005.

59 Gastrointestinal Tract Infections

OBJECTIVES

Upon completion of this chapter, the reader should be able to:

1. Explain the role of normal gastrointestinal (GI) flora in protecting the body against disease
2. Describe the three pathogenic mechanisms that cause acute diarrhea.
3. Differentiate between a diarrheal stool and dysentery.
4. List the most common bacterial enteric pathogens.
5. List the most common viral and parasitic enteric pathogens.
6. Differentiate between an infection and intoxication.
7. Explain specimen collection and handling for GI infections.
8. Describe bacterial culture media and methods.

SUMMARY OF KEY POINTS

A hundred years ago the most common food-borne diseases were cholera and typhoid fever. Today, the most common bacterial food-borne infections are due to *Campylobacter, Salmonella,* and *E. coli* O157:H7. The most common viral food-borne infection is caused by the noroviruses (formerly known as the Norwalk-like viruses). Because we consume food items shipped here from all over the world, the nature of the food-borne pathogens we see will most likely continue to change. In the late 1990s, there were several outbreaks of cyclosporiasis most probably associated with fresh raspberries from Guatemala. Other *Cyclospora cayetanensis* outbreaks have been associated with mesclun and fresh basil.

The gastrointestinal (GI) tract can be divided into two broad regions, upper and lower. Upper intestinal infections would involve the esophagus, stomach, and upper duodenum. Esophagitis is characterized by pain or difficulty swallowing. *Candida albicans* and herpes simplex virus can cause erosive disease. Because of the very low gastric pH, most ingested bacteria are killed soon after reaching the stomach. Gastric acid helps protect the lower GI tract from bacterial infection. One organism is capable of surviving this harsh environment and has emerged as a gastric pathogen associated with peptic ulcer disease. *Helicobacter pylori* rapidly hydrolyzes urea and releases ammonia. The bacteria become surrounded by this alkaline pH zone, or cloud, and are able to survive the acidic environment of the stomach.

Infections of the lower GI tract are typically characterized by diarrhea. The word *diarrhea* derives from the ancient Greek word that means "to run through." Diarrhea results when insufficient water is reabsorbed by the colon. *Dysentery* is a term that describes diarrhea with mucus, blood, and leukocytes accompanied by abdominal cramping and tenesmus. For centuries, urine and feces have been studied and described as indicators of human health. The composition of fecal material in the intestinal tract represents a complex microbial system composed mostly of obligate anaerobes. These resident normal flora provide colonization protection. Antimicrobial therapy can shift these resident populations and allow pathogens to overgrow. Such is the case with antibiotic-associated diarrhea and pseudomembranous colitis. After antimicrobial treatment, this organism flourishes and produces toxins that lead to the development of the pseudomembrane. The best way to diagnose this condition is to look for *C. difficile* toxins A and B in stool. Almost half of all healthy neonates carry *C. difficile;* this carriage rate decreases as the child ages. It is unclear why these infants do not develop diarrhea, but some possible explanations include neutralizing maternal antibodies and the immaturity of the neonatal immune system.

Enteric pathogens cause disease in one of three ways:

- A noninflammatory process that affects the water and electrolyte balance resulting in fluid loss and a cholera-like diarrhea. This process is mediated by enterotoxins. There is no fever or blood or leukocytes in the stool. Organisms associated with enterotoxin-mediated diarrhea include *Vibrio cholerae, Clostridium perfringens, Bacillus cereus, S. aureus,* enterotoxigenic *E. coli,* noroviruses, and enteric adenoviruses. The noninvasive parasites *Giardia lamblia, Cryptosporidium parvum, Isospora belli,* and *Cyclospora cayetanensis* also produce an afebrile, watery diarrhea.
- An inflammatory process caused by invasion of host cells and possible cytotoxin production. There is a true dysentery syndrome with blood and pus in the stool Organisms associated with invasion of the mucosal surface include *Shigella* spp., enteroinvasive and enterohemorrhagic *E. coli, Salmonella enteritidis, Campylobacter jejuni, Clostridium difficile, Vibrio parahaemolyticus,* and *Entamoeba histolytica.*
- A systemic infection with penetration of the intestinal mucosa and spread to the lymphatics. There may be leukocytes in the stool. Organisms associated with invasion and lymphatic spread include *Salmonella typhi* and *Yersinia enterocolitica.*

Stool specimens for culture should not be contaminated with urine and should be transported to the laboratory soon after collection. If there is to be a delay in processing, the specimens should be placed in an enteric transport media such as Cary-Blair. Stool specimens should not be refrigerated. Routine cultures should include media for the recovery of *Campylobacter, Salmonella,* and *Shigella.* There is agar to screen for *E. coli* O157:H7; these organisms are sorbitol-negative and will appear colorless on sorbitol-MacConkey agar. There is debate whether culture screening methods can be replaced with tests for Shiga toxin production as well as debate over the use of enrichment broths such as Gram-negative broth. It may also be the practice in certain high-risk areas to include media for the recovery of *Yersinia* and *Vibrio*.

Stool for ova and parasites should be in preservative. There is also a Giardia antigen test that can be performed. Special stains for parasites include a modified acid-fast stain for *Isospora, Cyclospora,* and *Cryptosporidium.*

INTEREST POINT

The CDC defines a food-borne-illness outbreak as an incident in which two or more people experience the same illness after eating the same food. The practice of reporting food-borne and waterborne disease in the United States began more than 60 years ago when state and territorial health officers became concerned about the high morbidity and mortality caused by typhoid fever and infantile diarrhea. They began investigating these cases to determine the role of food, milk, and water in the outbreak of these intestinal diseases. In 1925, the Public Health Service began publishing information about outbreaks attributable to milk. This information eventually led to public health legislation, for example, the Pasteurized Milk Ordinance. In 1961 the CDC took over these surveillance and reporting duties.

The most commonly reported causes of food-borne illnesses are due to failure to cool food properly, failure to cook and hold food at the proper temperature, and poor personal hygiene. The FDA writes the Food Code and shares responsibility with the U.S. Department of Agriculture for inspecting food processing plants to ensure the highest standards of compliance for safe food production. A food safety system known as HACCP (Hazard Analysis Critical Control Point) has been put into place to monitor techniques and do hazard analysis at specific points within the flow of food preparation. Here's one instance where food handling practices failed to meet the safety standards:

A day care center catered a lunch for its children and their parents. Of the 67 people who ate the lunch, 14 developed an acute GI illness that included vomiting and diarrhea within 1 hour of eating. The local health department launched an investigation; *Bacillus cereus* was isolated from the fried rice and from the vomitus of one of the children. The restaurant worker had left the cooked rice dish on the countertop to cool to room temperature the night before the luncheon. The rice was left unrefrigerated for 5 hours. On the day of the luncheon, the rice dish was reheated at 9 AM, delivered to the day care center at 10:30, and left at room temperature until noon. Because the onset of symptoms was so sudden, this was considered food intoxication rather than infection. Intoxication occurs when preformed toxins are ingested and there is rapid onset of symptoms. Food-borne infection refers to the ingestion of the pathogen with microbial replication in the human GI tract and delayed onset of symptoms. Fried rice is a leading cause of *B. cereus* food-borne illness in the United States. More information can be found at *www.cdc.gov/mmwr/preview/mmwrhtml/00025744.htm.*

KEY TERMS AND ABBREVIATIONS

Match the term in the left column with the definition on the right.

1. _____ colon
2. _____ Peyer's patches
3. _____ pseudomembranous colitis
4. _____ peristalsis
5. _____ tenesmus
6. _____ dysentery
7. _____ diarrhea
8. _____ gastritis

A. wavelike movement
B. large bowel
C. diarrhea with blood and mucus
D. *H. pylori* infection
E. inflammation caused by *C. difficile*
F. special areas of the small intestine that secrete IgA
G. straining during bowel movement
H. multiple stools that conform to the shape of the container

TRUE OR FALSE

1. _____ Food poisoning is actually intoxication because preformed toxins are ingested.
2. _____ Infant botulism has been associated with the ingestion of rice products in infants younger than 9 months of age.
3. _____ The specimen of choice for testing for *H. pylori* infection is a stool sample.
4. _____ The medium of choice for the transport of stool specimens for culture is Cary-Blair.
5. _____ XLD medium inhibits the growth of most *Enterobacteriaceae*, allowing *Salmonella* and *Shigella* spp. to be seen.

Multiple Choice

1. _____ The best way to diagnose *C. difficile* disease is
   A. stool culture.
   B. latex agglutination.
   C. toxin assay.
   D. modified acid-fast stain.
2. _____ Parasitic pathogens associated with diarrheal disease include
   A. *Giardia lamblia.*
   B. *Isospora* spp.
   C. both A and B.
   D. *Toxocara* spp.

3. _____ Which of the following foods is commonly associated with an outbreak of *Vibrio* spp.?
   A. undercooked eggs
   B. unpasteurized milk
   C. raw oysters
   D. canned beans
4. _____ Detection methods for *E. coli* O157:H7 include
   A. sorbitol-MacConkey agar
   B. Hektoen enteric agar
   C. XLD agar
   D. CNA agar
5. _____ Culture conditions that favor isolation of *Campylobacter jejuni* include
   A. 35° C in 5% CO_2.
   B. 42° C in 5% CO_2.
   C. 25° C in ambient air.
   D. 35° C in anaerobic conditions.

CASE STUDY

A 20-year-old man presented to the local emergency department with complaints of diarrhea for 2 days and bloody stool. Blood was collected for a CBC and comprehensive chemistry panel. A stool specimen was also collected; test orders included a stool culture, occult blood, fecal leukocytes, and an ova and parasites examination. There was not sufficient stool to do all the ordered tests; the emergency department physician canceled the ova and parasites test. Test results were as follows:

Test	Patient Result	Reference Range
Sodium	139	135-145
Potassium	4.0	3.6-5.0
Chloride	99	101-111
Occult blood	Positive	Negative
Fecal leukocytes	Moderate	None seen
Segmented neutrophils	74%	49%-69%
Lymphocytes	20%	25%-55%
Monocytes	6%	1%-8%
Stool culture	*Campylobacter jejuni* subsp *jejuni.* Organism sent to state laboratory for confirmation testing. No *Salmonella, Shigella, E. coli* O157, or *Yersinia* isolated.	

1. The fecal leukocytes and occult blood on stool test results were available within 1 hour of specimen collection. Both were positive. What information about disease processes does this give the physician?

2. In order to recover *Salmonella, Shigella, Campylobacter, E. coli* O157, and *Yersinia*, what media should be included in the battery of culture media?
3. Three days after this patient was in the emergency department, another patient presented with similar symptoms and was also febrile. Occult blood and fecal leukocytes were also both positive and the stool culture yielded *C. jejuni*. Per protocol, the isolates were sent to the state health department laboratory for confirmatory testing. Culture information was also reported to the local health department. According to the CDC, does this situation meet the criteria for a food-borne-illness outbreak?

ANSWERS

Key Terms and Abbreviations
1. B
2. F
3. E
4. A
5. G
6. C
7. H
8. D

True or False
1. T
2. F
3. F
4. T
5. T

Multiple Choice
1. C
2. C
3. C
4. A
5. B

Case Study
1. The presence of blood in the stool could mean there is an enterohemorrhagic process. Blood, however, could enter the GI tract at any point between the mouth and rectum and be present due to such diverse factors as peptic ulcer disease or bleeding gums. The presence of leukocytes signals an inflammatory process.
2. Stool culture media should include a nonselective medium, such as a blood agar plate, and several selective media such as Hektoen enteric or XLD agar for recovery of *Salmonella* spp. and *Shigella*, MacConkey agar, CIN agar for recovery of *Yersinia* spp., sorbitol-MacConkey agar for the detection of *E. coli* O157, and a Campylobacter blood agar plate. *Campylobacter* spp. grow best when incubated at 42° C, and *Yersinia* spp. grow well at 25° C.
3. The CDC definition of a food-borne illness outbreak is an incident in which two or more people experience the same illness after eating the same food. The two patients

experience the same illness, but it is incumbent on the local health department to question the patients to determine whether there is a common food source. The state laboratory will test and save the isolates sent for confirmatory testing. If additional testing becomes required for epidemiologic purposes, the specimens will be available. Pulsed field gel electrophoresis can be done to fingerprint the organisms in an investigation.

REFERENCES

Centers for Disease Control and Prevention: Diagnosis and Management of Foodborne Illnesses: A primer for physicians, *Morb Mortal Wkly Rep* 50(RR02):1, 2001.

Centers for Disease Control and Prevention: Epidemiologic notes and reports *Bacillus cereus* food poisoning associated with fried rice at two child day care centers—Virginia, 1993, *Morb Mortal Wkly Rep* 42:177, 1994.

60 Skin, Soft Tissue, and Wound Infections

OBJECTIVES

Upon completion of this chapter, the reader should be able to:

1. Describe the anatomy and function of the skin.
2. Describe the differences between infections of the skin and deeper infections of the subcutaneous tissues and muscle fascia and muscles.
3. List the various pathogens associated with bite wounds and burns.
4. Describe deep-seated infections that develop sinus tracts and the pathogens associated with these conditions.
5. Describe optimal culture methods for specimen collection and processing.
6. Explain terminology used to describe skin conditions: necrotizing fasciitis, folliculitis, furuncle, cellulitis, erysipelas, erysipeloid, decubitus ulcer, myositis, myonecrosis, petechiae.

SUMMARY OF KEY POINTS

Skin is part of the integumentary system and is the largest organ in the body. Skin is composed of three layers and contains the accessory structures of hair follicles, nails, and glands. The skin functions in homeostasis. Intact skin is the first barrier against the entry of microorganisms. The skin also helps maintain body temperature, decrease fluid loss, synthesize vitamins and hormones, and receive sensory information. A water-repellent protein, keratin, is found in keratinocytes in the epidermis. The surface of the skin is colonized with an array of flora that takes up residence shortly after birth. The concept of normal flora does not extend to viruses and parasites because they are not commensals and do not aid the host. The resident microbial population competes with invading microbes and protects the host by creating minienvironments unsuitable to many potential pathogens. Some studies have estimated that *Staphylococcus epidermidis* constitutes 90% of the local skin flora. Micrococci and diphtheroids are present as normal skin flora. *Propionibacterium acnes* is not seen on children younger than 10 years of age but becomes resident flora when sebaceous gland production changes. Beta-hemolytic streptococci are not seen on normal skin. Gram-negative bacilli can make up a small percentage of the skin flora, particularly in moist areas such as the axilla. Fungi can be found around and under nails.

Bacterial skin infections can occur if there is trauma, preexisting skin conditions, or poor hygiene. Impetigo is a superficial infection usually caused by *S. aureus* or *S. pyogenes*. The lesions are superficial, typically produce a yellow crust, and are easily spread by scratching.

Folliculitis is an inflammation of the hair follicle. The beard, neck, and axilla are typically affected. The most common cause of infection is *S. aureus* but *Pseudomonas aeruginosa* has been acquired after hot tub and swimming pool use. Folliculitis may develop into a deeper infection causing a nodule known as a *furuncle*. If the infection spreads even deeper into subcutaneous tissue, it can become a *carbuncle*. The most common agent of these infections is *S. aureus*.

Erysipelas is a superficial skin infection common in young children and older adults. Diabetes, venous insufficiency, and alcoholism are predisposing factors for this condition. Erysipelas is usually associated with *S. pyogenes* and *S. aureus*. It presents as a tender, erythematous, well-defined area and may be associated with fever and localized lymphadenopathy. Erysipelas can progress to a cellulitis. Cellulitis is a diffuse, spreading infection of the skin that extends into the subcutaneous tissue. It presents as a warm, erythematous, painful inflammation with poorly defined borders. Untreated cellulitis can evolve into a more serious systemic illness.

Necrotizing fasciitis is a rare but serious infection of the fascia and subcutaneous tissue. The site most commonly affected is the legs. Infection spreads rapidly both horizontally and vertically because at the fascia level there is no barrier to infection. Tissue damage progresses within hours to necrosis and gangrene. *S. pyogenes* is typically isolated from these infected sites, but there may be mixed infection with *Clostridium* spp. or other beta-hemolytic streptococci. Prompt surgical intervention is vital. Debridement, fasciotomy, and sometimes amputation are necessary to stop progression to myonecrosis. Organ failure, shock, and death may occur.

Fungi and viruses may also cause skin infections. Dermatophytes have a high affinity for keratinized tissue such as skin, hair, and nails. The three genera most commonly implicated in these infections are *Trichophyton, Microsporum,* and *Epidermophyton*. Cutaneous yeast infections are usually caused by *Candida albicans* and are commonly seen in the immunocompromised patient, the patient receiving antibiotics, and diabetics.

Viral infections of the skin can be caused by the papillomaviruses (warts), varicella-zoster virus (chicken pox and shingles), herpes simplex virus, poxvirus (molluscum contagiosum), paramyxovirus (rubeola), rubella virus (German measles), and others.

Wound infections occur because of trauma, surgery, or bites. The types of organisms infecting these wounds can vary greatly depending on the site, indigenous flora, and cause of the wound. Infected abdominal wounds frequently are caused by intestinal flora such as *E. coli, Bacteroides fragilis* group, anaerobic organisms, and streptococci.

S. aureus is also a frequently isolated pathogen from wounds. Human bite wounds are caused by oral flora such as alpha-hemolytic streptococci, *Eikenella corrodens, S. pyogenes,* and anaerobes. Animal bite wounds can be infected with *Pasteurella multocida, Enterobacter cloacae,* alpha-hemolytic streptococci, *Capnocytophaga canimorsus,* and others.

The best specimens for culture are pieces of tissue, aspirated fluid or pus, and debrided tissue. Superficial lesions can be cultured by scraping the active border of the lesion. If a fungal infection is suspected, skin and nail scrapings can be treated with 10% potassium hydroxide to visualize the fungal elements. Bacterial culture media should include a sheep blood agar plate, and chocolate and MacConkey agar. A Gram stain should be performed and a broth tube may also be inoculated. If the patient has blisters and herpes infection is suspected, several tests can be done to confirm the diagnosis. The blister should be unroofed and the skin scraped to collect cells from the base and edge of the lesion. The cells can be gently spread on a slide for a Tzanck prep, the swab can be used for antigen detection by direct immunofluorescence (DFA), or the cells can be cultured. The Tzanck prep is stained with a Papanicolaou (Pap) stain; if the herpes virus is present, multinucleate giant cells with nuclear molding will be seen. Varicella zoster virus will also produce these giant cells. Because of its lack of specificity, this test is being replaced by DFA, which is 100% specific for the herpes or varicella virus antigen.

INTEREST POINT

An article in the August 2004 edition of *CAP Today* (published by the College of American Pathologists) discussed the quality of swabs for culture compared to actual pieces of tissue or aspirated fluids. One of the three microbiologists interviewed found that a mini-tip swab could hold 15 μL of fluid and a regular culture swab could absorb 150 μL of fluid. For every 100 bacteria absorbed onto a swab, only 3 are recovered in culture. A wound culture will typically entail a minimum of two agar plates, possibly a thioglycolate broth tube, and a Gram stain. If a wound swab were to yield only three bacteria, it is unlikely that this culture would recover the pathogens. Swabs are never acceptable specimens for acid-fast bacilli or fungal cultures because these organisms are not present in tissue in the high concentrations typical of bacterial infections. Swabs can also make it difficult to detect anaerobes, even if an anaerobic Culturette system is used. The specimens of choice are pieces of tissue in wide-mouth sterile containers and aspirates of fluid or pus.

Burn wound management requires special techniques. Burn wound infection cannot be diagnosed on clinical signs alone; burn wound infection surveillance must be done to differentiate colonization from infection. The "gold standard" for identifying a burn wound infection has been quantitative culture of tissue biopsy samples and histologic observation of microbial invasion of the viable tissue beneath the necrotic tissue or eschar. The most common pathogens are *Pseudomonas aeruginosa* and *S. aureus* from the patient's own endogenous cutaneous and gastrointestinal flora. In electrical burns, anaerobic infections are more typical.

KEY TERMS AND ABBREVIATIONS

Match the term in the left column with the definition on the right.

1. _____ dermis	A. covering
2. _____ epidermis	B. common skin infection in children
3. _____ fascia	
4. _____ sebaceous	C. outermost skin layer
5. _____ keratin	D. removal of dead and infected tissue
6. _____ integument	
7. _____ necrotizing fasciitis	E. sheets of tissue that cover muscles
8. _____ erysipelas	F. death of tissues
9. _____ gangrene	G. oil producing
10. _____ myositis	H. water-repellent substance
11. _____ eschar	
12. _____ decubitus ulcer	I. layer containing blood vessels and nerves
13. _____ petechiae	J. spreading infection of the fascia
14. _____ debridement	
15. _____ cellulitis	K. inflammation of a muscle
	L. scab
	M. small hemorrhagic spots
	N. soft tissue infection that spreads through connective tissue
	O. bedsore

TRUE OR FALSE

1. _____ In staphylococcal scalded-skin syndrome, *S. aureus* produces an exfoliative toxin that causes the skin to peel off in sheets.
2. _____ Dermatophytes utilize keratin, which is found in hair and nails.
3. _____ If necrotizing fasciitis is suspected, cultures should be taken from the central portion of the wound.
4. _____ In a burn patient, if the bacterial wound counts are greater than 10^5 microorganisms per gram of tissue, risk of wound infection is great and skin graft survival is decreased.
5. _____ Intestinal flora are commonly isolated from decubitus ulcers.

MULTIPLE CHOICE

1. _____ Organisms isolated from dog and cat bite wounds include
   A. *E. coli.*
   B. *Pasteurella* spp.
   C. *Mycobacterium fortuitum*
   D. *Candida* spp.
2. _____ Functions of the skin include
   A. excretion.
   B. temperature regulation.
   C. synthesis.
   D. all of the above.
3. _____ An organism associated with human bite wounds is
   A. *Eikenella corrodens.*
   B. *Pasteurella multocida.*
   C. *Pseudomonas aeruginosa.*
   D. *Capnocytophaga canimorsus.*
4. _____ Which statement about diabetic foot infections is true?
   A. Foot infections can begin with a blister caused by ill-fitting shoes.
   B. They are the most common nontraumatic cause of amputation.
   C. *S. aureus* and beta-hemolytic streptococci are the most commonly isolated pathogens.
   D. All of the above are true.
5. _____ Anaerobes should be suspected in
   A. deep puncture wounds.
   B. folliculitis.
   C. draining sinuses.
   D. A and C.

CASE STUDY

A 36-year-old woman presented to the local emergency department with an open wound on her forearm that was red and painful. She said she was bitten by her cat several days ago. When bitten, she washed the wound with soap and water and put a bandage on it. The doctor inserted a swab into the wound and collected a small amount of pus and fluid. This specimen was sent for culture. A CBC and blood culture were also ordered. The woman's WBC count was slightly elevated at 12.4 $10^3/\mu L$ (reference range 4.8 to 10.8 $10^3/\mu L$). The differential was shifted with 80% segmented neutrophils, 2% bands, 15% lymphocytes, and 3% monocytes. The wound culture Gram stain showed few WBCs and few gram-positive cocci.

The next day the wound culture plates were examined. There was moderate growth on the blood agar and chocolate plates and no growth on the MacConkey plate. The colonies were grayish, nonhemolytic, and catalase-positive. A Gram stain was done using the colonies on the blood agar plate; there were gram-negative coccobacilli.

1. What organisms are frequently isolated from dog and cat bite wounds?
2. How can you explain the difference in Gram reaction between the clinical specimen and colonial growth?

3. The laboratory set up gram-negative identification and susceptibility panels for the Vitek II analyzer. The organism identification was *Pasteurella multocida* with a 97% confidence level. This is a gram-negative organism; why didn't it grow on the MacConkey plate? What are the drugs of choice for this organism?

ANSWERS

Key Terms and Abbreviations

1. I
2. C
3. E
4. G
5. H
6. A
7. J
8. B
9. F
10. K
11. L
12. O
13. M
14. D
15. N

True or False

1. T
2. T
3. F
4. T
5. T

Multiple Choice

1. B
2. D
3. A
4. D
5. D

Case Study

1. Normal oral flora in dogs and cats include *Pasteurella* spp., *Capnocytophaga canimorsus, S. aureus, Weeksella* spp., and *Enterobacteriaceae.* In one study of infected dog and cat bites, the most frequent isolates were *Pasteurella* spp. Other common aerobes included streptococci, staphylococci, *Moraxella,* and *Neisseria* species. Anaerobes included *Fusobacterium, Bacteroides, Porphyromonas,* and *Prevotella* species. Oral flora in both humans and animals is a complex microbiologic mix, and cultures of wound infections typically yield more than one pathogen. Empiric antibiotic therapy should be broad spectrum to cover both aerobes and anaerobes.
2. *Pasteurella multocida* is a gram-negative coccobacillus that often shows bipolar staining. Bipolar staining is described as a "closed safety pin" appearance. Because of this staining characteristic and the short rounded bacilli, it can be misidentified as a coccus.

If the clinical specimen were thick on the slide, it would have been more difficult to decolorize. If the slide were under-decolorized, the organisms would appear gram-positive.

3. *Pasteurella multocida* grows well on chocolate and blood agars (BAP), but does not grow on MacConkey, EMB, or other enteric media. In a clinical laboratory, if there is a gram-negative bacillus isolated from a dog or cat bite wound that grows on BAP and chocolate but not MacConkey and is oxidase-, catalase-, and spot indole–positive, a presumptive identification of *P. multocida* can be made. The organism is typically susceptible to penicillin and the expanded-spectrum cephalosporins.

REFERENCES

Brook I: Human and animal bite infections, *J Fam Pract* 28:713, 1989.

Church D, Elsayed S, Reid O, et al: Burn wound infections, *Clin Microbiol Rev* 19:403, 2006.

Paxton A: Swapping swabs for syringes and scalpels, *CAP Today*, vol 1, 2004.

Talan DA, Citron DM, Abrahamian FM, et al: Bacteriologic analysis of infected dog and cat bites. Emergency Medicine Animal Bite Infection Study Group, *N Engl J Med* 340:85, 1999.

Weedon D: Viral disease—Herpesviridae. In Weedon D, author: *Skin pathology,* ed 2, 2002, London, Churchill Livingstone.

61 Normally Sterile Body Fluids, Bone and Bone Marrow, and Solid Tissues

OBJECTIVES

Upon completion of this chapter, the reader should be able to:

1. Describe the compartmentalization of the body and the membranes and fluids associated with each cavity.
2. Explain the difference between thoracentesis and paracentesis.
3. Define pleural fluid, pericardial fluid, peritoneal fluid, joint fluid, and dialysis fluid, and explain how to process the various fluids for culture.
4. Describe how to process bone for culture.
5. Describe how to process solid tissue for culture.
6. List common pathogens associated with each specimen type.

SUMMARY OF KEY POINTS

The human body is divided into five main body cavities: cranial, spinal, thoracic, abdominal, and pelvic. These body cavities are lined with thin membranes. Small spaces are formed between these membranes and the body wall and between organs and the membranes surrounding them. Small amounts of fluid fill these spaces. This fluid bathes the membranes and organs and reduces friction between organs. The body tries to maintain a balance (homeostasis) during constant physiologic change. When the balance cannot be maintained, extra fluids are formed (effusions). These membranes and fluids can become infected with a variety of organisms.

Pleural fluid is the small amount of fluid that is in the pleural space in the chest. Its function is to lubricate the surfaces of the pleura, the membrane that surrounds the lungs and lines the chest cavity. Under normal conditions, there is an equilibrium across these pleural membranes. But in certain disease states or conditions, there is an abnormal fluid production and accumulation in the pleural space. This abnormal accumulation of fluid is known as a *pleural effusion*.

Pleural effusions can be exudative or transudative. Exudative effusions are due to inflammation, infection, and cancer. Transudative effusions are due to systemic factors and pressure changes, such as congestive heart failure.

These specimens are usually collected by thoracentesis. During this procedure, a needle is inserted through the chest wall into the pleural space. The excess fluid is aspirated. Effusions can be analyzed for cell count, total protein, glucose, lactate dehydrogenase, amylase, cytology, and culture. Total protein and glucose evaluations are useful for differentiation of transudates from exudates. If pus is present in the effusion, it is called an *empyema*. It has been estimated that 50% to 60% of patients develop empyema as a complication of pneumonia.

Pericardial fluid acts as a lubricant in the pericardial space surrounding the heart. Excess fluid can accumulate because of obstruction of drainage or because of malignant or infectious processes. Pericarditis is an inflammation of the pericardium. The leading cause of pericarditis is viral infection, especially coxsackievirus. The normal amount of fluid is approximately 20 mL, but in infections up to 500 mL of fluid may accumulate. Large amounts of pericardial fluid may seriously compromise cardiac function.

Myocarditis may accompany or follow pericarditis. In myocarditis, the heart muscle is inflamed. Common causes are viral infections with coxsackievirus, echoviruses, or adenovirus. Myocarditis may also be associated with bacterial and parasitic infections. Any organism causing bacteremia can cause myocarditis.

The peritoneum is a thin membrane that lines the abdominal and pelvic cavities. Peritoneal fluid acts as a lubricant between organs lying in the cavity such as bowel and the inner abdominal and pelvic side walls. When there is excess fluid in the peritoneal cavity, it is called *ascites*. Most cases of ascites are due to liver disease. In severe cases the abdomen is distended. This fluid can be collected for testing by paracentesis (the insertion of a needle into the abdomen and removal of fluid). As much as 10 L of fluid may be drained during this procedure. Tests typically performed on peritoneal fluid include amylase, protein, albumin, cell count, culture, and cytology.

Peritonitis results when this membrane becomes inflamed. There are two types of peritonitis. Primary peritonitis is rare and results when infection spreads from the blood and lymph nodes. When bacteria enter the peritoneum from the gastrointestinal or biliary tract, such as from a ruptured appendix, secondary peritonitis results. Secondary peritonitis is often polymicrobial. Because anaerobic bacteria are numerous in the bowel, anaerobes play a prominent role in intraabdominal infection.

Peritoneal dialysis has been used as treatment for renal disease for more than 60 years. Because this process requires injection into and removal of fluid from the peritoneal cavity via catheter, there is a high incidence of infection. Peritonitis is a major complication of continuous ambulatory peritoneal dialysis (CAPD). The majority of these infections are due to gram-positive organisms, such as *Staphylococcus epidermidis* and *S. aureus*. There are, however, a significant percentage of cases of peritonitis that are culture-negative. This may be due to the fact that the concentration of organisms in the CAPD effluent is very low. Many recent studies show that improved sensitivity can be achieved by using automated blood culture systems in which 10 mL of fluid is inoculated into culture bottles.

176

Arthritis is an inflammation in a joint space. Bacterial invasion usually involves only one joint (monarticular). Hematogenous seeding during bacteremia may involve multiple joints. In bacterial arthritis, the knee and hip are the most commonly affected joints in all age groups. The most frequently isolated bacteria in septic arthritis include *S. aureus, H. influenzae,* streptococci, and *Bacteroides* spp. Chronic monarticular arthritis is frequently due to mycobacteria, *Nocardia asteroides,* and fungi. Diagnosis is made by aspiration of joint fluid for culture and microscopic examination. To prevent the fluid from clotting, it may be inoculated directly into blood culture bottles. Some fluid should be saved for Gram stain and inoculation of sheep blood agar, chocolate agar, and anaerobic media. AFB and fungal culture may also be warranted.

Osteomyelitis is infection of the bone. This may occur by hematogenous spread, by spread from a contiguous site of infection, or by trauma or surgery. Acute osteomyelitis may progress to chronic inflammation. Chronic infection cannot be cured without removal of the nidus. Some factors that can affect infection include the underlying conditions of diabetes, malnutrition, malignancy, immunosuppression, and tobacco abuse. Diagnosis of bone infection is made by biopsy of the bone. Small pieces need to be ground to release the microorganisms. Surrounding tissue may also be cultured. Aerobic and anaerobic media should be included. Common isolates include *S. aureus, Enterobacteriaceae, P. aeruginosa, E. corrodens, Actinomyces* spp., *Prevotella, Porphyromonas,* and other anaerobes.

Pieces of solid tissue are processed in a manner similar to that for bone. Aerobic and anaerobic media should be included. It should be emphasized that pieces of tissue or several milliliters of fluid or aspirate are superior to swabs for culture. Body fluids should be concentrated by centrifugation and the sediment used for culture. Cytocentrifugation of fluids for Gram stain can concentrate organisms up to 1000-fold.

KEY TERMS AND ABBREVIATIONS

Match the term in the left column with the definition on the right.

1. _____ pleural fluid
2. _____ effusion
3. _____ synovial fluid
4. _____ transudate
5. _____ exudate
6. _____ thoracentesis
7. _____ empyema
8. _____ peritonitis
9. _____ ascites
10. _____ pericardial space
11. _____ CAPD
12. _____ osteomyelitis

A. collection of pus in pleural space
B. inflammation of the bone
C. fluid in the peritoneal cavity
D. continuous exchange of fluid in the peritoneal cavity
E. fluid that filters from circulatory system to an area of inflammation
F. escape of fluid into body cavities

G. space between the membranes surrounding the heart
H. fluid filtrate of blood produced due to osmotic pressure changes
I. fluid from the space between the lung and chest wall
J. needle aspiration of the pleural cavity
K. inflammation of the peritoneum
L. joint fluid

TRUE OR FALSE

1. _____ Empyema usually occurs as a complication of pneumonia.
2. _____ Thoracentesis is the insertion of a needle into the abdomen with the aspiration of fluid.
3. _____ Among sexually active women, *N. gonorrhoeae* is a common cause of peritoneal infection.
4. _____ Coagulase-negative staphylococci are common pathogens in patients undergoing dialysis.
5. _____ The most common cause of prosthetic joint infection in adults younger than 30 years of age is *N. gonorrhoeae.*

MULTIPLE CHOICE

1. _____ Osteomyelitis of the jaw associated with poor oral hygiene can be caused by
   A. *M. avium* complex.
   B. *Pasteurella* spp.
   C. *Actinomyces* spp.
   D. *Candida* spp.
2. _____ A common cause of pericarditis is
   A. coxsackievirus.
   B. *N. gonorrhoeae.*
   C. *S. pyogenes.*
   D. *H. influenzae.*
3. _____ A 5-year-old child developed a swollen painful knee, but there was no evidence of trauma or fracture. This symptom came on suddenly. She also had a mild cough and sore throat for the previous few days. Fluid was aspirated from the knee but no bacteria were recovered from culture. Her pediatrician gave her a course of amoxicillin for the cough. The sore knee resolved and the child was completely well within 2 weeks. The probable cause of the joint inflammation was
   A. viral.
   B. inflammatory response to *S. pyogenes* infection.
   C. Lyme disease.
   D. reactive arthritis due to *Salmonella* spp.

4. _____ Proper handling of CAPD fluid would involve
   A. inoculating aerobic and anaerobic blood culture bottles.
   B. concentrating by centrifugation and plating the sediment.
   C. only process A.
   D. both A and B.
5. _____ Tissue for culture may be obtained during autopsy. If studies are being performed on a stillborn premature infant, an organism that should be cultured for is
   A. *Listeria.*
   C. *Chlamydia.*
   B. CMV.
   D. *N. gonorrhoeae.*

CASE STUDY

A 63-year-old woman sought treatment from her dentist when she noticed pus on the gumline that had been irritated by a bridge. The x-rays were consistent with osteomyelitis. The patient was put on oral antibiotics. The patient's condition did not improve significantly, so she was admitted for intravenous antibiotic therapy. The patient had a history of COPD and admitted to smoking a pack of cigarettes each day. The patient was taken to surgery for debridement of the mandible. During surgery, bone and soft tissue specimens of the mandible were taken and sent for culture. The Gram stains of both specimens showed few WBCs and no organisms. After 3 days, there was no aerobic or anaerobic growth from the soft tissue. But the bone culture had polymicrobic growth that included *Eikenella corrodens*, *Streptococcus constellatus*, and *Prevotella buccae*.
1. What do these three organisms have in common?
2. What are some unique morphology characteristics of *E. corrodens?*
3. What is the clinical significance of *E. corrodens* osteomyelitis?
4. How can *E. corrodens* osteomyelitis be treated?

ANSWERS

Key Terms and Abbreviations
1. I
2. F
3. L
4. H
5. E
6. J
7. A
8. K
9. C
10. G
11. D
12. B

True or False
1. T
2. F
3. T
4. T
5. F

Multiple Choice
1. C
2. A
3. B
4. D
5. A

Case Study
1. All are normal oropharyngeal flora. *S. constellatus* is a viridans streptococcus in the Anginosus group.
2. *E. corrodens* produces small colonies on the sheep blood agar plate and chocolate agar but not on MacConkey. The colonies frequently pit the agar and growth has been described as smelling like bleach.
3. *E. corrodens* has been isolated from a variety of head and neck infections. If there is poor oral hygiene, *E. corrodens* may cause oral infections such as gingivitis, root canal infections, and other mandibular abscesses. It has also been isolated from human bite wounds and hand wounds related to fist fights. Infection can spread from the subcutaneous tissue to the bones and joints causing osteomyelitis and septic arthritis.
4. Susceptibility testing of this organism is not routinely done. Due to its fastidious nature, susceptibility testing is difficult to perform. There are no standard interpretive guidelines published by the Clinical and Laboratory Standards Institute (formerly NCCLS). The drugs of choice are penicillin, ampicillin, and amoxicillin/clavulanate.

REFERENCES

Alfa MJ, Degagne P, Olson N, Harding GKM: Improved detection of bacterial growth in continuous ambulatory peritoneal dialysis effluent by use of BacT/Alert FAN bottles, *J Clin Microbiol* 35:862, 1997.

Bourbeau P, Riley J, Heiter BJ, et al: Use of the BacT/Alert Blood Culture System for culture of sterile body fluids other than blood, *J Clin Microbiol* 36:3273, 1998.

Marinella MA: Electrocardiographic manifestations and differential diagnosis of acute pericarditis, *Am Fam Physician* 15:699, 1998.

62 Laboratory Physical Design, Management, and Organization

OBJECTIVES

Upon completion of this chapter, the reader should be able to:
1. Differentiate between sensitivity and specificity.
2. Differentiate between accuracy and precision.
3. Explain federal regulations regarding transmission of patient reports via fax and medical necessity coding.
4. Explain CLIA '88 and how it affects laboratory operations.
5. Explain the role of CAP in laboratory operations.
6. Explain what an antibiogram is and how it can be used.
7. List some safety features that are required to be in all laboratories.

SUMMARY OF KEY POINTS

The management of a clinical laboratory entails oversight of a varied group of functions and activities. Some elements of laboratory management are the design and maintenance of the physical space, regulatory compliance, technology, finance, personnel standards, and customer service. To complicate this further, health care practices are not static; there is remarkably rapid change in the way health care is provided. In the 1990s, laboratory services were decentralized so that there was more alternate-site testing, such as in physician's office laboratories. Testing was brought to the patient's bedside with point of care testing (POCT). As always, there is pressure to reduce costs, which places laboratories in the dilemma of reducing expenses without sacrificing quality. Another trend has been the consolidation of microbiology laboratories within health systems. Other areas of the laboratory that lend themselves to automation, such as chemistry, are being redesigned to maximize efficient workflow by using robotics and autoverification. Microbiology, however, has always been a more manual area of testing.

The microbiology laboratory must utilize space efficiently while maintaining compliance with the safety directives from a variety of organizations. Space must be allotted for the various activities typically performed in a microbiology laboratory, for example, separate rooms are needed for fluorescent microscopy and for waste disposal, a sink is needed for staining, and so on. The Centers for Disease Control and Prevention (CDC) has published recommendations that allow 200 square feet per two to three technologists. Laboratory safety is addressed by the Occupational Safety and Health Administration (OSHA). There must be emergency shower and eye wash stations located throughout the laboratory and no more than 100 feet from each work area. Cold water should be used to flush the eyes and skin in the event of a chemical splash.

The National Fire Protection Agency (NFPA) publishes guidelines on the safe storage of chemicals. Flammables should be stored in a special cabinet; acids and bases should not be stored on the same shelf. There must be fire extinguishers and blankets and two means of exit in case of fire. Electrical outlets should be grounded and critical equipment should be on dedicated circuits. Hospitals must have emergency generators to provide an uninterrupted source of power.

Laboratory doors should be self-closing. If radionuclides are used in the microbiology laboratory, state radiation safety offices should be consulted. The heating, ventilation, and air conditioning (HVAC) systems must maintain a constant temperature in a narrow range. The relative humidity and room temperatures are generally specified by instrument manufacturers. Air flow is an important consideration. Negative pressure should be maintained in administrative areas to prevent fumes or pathogens from escaping the work area. Air can be exhausted directly out of the building without passing through HEPA or charcoal filters except in biosafety 3 or 4 facilities. There should be 10 to 15 air exchanges per hour in laboratory work areas; office spaces do not require this high exchange rate.

Laboratories became federally regulated by passage of the Clinical Laboratory Improvement Act of 1967. The Health Care Financing Administration (HCFA) was created to implement and oversee these new laboratory regulations as well as the Medicare and Medicaid programs. HCFA is now the Centers for Medicare and Medicaid Services (CMS). In 1988, this act (CLIA '88) was amended and expanded to encompass all testing on human specimens. CMS has granted the College of American Pathologists (CAP) Laboratory Accreditation Program deeming authority. This means CAP has been judged by CMS to have requirements equivalent to or more stringent than CMS's regulatory requirements. CAP can inspect a laboratory in lieu of CMS. In addition to federal regulations, many states have their own regulations governing laboratory practices. Another federal agency that plays a role in laboratory testing and management is the CDC. The CDC writes the regulations for enforcement of CLIA. The CDC also works closely with OSHA to ensure safe work place practices. The Food and Drug Administration (FDA) evaluates new tests and technologies and determines whether they can be used for diagnostic testing. The FDA also has the power to remove test systems from production if there are serious quality issues.

CLIA '88 has published minimum standards that apply to all sites where human testing is being performed. This includes the physician office laboratory (POL). CLIA '88 defined four categories of laboratory testing based on complexity. The simplest of tests are the waived tests. These are typically tests that can be performed at the bedside as POCT. This group includes fingerstick glucose testing and many rapid group A streptococcal antigen tests. The majority of laboratory tests performed fall into the moderate and high complexity categories. The processes involved in isolating and identifying an anaerobe would be considered high complexity testing. Moderate and high complexity laboratories must have on-site inspections as well as compliance with more stringent personnel qualifications, QC, and proficiency testing (PT) requirements. PT involves the analysis of unknown samples and provides a way to assess the accuracy of test systems as well as the competency of personnel. CAP both produces PT materials and performs on-site inspections.

In 1996 legislation was passed to maintain security and privacy of information found in patient records. Title II of the Health Insurance Portability and Accountability Act (HIPAA) addresses national standards for electronic health care transactions and national identifiers for providers, health insurance plans, and employers. Secure phone and fax lines must be used for the transmission of laboratory data, and access to information must be on a need-to-know basis.

Quality assessment (QA) and quality control (QC) standards changed with CLIA '88. The responsibility to determine appropriate control procedures that monitor the complete analytical process rests with the laboratory director. The purpose of control procedures is to assess the accuracy and precision of test performance and to verify that the testing system has not been affected by variations in the environment or operator. *Accuracy* is correctness; it is a comparison of the test result to the reference method ("gold standard"). *Precision* refers to the reproducibility of the test. Precision studies are typically done by testing the same specimen 10 times and measuring the variability of results. Precision does not necessarily imply accuracy. An analogy would be in firing 10 shots at a target. The 10 bullets may be grouped in a tight circle (precision) but they are outside the target perimeter (poor accuracy).

Laboratories must determine the tests they will offer that will best meet the needs of their clients (physicians and patients) weighed against cost and many other considerations. Although the developing standard for mycobacterial identification is DNA sequencing, most hospital laboratories will not be able to implement this process. Factors to consider include prevalence of disease, space, equipment, personnel, cost, PT materials, QC required, and specimen collection and storage requirements, to name a few. Tests must also be evaluated for their performance regarding accuracy, precision, sensitivity, and specificity. Accuracy and precision have already been discussed. Analytical sensitivity refers to the detection limits of the test; this is how much of a substance needs to be present for detection by the test. Clinical sensitivity is the percentage of true-positive results. If a test has a sensitivity of 99.7%, a negative result can exclude the disease. Analytical specificity is a measure of cross reactivity. Clinical specificity is the percentage of true negative results. If a bacterial antigen test has a specificity of 76%, then 24% of results will be false positives.

Once a decision has been made to institute a new test, the test must be verified for precision and accuracy before it can be used to test patient samples. Verification is a one-time process that demonstrates that the laboratory can reproduce manufacturer's claims and test results are statistically comparable to the reference method. Validation is a continuous process ensuring that the test is performing correctly based on QC data and PT results.

The financial aspect of laboratory management involves balancing revenue (income) against expenses in a budget. *Expenses* include costs for consumables and indirect costs, such as license fees, continuing education programs, equipment maintenance, repairs, and so on. *Capital equipment* refers to instruments that will need to be periodically replaced. *Revenue* involves reimbursement for tests performed. Outpatient reimbursement is based on Current Procedure Terminology (CPT) codes that are part of the code set standard selected by HIPAA. CPT codes are used to describe health care services. The medical necessity for the test is justified by the International Classification of Diseases, Clinical Modification (ICD-9-CM) codes. A urine culture for suspected urinary tract infection (ICD-9-CM code 599.7) will not be reimbursed if a code of 496 designating COPD is used.

A laboratory manager will need to handle personnel issues. This includes interviewing and hiring employees. The manager must not ask personal questions. Interview questions should revolve around the job description, the candidate's qualifications, career goals, holiday and shift work, and so on. Candidates with disabilities should not be discriminated against and are protected under the Americans with Disabilities Act. The job description is also used as an evaluation tool to assess an employee's job performance. Certain documents are required by accrediting agencies to be in the personnel records; refer to specific agency regulations.

It is the manager's responsibility to provide a procedure manual for employees. Procedures must be written in the format outlined by the Clinical and Laboratory Standards Institute (CLSI). Elements that should be in every procedure are the title and principle of the test, specimen requirements, reagent list, the procedure itself, quality control, test interpretation, and references.

The laboratory must also provide a handbook for its clinician clients. The handbook should provide a list of tests with specimen and transportation requirements, CPT codes, reference ranges, and special instructions. Another useful tool is an antibiogram. An antibiogram is a picture of the in vitro susceptibility testing results for a particular organism. The microbiology department should periodically collect this patient data and produce a cumulative report for that laboratory and geographic area. Physicians can refer to this chart of common isolates if treating a patient empirically, that is, using general observations on susceptibility patterns rather than test data on that particular isolate.

KEY TERMS AND ABBREVIATIONS

Match the term in the left column with the definition on the right.

1. _____ verification	A.	sets the workplace safety standards
2. _____ POCT	B.	reproducibility
3. _____ NFPA	C.	ensures patient confidentiality
4. _____ CDC	D.	one-time assessment of accuracy and precision
5. _____ OSHA	E.	number that describes the service performed
6. _____ CAP	F.	continuing process of test assessment
7. _____ HIPAA	G.	cumulative susceptibility data
8. _____ accuracy	H.	writes enforcement regulations for CLIA
9. _____ precision	I.	detection limit
10. _____ sensitivity	J.	has deeming authority to inspect laboratories
11. _____ specificity	K.	no interference from similar substances
12. _____ validation	L.	sets safe practices for chemical handling
13. _____ ICD-9-CM code	M.	conformity to the "gold standard"
14. _____ CPT code	N.	bedside testing
15. _____ antibiogram	O.	describes medical necessity

TRUE OR FALSE

1. _____ The emergency shower must be within 100 feet of each work area.

2. _____ If the laboratory were to change blood culture systems, it needs to do parallel testing with the same specimens on both analyzers.

3. _____ OSHA protects worker safety by setting the standards for chemical storage.

4. _____ Some antigen detection tests have a high incidence of false negatives. These tests have a high sensitivity.

5. _____ If a specimen is tested three times by the same person and different results are obtained each time, the test system lacks precision.

ANSWERS

Key Terms and Abbreviations

1. D
2. N
3. L
4. H
5. A
6. J
7. C
8. M
9. B
10. I
11. K
12. F
13. O
14. E
15. G

True or False

1. T
2. T
3. F
4. F
5. T

63 Quality in the Clinical Microbiology Laboratory

OBJECTIVES

Upon completion of this chapter, the reader should be able to:
1. Explain the difference between QC and QA.
2. Explain the difference between preanalytic, analytic, and postanalytic variables.
3. List some elements of a basic QC program.
4. Explain the hierarchy of organization regarding laboratory quality standards.
5. Explain proficiency testing.
6. List some basic regulations regarding the performance and frequency of quality control testing.

SUMMARY OF KEY POINTS

Several organizations are involved in setting the standards of quality that laboratories must achieve. The preeminent organization is the Centers for Medicare and Medicaid Services (CMS), administered by the United States Department of Health and Human Services (DHHS). Federal regulations governing laboratory testing were issued in 1967 and 1988. The Clinical Laboratory Improvement Act of 1967 was amended in 1988 and has become known as CLIA'88. The Joint Commission on Accreditation of Healthcare Organizations (JCAHO) and the College of American Pathologists (CAP) have deemed status under CLIA to inspect and accredit laboratories.

The patient test results generated by clinical laboratories are useful to clinicians only if they are accurate. The concepts of quality management, quality assessment, and quality control are vital to laboratory operation. Quality systems in health care have evolved over the years. Quality assurance terminology has been removed from CLIA and replaced by the term quality assessment (QA). "Assurance" requires that the cause of the problem be identified and eliminated, whereas "assessment" implies a broader approach to monitor, identify, and improve practices by preventing errors from happening. Quality control (QC) is another concept inherent in laboratory operations. Quality control refers to internal monitors that evaluate performance and identify problems within the test process.

In assessing all the components of the process to generate accurate and timely test results, the processes can be divided into three phases: preanalytical, analytical, and postanalytical. A problem can arise before or after testing of the specimen, as well as during the test process itself. Table 63-1 outlines some basic elements from a quality assessment program as it follows a specimen through the microbiology laboratory to patient outcome.

Table 63-1 Basic Elements of a Quality Assessment Program

Process Point	Variables
Preanalytic	Test order
	Processing of order
	Specimen collection
	Specimen transport
	Specimen processing
Analytic	Examination of culture and workup
	Interpretation of test results
Postanalytic	Formulation of written report
	Communication of results to clinician
	Interpretation of report
	Institution of appropriate therapy

Quality control can be thought of as a set of practices within a QA program. QC begins with specimen collection and transport. A common adage among laboratory professionals is that the test results can only be as good as the quality of the specimen. Mislabeled specimens, specimens submitted in an inappropriate transport medium, or specimens transported at the improper temperature are examples of factors that affect test results.

Laboratories follow practice guidelines set forth by the Clinical and Laboratory Standards Institute (CLSI), formerly known as NCCLS. Laboratories are required to have a complete set of operating procedures available at all times for reference by staff. Procedures should be in a standardized format delineated by CLSI. Retired procedures must be retained for 2 years.

Laboratories are required to participate in external proficiency testing programs for each test performed within the laboratory. Proficiency testing (PT) involves analyzing a series of unknown samples that represent patient specimens. The laboratory must handle these PT specimens exactly as it would any other patient specimen. There can be no interlaboratory communication. This PT process checks personnel competency, reagents, equipment, and procedures. Results are reviewed and graded and compared with those from other program participants. Failure to produce acceptable results requires an investigation with documentation of corrective action. A laboratory that has continuing PT failures may have sanctions imposed.

Media, reagents, and methods must all be tested following standardized protocols using specific strains of bacteria. The American Type Culture Collection (ATCC [Rockville, Md]) maintains reference strains of these QC organisms. Each susceptibility test system must be tested each day of patient testing using these ATCC strains. Susceptibility QC may be reduced to a weekly schedule as long as the laboratory achieved adequate performance during a 20- to 30-day daily testing protocol. QC records must be retained for a minimum of 2 years.

Instrument maintenance must be documented and records should be maintained for the life of the instrument. Table 63-2 lists some elements of a basic QC program.

Table 63-2 Elements of a Quality Control Program to Detect and Correct Analytic Errors

Basic Elements	Specific Processes
Test methods and procedure	Specimen collection, quality, and transport
	Reagents and media (e.g., storage, expiration)
	QC stocks and QC records
	Equipment maintenance and function checks
	Daily temperature logs
	Turnaround time monitors
Verification and validation of tests	Validation of new test methods
	Verification of performance of new shipments
	Instrument-to-instrument correlation studies
Procedure manuals	Standard operating procedures and forms
Personnel competency	Initial training checklists
	Yearly competency evaluation
	Direct observations of personnel perform testing
Proficiency testing	Outside proficiency testing program

KEY TERMS AND ABBREVIATIONS

Match the term in the left column with the definition on the right.

1. _____ quality control
2. _____ quality assessment
3. _____ proficiency testing
4. _____ SOPM
5. _____ corrective action
6. _____ CLSI
7. _____ CAP
8. _____ ATCC
9. _____ preanalytic
10. _____ analytic
11. _____ postanalytic
12. _____ benchmark-ing
13. _____ CLIA '88

A. steps taken to resolve a problem
B. sources of error after testing has been done
C. standard procedures
D. process of seeking best practices by communication with other laboratories
E. laboratory accrediting organization
F. federal law governing laboratories
G. problem areas before testing occurs
H. prepares and stores reference organisms
I. sets susceptibility breakpoints
J. potential problems within the test process
K. program to monitor and improve processes
L. measures to evaluate and control testing performance
M. testing of unknown samples to assess competency and processes

TRUE OR FALSE

1. _____ The interpretation of an oxidase test is a post-analytical variable.
2. _____ When identifying an isolate, it is important to document each step in the testing process. Both electronic and paperwork cards must be saved for 2 years.
3. _____ Proficiency testing evaluates the reporting process and communication of results to the clinician.
4. _____ As part of the continuous monitoring process, it is important to compare culture results to Gram stain results.
5. _____ To monitor shipping temperatures, each shipment of kits must be tested even if the lot number is the same as a previous shipment.

ANSWERS

Key Terms and Abbreviations

1. L
2. K
3. M
4. C
5. A
6. I
7. E
8. H
9. G
10. J
11. B
12. D
13. F

True or False

1. F
2. T
3. F
4. T
5. T

REFERENCES

Lasky FD: Technology variations: strategies for assuring quality results, *Lab Med* 36:617, 2005.

Westgard JO, Klee GG: Quality management. In Burtis CA, et al, editors: *Tietz textbook of clinical chemistry and molecular diagnostics,* St Louis, Saunders, 2006.

64 Infection Control

OBJECTIVES

Upon completion of this chapter, the reader should be able to:
1. Explain what a nosocomial infection is and list the patient risk factors.
2. Explain Standard Precautions.
3. Explain the difference between droplet precautions and airborne precautions.
4. Describe contact precautions.

SUMMARY OF KEY POINTS

Nosocomial (hospital-acquired) infections are an important problem in health care. Every year, as many as 10% of the patients admitted to acute care facilities develop an infection as a result of their hospitalization. This is costly, adds days to the length of stay, and can result in death.

Handwashing has long been regarded as desirable for personal hygiene. However, it wasn't until the mid-1800s that the connection between handwashing and spread of disease was clearly made. There was a high rate of puerperal sepsis. Two physicians, Semmelweis and Holmes, made independent observations that puerperal fever was transmitted by the hands of health care personnel. Semmelweis insisted that physicians and students clean their hands with a chlorine solution after seeing one patient and before seeing another at the clinic. Other physicians at the time were reluctant to accept this new concept and practice, but Pasteur proved the existence of germs and their role in disease transmission. Another physician, Lister, reduced surgical wound infections by spraying carbolic acid and cleaning surgical instruments. Handwashing is still the single most effective means of preventing the spread of infection.

The Centers for Disease Control and Prevention (CDC) monitors the incidence of nosocomial infections in the United States through the National Nosocomial Infections Surveillance (NNIS) program. Data collected through this program shows the most common infections are urinary tract infections, then, in decreasing frequency, pneumonia, surgical site infections, and bloodstream infections. Bloodstream infections have a high morbidity and mortality; as many as 60% of patients with nosocomial bloodstream infections or lung infections die each year.

Hospitalized patients, by virtue of their hospitalization, are at increased risk for infection. An underlying disease or chemotherapy may suppress their immune responses, which may in turn alter their normal microbiota. Patients are frequently having invasive procedures done that include the placement of indwelling catheters. The natural defense of the skin is breached and foreign objects provide a route

for opportunistic pathogens to directly enter the bloodstream. But pathogens can be transmitted by less obvious routes, such as direct contact with a contaminated object (fomite) or contaminated food, water, or medications. Pathogens can also be airborne. Typical risk factors that predispose patients to infection include advanced age, an underlying disease, and prolonged hospital stays. Other specific risk factors include (1) aspiration or chest surgery that can lead to a lung infection; (2) diabetes, malnutrition, or extended surgery time can lead to a surgical site infection; (3) immunosuppressive therapy, stay in the intensive care unit, or malnutrition can lead to a bloodstream infection.

The number of vancomycin-resistant enterococci (VRE) has been increasing and a handful of cases of vancomycin-resistant *Staphylococcus aureus* have been reported. The widespread use and misuse of antibiotics have promoted the emergence of more resistant strains. Nursing home residents and health care workers are frequently colonized with resistant strains of *S. aureus,* known as methicillin-resistant *S. aureus* (MRSA). Facilities may now screen patients before admission so that those with MRSA can be isolated.

To prevent the spread of infection within health care facilities, the CDC has published a series of guidelines. Terminology and practices have evolved over the years, but in 1996 the system of Standard Precautions was published. Standard Precautions apply to blood, all body fluids, secretions, and excretions (except sweat), nonintact skin, and mucous membranes. Standard Precautions are designed to reduce the risk of transmission of microorganisms from both recognized and unrecognized sources of infection in hospitals. Handwashing and the use of gloves are vitally important to break the chain of infection. Gloves must be removed and hands washed after seeing each patient and before seeing another. Gloves should be changed between tasks on the same patient if there is contact with areas with high concentrations of microorganisms. Gloves should also be removed before contact with inanimate objects within a room; bedrails, door knobs, and light switches can harbor viable organisms for extended periods of time. Standard Precautions may also include the use of gowns and masks, as needed.

The need for additional guidelines based on specific routes of transmission led to the following precaution categories: contact, droplet, and airborne. Contact precautions apply when the infectious agent is in wounds or when close physical contact with the patient can result in transmission of the organism to another person or object. It also applies to patients known or suspected of being colonized (presence of microorganism in or on a patient but without clinical signs and symptoms of infection) with epidemiologically important microorganisms that can be transmitted by direct or indirect contact. Gloves and gown are usually the only personal protective equipment (PPE) needed. When organisms are dispersed via air currents, droplet precautions or airborne precautions may apply. Droplet transmission involves contact of the mucous membranes of the eye, nose, or mouth with large-particle droplets (larger than 5 μm in size) that contain microorganisms generated from a person who is either infected or colonized with an infectious organism. Droplets are generated from the source person during coughing, sneezing, or talking and during certain procedures such as suctioning and bronchoscopy. Transmission via large-particle droplets requires close contact between source and recipient persons, because droplets do not remain suspended in the air and generally cannot travel further than 3 feet. Organisms that require droplet precautions include *N. meningitidis, C. diphtheriae, M. pneumoniae,* and the mumps virus. Droplet precautions should be used whenever an infectious organism, such as MRSA or a multidrug resistant gram-negative bacillus, is present in respiratory secretions. Airborne precautions apply when airborne droplet nuclei are small (5 μm or smaller in size). Evaporated droplets or dust particles containing infectious organisms may remain suspended for long periods of time. Organisms in this category include mycobacteria and the varicella and rubeola viruses. Patients need to be in a single room with negative air pressure. PPE necessary for contact with these patients includes an N95 respirator, gown, and gloves. These masks must be fit-tested on personnel.

The infection control practitioner and microbiology laboratory need to work closely together both in surveillance activities and in the characterization of an outbreak situation. If an outbreak is identified, isolates must be saved. It may be necessary to culture additional patients or personnel and to perform strain typing. Health departments can offer biotyping, serotyping, bacteriocin typing, bacteriophage typing, as well as molecular fingerprinting. Environmental surveillance cultures are generally considered to be of little value and should not be performed unless part of an epidemiologic investigation.

INTEREST POINT

A VRE-free patient was admitted to a hospital room that had previously been occupied by a patient who was colonized with VRE. The VRE-free patient acquired VRE from his hospital environment. There are documented nosocomial outbreaks that involved objects such as stethoscopes and electronic ear-probe thermometers. It is also well documented that viruses and bacteria can survive wash cycles and be recovered from fabrics. A variety of organisms have been recovered from the garments of health care workers, including *Enterobacteriaceae* from physicians' ties. An infection control program must specify the cleaning process for isolation rooms that includes ceiling to floor disinfection. An interesting recent situation of environmental contamination occurred in a microbiology laboratory

when VRE control strains were documented to have contaminated several clinical specimens. The VRE strains in question were isolated from a computer keyboard, chair back, wire rack, and workbench surface in the laboratory. But no break in procedure could be identified as the cause of this cross-contamination.

KEY TERMS AND ABBREVIATIONS

Match the term in the left column with the definition on the right.

1. _____ morbidity
2. _____ mortality
3. _____ nosocomial
4. _____ NNIS
5. _____ fomite
6. _____ contact precautions
7. _____ droplet precautions
8. _____ airborne precautions
9. _____ vector-borne
10. _____ standard precautions
11. _____ MRSA
12. _____ VRE
13. _____ cohorting

A. requires a negative air pressure room
B. objects capable of transmitting disease
C. transmitted by mosquitoes
D. two patients with same disease in same room
E. incidence of disease
F. vancomycin-resistant *E. faecium*
G. gown and gloves required, no mask
H. oxacillin-resistant *S. aureus*
I. handwashing
J. death rate
K. CDC's surveillance and reporting system
L. hospital-acquired
M. wear mask within 3 feet of patient

TRUE OR FALSE

1. _____ It is the infection control practitioner's job to identify all cases of an outbreak, but it is the role of the microbiology laboratory to report infectious diseases to the health department.
2. _____ A college student admitted for meningococcal meningitis should be placed in airborne isolation.
3. _____ Contact precautions should be used when bathing a nursing home patient with MRSA in her sputum.
4. _____ Infectious organisms can be inadvertently spread among patients if tourniquets used to draw blood are reused rather than discarded between patients.
5. _____ Handwashing is the single most important means of preventing the spread of infection.

CASE STUDY

A new medical and postsurgical wing was added to a hospital. As part of this expansion and modernization, wireless mobile phones were issued to the nurses and the patient rooms were equipped with cabinets that were accessible both from inside the room and from the hallway outside the room. After several months of operation, the microbiology department noticed an increase in the number of resistant *S. aureus* isolates from these two nursing units. The infection control nurse was alerted; she did a "look-back" to gather data to plot a timeline and locations. There was a definite increase in the number of methicillin-resistant *S. aureus* (MRSA) isolates, especially from wound cultures, but the patients had all been assigned to different rooms. The contact isolation protocol was reviewed and charts were reviewed; in all cases the patients were isolated as soon as the resistance pattern was determined. Fortunately, the microbiology department had been following its protocol of freezing very resistant isolates. After consultation with the state health department laboratory, eight of these isolates were sent for DNA fingerprinting. The state laboratory did pulsed-field gel electrophoresis and found that four of the eight MRSA isolates were identical. Each isolate was from a different patient.

1. What is the implication to the patient for the presence of MRSA in a wound culture?
2. What is pulsed-field gel electrophoresis? How is it applicable to this situation?
3. Given that four of the eight isolates were genetically identical, what does this mean in terms of infection control? What changes needed to be instituted in these two nursing areas?

ANSWERS

Key Terms and Abbreviations

1. E
2. J
3. L
4. K
5. B
6. G
7. M
8. A
9. C
10. I
11. H
12. F
13. D

True or False

1. T
2. F
3. F
4. T
5. T

Case Study

1. Patients in a hospital setting who have MRSA isolated in culture must be isolated from other patients to prevent transmission. MRSA outbreaks occur when this resistant bacterium is transferred from person to person. Health care workers can transfer the MRSA on their hands, clothes, and equipment. Treatment options are limited; vancomycin is the drug typically used but it must be administered intravenously and is expensive.

2. To determine strain relatedness, molecular methods for genotyping are used. One such method that is widely used is pulsed-field gel electrophoresis (PFGE). The bacterial plasmid is extracted and then cleaved using restriction endonucleases. The chromosomal DNA fragments are separated by electrophoresis and the restriction patterns are compared. In this situation there would have been eight lanes set up on the gel plate; four of these eight lanes had identical restriction patterns.

3. These genotypic patterns indicated that four of the patients were infected with the identical strain of *S. aureus*. It is highly unlikely they had acquired this exact same strain from the community. These were nosocomial infections acquired after admission to these nursing units and transfer had to have happened via health care personnel. If all isolates had been associated with the same room, environmental cultures could have been done to determine whether the organisms were surviving on surfaces in the room. But given the fact that different patient rooms were involved, it is more likely that personnel were transferring the organism horizontally throughout the unit. Because there was documentation that every patient was put on a contact isolation protocol, there had to have been a break in that protocol. The mobile phones were new to everyone; when questioned, the nurses did admit to bringing the phones into isolation rooms. They were properly gowned and gloved, but did not think about the phones as a source of contamination. The phones were all disinfected and new plastic covers were purchased. All nurses and support staff were reeducated on infection control. The remedial plan was successful; there were no further nosocomial outbreaks involving MRSA.

REFERENCES

Centers for Disease Control and Prevention: Guideline for hand hygiene in healthcare settings. Recommendations of the Healthcare Infection Control Practices Advisory Committee and the HIPAC/SHEA/APIC/IDSA Hand Hygiene Task Force, *Morb Mortal Wkly* 51(RR16):1, 2002.

Katz KC, McGeer A, Low DE, Willey BM: Laboratory contamination of specimens with quality control strains of vancomycin-resistant enterococci in Ontario, *J Clin Microbiol* 40:2686, 2002.

Neely AN, Maley MP: Survival of enterococci and staphylococci on hospital fabrics and plastic, *J Clin Microbiol* 38:724, 2000.

Neely AN, Orloff MM: Survival of some medically important fungi on hospital fabrics and plastics, *J Clin Microbiol* 39:3360, 2001.

Sidwell RW, Dixon DJ, Westbrook L, Forziati FH: Quantitative studies on fabrics as disseminators of viruses. V. Effect of laundering on poliovirus-contaminated fabrics, *Appl Microbiol* 21:227, 1971.

65 Sentinel Laboratory Response to Bioterrorism

OBJECTIVES

Upon completion of this chapter, the reader should be able to:

1. Explain the concept of bioterrorism.
2. Describe some legislation that deals with biosecurity.
3. Explain the Laboratory Response Network (LRN).
4. Explain the role of the clinical laboratory in the LRN.
5. Describe select agents and list several.
6. Differentiate between dangerous goods, infectious substances, and clinical specimens.
7. Access current bioterrorism preparedness information from the ASM website.

SUMMARY OF KEY POINTS

Bioterrorism involves the use of biologic agents as weapons. Biowarfare actually has a long history. Before the germ theory of disease was formulated, disease was associated with foul odors. The Greeks and Romans sought to pollute the drinking water of their enemies by throwing dead animals into their water supplies. The British tried to infect Native Americans with smallpox in 1763 by giving them blankets used by smallpox victims. Chemical weapons were used during World War I and there was research into biowarfare by both sides during World War II. In 1984, food was deliberately contaminated with *Salmonella* by a cult group; in 1995, sarin gas was released into the Tokyo subway system. In 2001, anthrax spores in mailed letters and packages infected 22 people and caused 5 deaths in the United States. These events changed microbiology in the clinical laboratory. Federal laws were quickly passed after the anthrax incidents to increase security and require laboratories to formulate a bioterrorism preparedness plan. The microbiology laboratory is a critical element in the detection of a biologic weapon.

The Centers for Disease Control and Prevention (CDC) created an organizational structure to facilitate communication between clinical and public health laboratories. The Laboratory Response Network (LRN) is currently a three-tiered system that has clinical laboratories as the base fulfilling the role of sentinel laboratories. Sentinel laboratories will be the first to recognize a potential problem. They should rule out biologic warfare agents and send isolates to a reference laboratory for confirmatory testing and identification. These reference laboratories would then communicate with the select national laboratories that have the capability to definitively characterize the suspect organism. The clinical microbiology laboratory should never accept for testing nonhuman specimens such as powders or specimens from animals or the environment. Sentinel laboratories must have a bioterrorism

response plan developed that allows rapid communication between them and infection control and public health laboratories. Sentinel laboratories do not make the determination that a bioterrorist event has occurred nor do they notify law enforcement.

Clinical microbiologists should be trained to be alert for those agents thought to be the most likely weapons of bioterrorism. Some bacteria and fungi on the select agent list that could be recovered in clinical specimens include *Bacillus anthracis, Brucella* spp., *Burkholderia mallei, Burkholderia pseudomallei, Clostridium botulinum, Coxiella burnetii, Francisella tularensis, Yersinia pestis,* and *Coccidioides immitis*. Laboratory workers who ship or transport specimens and isolates are required to be trained in the packing and shipping of those agents. Dangerous goods are any materials that pose a risk to health and safety; these include infectious substances and chemicals. There are distinctions made between diagnostic clinical specimens (e.g., swabs, tissues, body fluids for testing) and infectious substances (e.g., cultures of *B. anthracis* or *M. tuberculosis*). The American Society for Microbiology has developed algorithms for organism identification and handling and has made these available on their website. This information can be accessed at *www.asm.org/policy/index.asp?bid=6342*.

KEY TERMS AND ABBREVIATIONS

Match the term in the left column with the definition on the right.

1. _____ biocrime
2. _____ overt crime
3. _____ covert crime
4. _____ select agents
5. _____ sentinel laboratory
6. _____ biosecurity
7. _____ dangerous goods
8. _____ infectious substance

A. all potential bioterrorism agents
B. material that poses a risk to health and safety when not handled properly
C. announced terrorist act
D. clinical diagnostic laboratory
E. event involving intentional use of a select agent
F. concealed act of terrorism
G. material expected to contain pathogens
H. laboratory security issues

TRUE OR FALSE

1. _____ The CDC created the Laboratory Response Network to establish an organized chain of communication in the event of a bioterrorist act.

189

2. _____ The contamination of the salad bar with *Salmonella* in Oregon in 1984 was an overt act of terrorism.
3. _____ Clinical laboratories are now required to have a bioterrorism response plan.
4. _____ Once a sentinel laboratory identifies *B. anthracis* in a clinical specimen, the laboratory director should immediately notify the police.
5. _____ The clinical laboratory has a responsibility to accept and test specimens such as powders brought to them by concerned citizens.

MULTIPLE CHOICE

1. _____ Which of the following bacteria is not on the select agent list?
   A. *Yersinia pestis*
   B. *Clostridium perfringens*
   C. *Bacillus anthracis*
   D. *Brucella abortus*
2. _____ A pure culture of *Shigella dysenteriae* is rated by IATA as
   A. a dangerous good.
   B. an infectious substance.
   C. a diagnostic specimen.
   D. both A and B.
3. _____ Which of the following statements about a sentinel laboratory is not true?
   A. Technologists should be vigilant to look for a single case of disease caused by an unusual organism.
   B. There should be a class III biosafety cabinet and splash guards.
   C. The laboratory should participate in a proficiency testing program.
   D. The algorithms established by ASM should be followed to rule out possible bioterrorism agent.
4. _____ In addition to bacteria, other identified select agents include
   A. yellow fever virus.
   B. botulinum toxins.
   C. *Coccidioides immitis.*
   D. all of the above.
5. _____ Which statement is false?
   A. *Brucella* and *Francisella* may be mistaken for *Haemophilus* in culture.
   B. If a clinical laboratory recovers *B. anthracis* from a clinical specimen, it must be sent to a public health laboratory or destroyed within 7 days of identification.
   C. The level A sentinel laboratory has access to special assays developed by the CDC to confirm identification of critical agents.
   D. To use *Coccidioides immitis* as a positive control in molecular assays, laboratories must register with the CDC.

CASE STUDY

A teenage boy and his friend shot two rabbits on his family's acreage in Missouri. The boys dressed the rabbits and froze them. Two days later, one of the boys complained of a fever; he had a lesion on his hand. By the next day, the other boy became febrile, complained of swollen lymph nodes, and also developed an ulcerative lesion on one of his fingers. At that point, both boys went to the local hospital. Both boys had blood cultures collected as well as blood for a CBC and chemistry tests. A culture of the one exudative lesion was done. Gram stain showed WBCs and tiny, poorly staining gram-negative coccobacilli. When the doctor questioned the boys about their activities over the last week, they told him they had gone rabbit hunting. Chest x-ray examinations were done on both boys, they were admitted to the hospital, and they were started on streptomycin. The doctor alerted the microbiology department to exercise caution when handling the cultures from these patients.

1. What are some possible causes for these symptoms in these two patients?
2. After 3 days, there were tiny colonies on the chocolate plate but no growth on any other media. The blood cultures from both boys were positive but only a few organisms were seen in the blood broth Gram stain. Per protocol, the blood cultures were plated to sheep blood agar, chocolate, and MacConkey plates. After 2 days, there were tiny colonies on the blood agar and chocolate plates but no growth was seen on the MacConkey plate. If these are gram-negative organisms, why aren't they growing on MacConkey agar?
3. What special precautions should be taken in the microbiology laboratory?
4. The boys were given antibiotics and recovered rapidly. These cases were reported to the local health department. The health department asked for the frozen rabbit meat. CDC was notified and the rabbits were sent to CDC for testing. Cultures from the rabbits' bone marrow grew *F. tularensis*. The health department recommended that antibody titers to *F. tularensis* be done on acute and convalescent sera from the boys. Why do antibody testing on the boys? Why did the CDC test the rabbits?

ANSWERS

Key Terms and Abbreviations
1. E
2. C
3. F
4. A
5. D
6. H
7. B
8. G

True or False
1. T
2. F
3. T
4. F
5. F

Multiple Choice

1. B
2. D
3. B
4. D
5. C

Case Study

1. The fever, lymphadenopathy, and hand sores coupled with the hunting activity would make the doctor suspicious of tick-borne illnesses or zoonoses such as brucellosis and tularemia.

2. *Brucella* and *Francisella* are tiny gram-negative coccobacilli. *Brucella* requires a prolonged incubation period to grow in commercial blood culture systems. *Francisella* is a slow grower but will produce colonies on agar in 2 to 4 days. *Francisella* is a fastidious organism that requires cystine and cysteine for growth. These nutrients are in blood; when the blood broth mixture was inoculated to agar plates, the organisms grew. A characteristic of *Francisella* is that it will not grow on sheep blood agar if subcultured from these plates because there is no cystine.

3. For both *Brucella* and *Francisella* cultures, biosafety level 3 precautions need to be followed. Clinical specimens should be handled in a biological safety cabinet following biosafety level 2 protocols. The inoculum amount required for infection is very small. Tularemia and brucellosis are two of the most common laboratory-acquired infections. Because of their infectiousness, they are on the select agent list.

4. *Francisella* is difficult to grow in the laboratory without special media such as cysteine heart agar. Sentinel clinical laboratories should not undertake the identification of these highly infectious organisms. They should do enough testing to rule out certain organisms. If further testing is required, it should be done by a specially equipped reference laboratory that is registered with the CDC. Because of the risk of infection to laboratory workers and the fastidious nature of the organism, diagnosis is usually made by serologic methods. *Francisella* is endemic in certain parts of the United States. The CDC tracks these infections and does epidemiologic typing of the organisms. Isolation of the organism from the rabbits establishes the source of the infection.

REFERENCES

Klietmann WF, Ruoff KL: Bioterrorism: implications for the clinical microbiologist, *Clin Microbiol Rev* 14:364, 2001.